CLINICAL CALCULATIONS MADE EASY

Solving Problems Using Dimensional Analysis

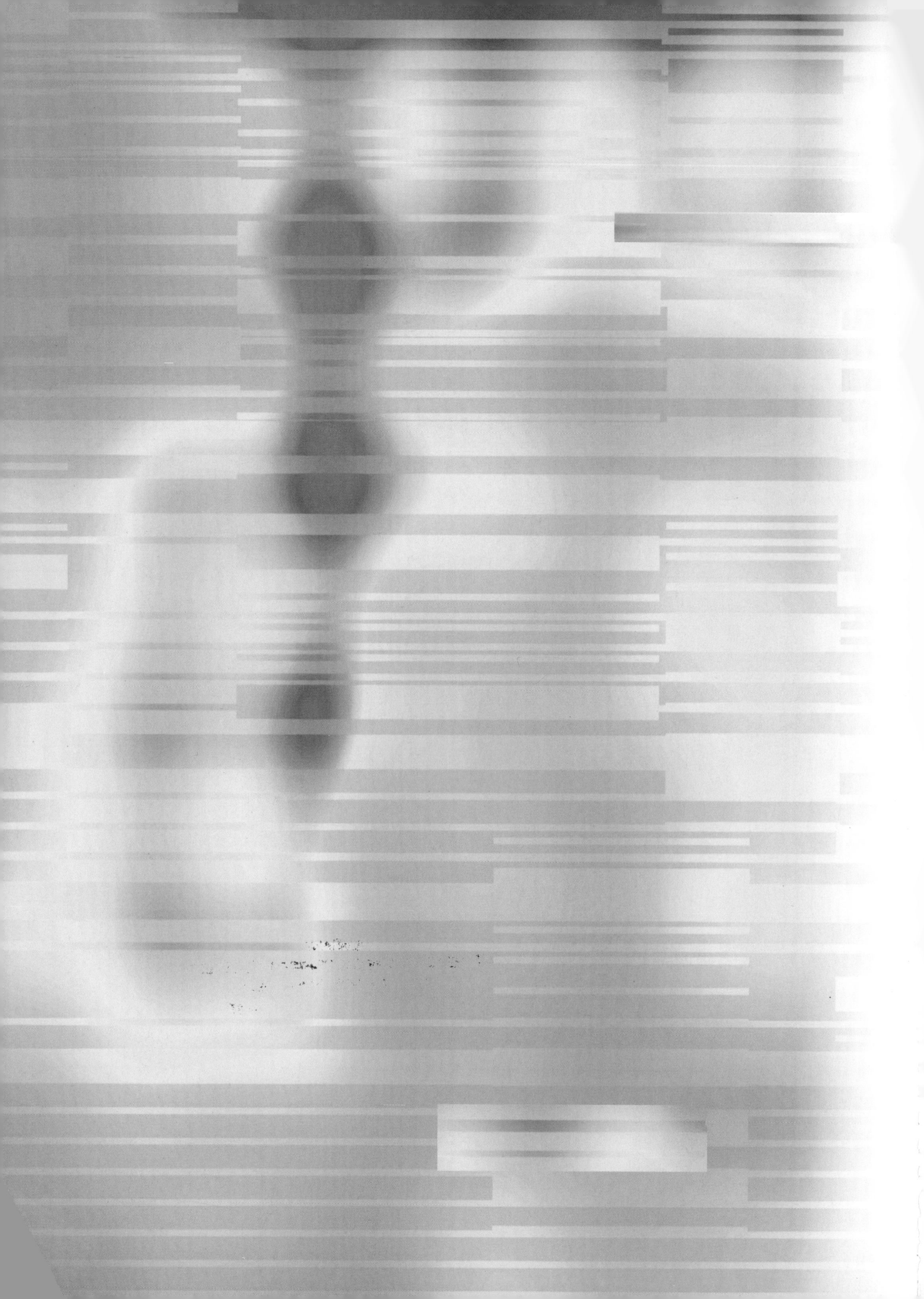

EDITION

2

CLINICAL CALCULATIONS MADE EASY

Solving Problems Using Dimensional Analysis

Gloria P. Craig, RN, MSN, EdD
Department Head, Nursing Student Services
Assistant Professor
South Dakota State University
College of Nursing
Brookings, South Dakota

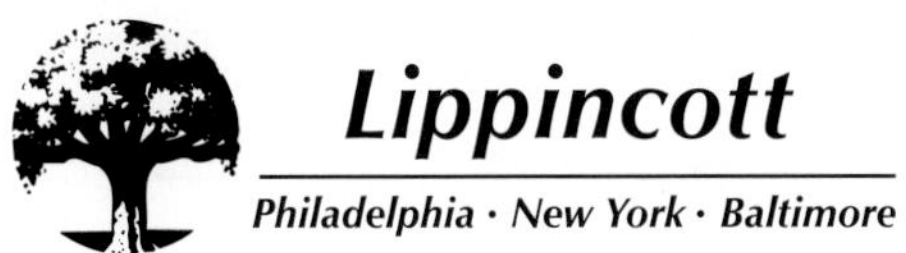

Acquisitions Editor: Margaret Zuccarini
Managing Editor: Claudia Vaughn
Editorial Assistant: Helen Kogut
Project Editor: Debra Schiff
Senior Production Manager: Helen Ewan
Senior Production Coordinator: Michael Carcel
Art Director: Carolyn O'Brien
Design: BJ Crim
Manufacturing Manager: William Alberti
Indexer: Lynne McCabe
Compositor: Circle Graphics
Printer: R. R. Donnelley-Willard

Edition 2

9 8 7 6 5 4 3

Library of Congress Cataloging-in-Publication Data

Craig, Gloria P., 1949-
Clinical calculations made easy : solving problems using dimensional analysis / Gloria P. Craig.—2nd ed.
p, ; cm.
Rev. ed. of: Clinical calculations using dimensional analysis. c1997.
Includes bibliographical references and index.
ISBN 0-7817-3099-6 (alk. paper)
1. Pharmaceutical arithmetic. 2. Dimensional analysis. 3. Nursing—Mathematics. I. Craig, Gloria P., 1949- Clinical calculations using dimensional analysis. II. Title.
[DNLM: 1. Pharmaceutical Preparations—administration & dosage—Nurses' Instruction. 2. Pharmaceutical Preparations—administration & dosage—Problems and Exercises. 3. Mathematics—Nurses' Instruction. 4. Mathematics—Problems and Exercises. 5. Problem Solving—Nurses' Instruction. 6. Problem Solving—Problems and Exercises. QV 748 C886ca 2001]
RS57.C73 2001
615′.14′0151—dc21 00-048750

Care has been taken to confirm the accuracy of the information presented and to describe generally accepted practices. However, the authors, editors, and publisher are not responsible for errors or omissions or for any consequences from application of the information in this book and make no warranty, express or implied, with respect to the content of the publication.

The authors, editors, and publisher have exerted every effort to ensure that drug selection and dosage set forth in this text are in accordance with the current recommendations and practice at the time of publication. However, in view of ongoing research, changes in government regulations, and the constant flow of information relating to drug therapy and drug reactions, the reader is urged to check the package insert for each drug for any change in indications and dosage and for added warnings and precautions. This is particularly important when the recommended agent is a new or infrequently employed drug.

Some drugs and medical devices presented in this publication have Food and Drug Administration (FDA) clearance for limited use in restricted research settings. It is the responsibility of the health care provider to ascertain the FDA status of each drug or device planned for use in his or her clinical practice.

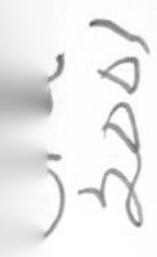

Margaret Cooper, RN, MS
Clinical Educator
Iowa Methodist Medical Center, Iowa Lutheran Hospital,
and Blank Children's Hospital
Des Moines, Iowa

Kari R. Lane, RN, BSN, MScN
Nursing Instructor
Clinton Community College
Eastern Iowa Community College District
Clinton, Iowa

Francine P. Pappalardo, BSN, MSN
Professor
Northern Essex Community College
Lawrence, Massachusetts

Terri M. Perkins, RN, MN
Instructor
Bellevue Community College
Bellevue, Washington

Peggy Anne Przybycien, RN, BSN, MSN, CNS
Assistant Professor
Onondaga Community College
Syracuse, New York

Alice Rasmussen, RN, MSN
Nursing Coordinator and Health Science Department Chair
Lake Michigan College
Benton Harbor, Michigan

Laura Sessions, RN, MScN
Instructor of Nursing
Howard Community College
Columbia, Maryland

Jo A. Voss, RN, MSN, CNS
Instructor
College of Nursing, West River Program
South Dakota State University
Rapid City, South Dakota

Many people experience stumbling blocks calculating math problems because of a lack of mathematical ability or associated "math anxiety." Even people with strong math skills often set up medication problems incorrectly, putting the patient at an increased risk for incorrect dosages and the ensuing consequences. However, dosage calculation need not be difficult if you use a problem-solving method that is easy to understand and to implement.

As a student, I experienced anxiety related to poor mathematical abilities and consequently had difficulty with medication calculations. However, a friend introduced me to a problem-solving method that was easy to visualize. By using this method, I was able to easily understand medication problems and thereby avoid the stumbling blocks that I had experienced with other methods of dosage calculations. Later, as a practicing nurse and nursing instructor, I realized that many of my colleagues and students shared my experience with "math anxiety," so I began sharing this problem-solving method with them.

During my baccalaureate nursing education, this problem-solving method became my teaching plan. During my master's education, it became my research. During my doctoral education, it became my dissertation. Now, I would like to share this method with anyone who ever believed that they were mathematically "challenged" or trembled at the thought of solving a medication problem.

The method, called dimensional analysis (also known as factor-label method or conversion-factor method), is a systematic, straightforward approach to setting up and solving problems that require conversions. It is a way of thinking about problems that can be used when two quantities are directly proportional to each other, but one needs to be converted using a conversion factor in order for the problem to be solved.

Dimensional Analysis as a Teaching Tool

Dimensional analysis empowers the learner to solve a variety of medication problems using just one problem-solving method. As a method of reducing errors and improving calculations, dimensional analysis has many possibilities. Whether it is used in practice or education, it is a strong approach when the goals are improving medication dosage-calculation skills, reducing medication errors, and improving patient safety. Ultimately, this improved methodology has the potential to reduce the medication errors that occur within the discipline of nursing.

Dimensional analysis helps the learner see and understand the significance of the whole process, since it focuses on how to learn, rather than what to learn. It provides a framework for understanding the principles of the problem-solving method and supports the critical thinking process. It helps the learner to organize and evaluate data, and to avoid errors in setting up problems. Dimensional analysis thus supports the conceptual mastery and higher-level thinking skills that have become the core of curricula at all levels of nursing education.

Organization of This Book

The book is divided into four sections: Section 1 provides instruction and explanation for students learning to solve clinical calculations problems by using dimensional analysis, Section 2 provides practice problems for students to strengthen their skills, Section 3 contains 20 case studies to help students relate their skills to clinical situations, and Section 4 contains a comprehensive Post-Test.

Section 1: Clinical Calculations

This text uses the simple-to-complex approach to teach students clinical calculations. The first chapter provides a review of basic arithmetic skills, while the second chapter reviews systems of measurement and common equivalents. The third chapter introduces students to dimensional analysis and allows them to build upon Chapter 2 by using common equivalents to practice their dimensional analysis skills. Finally, Chapters 4 to 6 teach clinical calculations, starting with One-Factor Conversions (Chapter 4), then Two-Factor Conversions (Chapter 5), and finally Three-Factor Conversions (Chapter 6).

Similarly, each chapter uses the simple-to-complex approach to the material. As the learner continues through the text, more complex concepts are presented. Each chapter contains numerous examples with detailed explanations, including a special **Thinking It Through** feature, to enhance student learning. **In-chapter exercises**, which occur after the presentation and explanation of each new concept, provide an opportunity for the learner to gain ability and build confidence in the material before proceeding to the next concept. To provide the learner with the clinically realistic examples, **actual drug labels** are liberally used as the basis of medication problems. Near the end of each chapter are **practice problems** where the students can practice their skills and assess mastery of the material, to identify any areas where more review is necessary.

The answers to all of the exercises and the practice problems are located at the end of each chapter in an **answer key**, for easy reference for students. The answer section also provides a complete explanation for each problem by showing exactly how the problem was set up and then solved.

Finally, each chapter concludes with a **post-test,** a resource for instructors to evaluate their students' understanding of the concepts presented in that chapter. The post-tests are designed so that the students may work on them, tear them out of the book, and hand them in. The answers to the post-tests are in the Instructor's Manual.

Section 2: Practice Problems

This section allow students to refine their skills in each area. The three parts are one-, two-, and three-factor practice problems, respectively, and a final section on comprehensive questions. An answer key at the end of this section contains answers and explanations for all of the problems.

Section 3: Case Studies

This section contains 20 case studies, related to different fields of nursing. The purpose of the case studies is to help students relate their clinical calculation skills to clinical situations.

Section 4: Comprehensive Post-Test

The last section of the book contains a post-test of 20 questions allowing the instructor to assess the students' mastery of solving clinical calculations using dimensional analysis. The answers to these questions are found in the Instructor's Manual.

New to This Edition

The focus of the revision of the second edition was enhancing the visual appeal of the book to make it more "user-friendly." To that end, we have designed the new edition in four colors. Not only does this make the text more visually interesting, but it allows us to reprint drug labels exactly, in order to more closely simulate the real clinical experience of the nurse. We have also changed the size of the book to a workbook size to allow students more room to work. Another goal of the revision was to provide more opportunity for students to practice their skills. To accomplish that, we have added post-tests, extra practice questions, and 10 new case studies.

It is my hope that this new edition will help nursing students and nurses find that clinical calculations can indeed be made easy using dimensional analysis.

Gloria P. Craig

Acknowledgments

There are many people who have assisted me with my professional growth and development including:

- **Pauline Callahan**, who believed that I would be a great nurse and nursing instructor when I could not believe in myself.
- **Jackie Kehm**, who introduced me to dimensional analysis and helped me pass the medication module that I was sure would be my stumbling block.
- **Dr. Sandra L. Sellers**, for her expertise and guidance throughout the process of writing my thesis and her encouragement to write a textbook.
- **Margaret Cooper**, for her friendship and editing support throughout the writing of this textbook.
- My students, colleagues, and reviewers for helping me develop my abilities to explain and teach the problem-solving method of dimensional analysis.
- The numerous pharmaceutical companies listed throughout this book that supplied medication labels and gave permission for the labels to be included in this textbook.
- The faculty at South Dakota State University, College of Nursing for allowing dimensional analysis to be integrated into the curriculum as the problem-solving method for medication calculation.
- The Lippincott editorial and production teams, for all of their hard work: **Margaret Zuccarini**, Senior Nursing Editor; **Helen Kogut**, Editorial Assistant; **Claudia Vaughn**, Managing Editor; **Debra Schiff**, Production Editor; **Mike Carcel**, Production Coordinator; and **Carolyn O'Brien**, Art Director.

To these people and many more, I would like to express my sincere appreciation for their mentoring, guidance, support, and encouragement that have helped to turn a dream into a reality.

CLINICAL CALCULATIONS MADE EASY

Solving Problems Using Dimensional Analysis

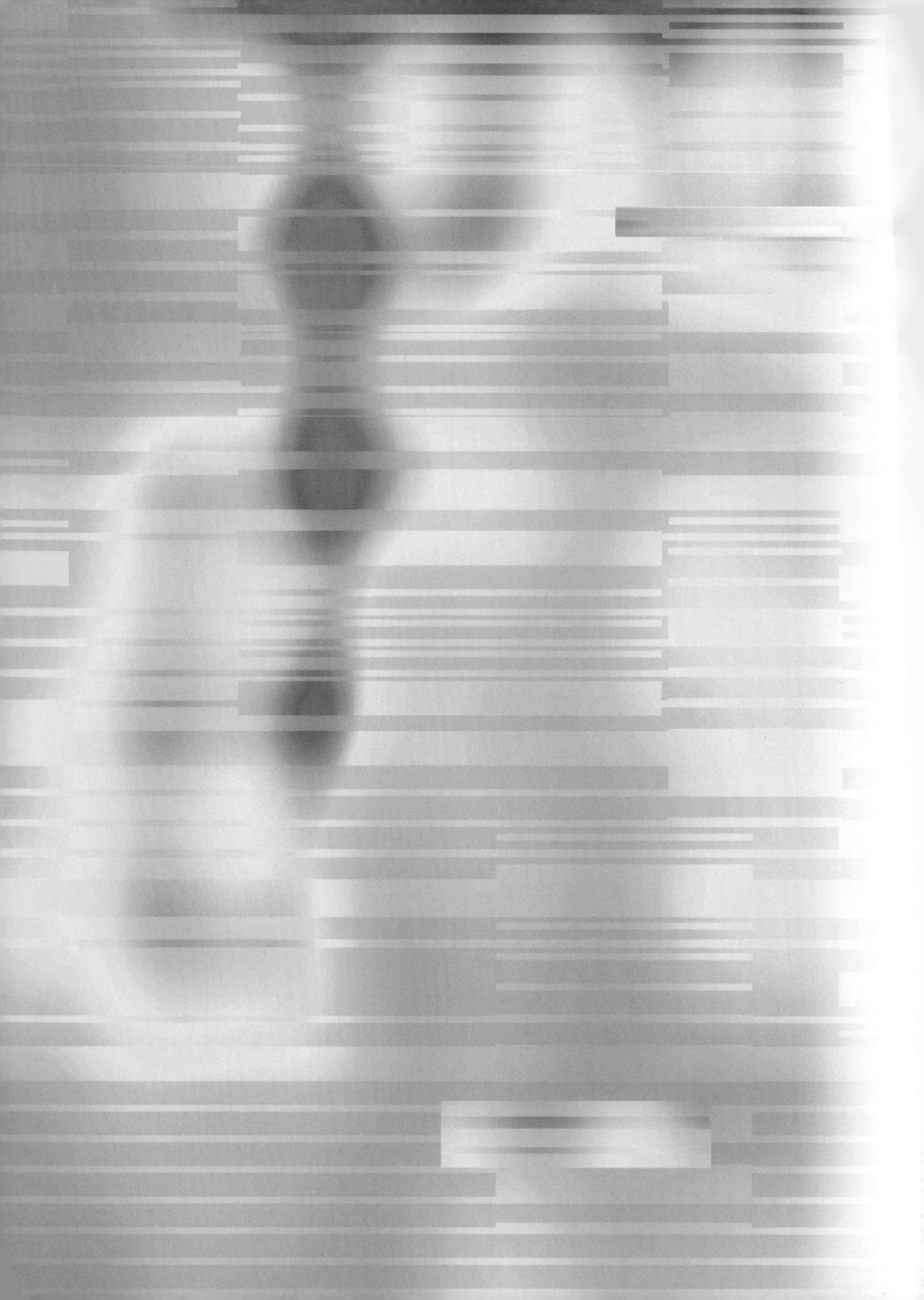

SECTION 1

CLINICAL CALCULATIONS

This chapter reviews basic arithmetic skills that will prepare you to calculate medication dosage problems using the problem-solving method of **dimensional analysis.**

1

ARITHMETIC REVIEW

Outline

Objectives

After completing this chapter, you will be able to:

1. Express Arabic numbers as Roman numerals.
2. Express Roman numerals as Arabic numbers.
3. Identify the numerator and denominator in a fraction.
4. Multiply and divide fractions.
5. Multiply and divide decimals.
6. Convert fractions to decimals.

ARABIC NUMBERS AND ROMAN NUMERALS

Most medication dosages are ordered by the physician in the metric and household systems for weights and measures using the Arabic number system with symbols called **digits** (ie, 1, 2, 3, 4, 5). Occasionally, orders are received in the apothecary system of weights and measures using the Roman numeral system with numbers represented by **symbols** (ie, I, V, X). The Roman numeral system uses seven basic symbols, and various combinations of these symbols represent all numbers in the Arabic number system.

Table 1-1 includes the seven basic Roman numerals and the corresponding Arabic numbers.

The combination of Roman numeral symbols is based on three specific principles:

1. Symbols are used to construct a number, but no symbol may be used more than three times. The exception is the symbol for five (V), which is used only once because there is a symbol for 10 (X) and a combination of symbols for 15 (XV).

EXAMPLE 1.1

III = (1 + 1 + 1) = 3

XXX = (10 + 10 + 10) = 30

2. When symbols of lesser value follow symbols of greater value, they are *added* to construct a number.

EXAMPLE 1.2

VIII = (5 + 3) = 8

XVII = (10 + 5 + 1 + 1) = 17

● TABLE 1.1 Seven Basic Roman Numerals

ROMAN NUMERALS	ARABIC NUMBERS
I	1
V	5
X	10
L	50
C	100
D	500
M	1000

3. When symbols of greater value follow symbols of lesser value, those of lesser value are *subtracted* from those of higher value to construct a number.

EXAMPLE 1.3

IV = (5 – 1) = 4

IX = (10 – 1) = 9

Exercise 1.1 Arabic Numbers and Roman Numerals

(See page 21 for answers)

Express the following Arabic numbers as Roman numerals.

1. 1 = ______
2. 2 = ______
3. 3 = ______
4. 4 = ______
5. 5 = ______
6. 6 = ______
7. 7 = ______
8. 8 = ______
9. 9 = ______
10. 10 = ______
11. 11 = ______
12. 12 = ______
13. 13 = ______
14. 14 = ______
15. 15 = ______
16. 16 = ______
17. 17 = ______
18. 18 = ______
19. 19 = ______
20. 20 = ______

(Exercise continues on page 6)

Although medication orders rarely involve Roman numerals higher than 20, for additional practice, express the following Arabic numbers as Roman numerals.

21. 43 = ______
22. 24 = ______
23. 55 = ______
24. 32 = ______
25. 102 = ______
26. 150 = ______
27. 75 = ______
28. 92 = ______
29. 64 = ______
30. 69 = ______

Express the following Roman numerals as Arabic numbers.

31. II = ______
32. IV = ______
33. VI = ______
34. X = ______
35. VIII = ______
36. XIX = ______
37. XX = ______
38. XVIII = ______
39. I = ______
40. XV = ______
41. III = ______
42. V = ______
43. IX = ______
44. VII = ______
45. XI = ______
46. XIV = ______
47. XVI = ______
48. XII = ______
49. XVII = ______
50. XIII = ______

To increase your abilities to use either system, convert the following Arabic numbers or Roman numerals.

51. 19 = ______
52. XII = ______
53. 7 = ______
54. IX = ______
55. IV = ______
56. 11 = ______
57. VIII = ______
58. 16 = ______
59. XX = ______
60. 5 = ______
61. I = ______
62. 18 = ______
63. VI = ______
64. 2 = ______
65. III = ______
66. 10 = ______
67. XIII = ______
68. 14 = ______
69. XV = ______
70. 17 = ______

FRACTIONS

Medication dosages with fractions are occasionally ordered by the physician or used by the pharmaceutical manufacturer on the drug label. A **fraction** is a number that represents part of a whole number and contains three parts:

1. **Numerator**—the number on the top portion of the fraction that represents the number of parts of the whole fraction.
2. **Dividing line**—the line separating the top portion of the fraction from the bottom portion of the fraction.
3. **Denominator**—the number on the bottom portion of the fraction that represents the number of parts into which the whole is divided.

$$\frac{3}{4} = \frac{\text{numerator}}{\text{denominator}}$$

To solve medication dosage calculation problems using dimensional analysis, you must be able to identify the numerator and denominator portion of the problem. You also must be able to multiply and divide numbers, fractions, and decimals.

Multiplying Fractions

The three steps for multiplying fractions are:

1. Multiply the numerators.
2. Multiply the denominators.
3. Reduce the product to the lowest possible fraction.

EXAMPLE 1.4

$$\frac{2}{4} \times \frac{1}{8} = \frac{2}{32} = \frac{1}{16}$$

or

$$\frac{2\ (\text{numerator})}{4\ (\text{denominator})} \times \frac{1\ (\text{numerator})}{8\ (\text{denominator})} = \frac{2\ (\text{numerator})}{32\ (\text{denominator})}$$

$$= \frac{1}{16}\ (\text{reduced to lowest possible fraction})$$

EXAMPLE 1.5

$$\frac{1}{2} \times \frac{2}{4} = \frac{2}{8} = \frac{1}{4}$$

or

$$\frac{1\ (\text{numerator})}{2\ (\text{denominator})} \times \frac{2\ (\text{numerator})}{4\ (\text{denominator})} = \frac{2\ (\text{numerator})}{8\ (\text{denominator})}$$

$$= \frac{1}{4}\ (\text{reduced to lowest possible fraction})$$

Exercise 1.2 Multiplying Fractions

(See pages 21–22 for answers)

To increase your abilities when working with fractions, multiply the following fractions and reduce to the lowest fractional term.

1. $\frac{3}{4} \times \frac{5}{8} =$

2. $\frac{1}{3} \times \frac{4}{9} =$

3. $\frac{2}{3} \times \frac{4}{5} =$

4. $\frac{3}{4} \times \frac{1}{2} =$

5. $\frac{1}{8} \times \frac{4}{5} =$

6. $\frac{2}{3} \times \frac{5}{8} =$

7. $\frac{3}{8} \times \frac{2}{3} =$

8. $\frac{4}{7} \times \frac{2}{4} =$

9. $\frac{4}{5} \times \frac{1}{2} =$

10. $\frac{1}{4} \times \frac{1}{8} =$

Dividing Fractions

The four steps for dividing fractions are:

1. Invert (turn upside down) the divisor portion of the problem (the second fraction in the problem).
2. Multiply the two numerators.
3. Multiply the two denominators.
4. Reduce answer to lowest term (fraction or whole number).

EXAMPLE 1.6

$$\frac{2}{4} \div \frac{1}{8} = \frac{2}{4} \times \frac{8}{1} = \frac{16}{4} = 4$$

or

$$\frac{2\ (\text{numerator})}{4\ (\text{denominator})} \div \frac{1\ (\text{numerator})}{8\ (\text{denominator})}$$

$$= \frac{2\ (\text{numerator}) \times \overset{(\text{inverted fraction})}{8\ (\text{numerator})} = 16}{4\ (\text{denominator}) \times 1\ (\text{denominator}) = 4}$$

$= 4$ (answer reduced to lowest term)

EXAMPLE 1.7

$$\frac{1}{2} \div \frac{2}{4} = \frac{1}{2} \times \frac{4}{2} = \frac{4}{4} = 1$$

or

$$\frac{1\ (\text{numerator})}{2\ (\text{denominator})} \div \frac{2\ (\text{numerator})}{4\ (\text{denominator})}$$

$$= \frac{1\ (\text{numerator}) \times 4\ (\text{numerator})\ \overset{(\text{inverted fraction})}{} = 4}{2\ (\text{denominator}) \times 2\ (\text{denominator}) = 4}$$

$= 1$ (answer reduced to lowest term)

Exercise 1.3 Dividing Fractions

(See page 22 for answers)

To increase your abilities when working with fractions, divide the following fractions and reduce to the lowest fractional term.

1. $\frac{3}{4} \div \frac{2}{3} =$

2. $\frac{1}{9} \div \frac{3}{9} =$

3. $\frac{2}{3} \div \frac{1}{6} =$

4. $\frac{1}{5} \div \frac{4}{5} =$

5. $\frac{3}{6} \div \frac{4}{8} =$

6. $\frac{5}{8} \div \frac{5}{8} =$

7. $\frac{1}{8} \div \frac{2}{3} =$

8. $\frac{1}{5} \div \frac{1}{2} =$

DECIMALS

Medication orders are often written using decimals, and pharmaceutical manufacturers may use decimals when labeling medications. Therefore, you must understand the learning principles involving decimals and be able to multiply and divide decimals.

- A decimal point is preceded by a zero if not preceded by a number to decrease chance of an error if the decimal point is missed.

EXAMPLE 1.8

0.25

- A decimal point may be preceded by a number and followed by a number.

EXAMPLE 1.9

1.25

- Numbers to the left of the decimal point are *units, tens, hundreds, thousands,* and *ten-thousands.*
- Numbers to the right of the decimal point are *tenths, hundredths, thousandths,* and *ten-thousandths.*

EXAMPLE 1.10

0.2 = 2 tenths

0.05 = 5 hundredths

0.25 = 25 hundredths

1.25 = 1 unit and 25 hundredths

110.25 = 110 units and 25 hundredths

Rounding Decimals

- Decimals may be rounded off. If the number to the right of the decimal is greater than or equal to 5 (≥5), round up to the next number.
- If the number to the right of the decimal is less than 5 (<5), delete the remaining numbers.

EXAMPLE 1.11

0.78 → 0.8

0.213 → 0.2

Exercise 1.4 **Rounding Decimals**
(See page 22 for answers)

Practice rounding off the following decimals to the tenth.

1. 0.75 =
2. 0.88 =
3. 0.44 =
4. 0.23 =
5. 0.67 =
6. 0.27 =
7. 0.98 =
8. 0.92 =

Multiplying Decimals

When multiplying with decimals, the principles of multiplication still apply. The numbers are multiplied in columns, but the number of decimal points are counted and placed in the answer counting places from right to left.

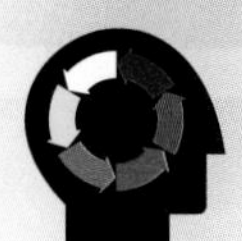

THINKING IT THROUGH

2 decimal points added to the answer counting 2 places from the right to left

EXAMPLE 1.12

```
  2.3 (1 decimal point)
×1.5 (1 decimal point)
  115
  230
 3.45
```

Exercise 1.5 **Multiplying Decimals**
(See page 22 for answers)

Practice multiplying the following decimals.

1. 2.5 × 4.6
2. 1.45 × 0.25

3. $\begin{array}{r} 3.9 \\ \times 0.8 \\ \hline \end{array}$

4. $\begin{array}{r} 2.56 \\ \times 0.45 \\ \hline \end{array}$

5. $\begin{array}{r} 10.65 \\ \times\ 0.05 \\ \hline \end{array}$

6. $\begin{array}{r} 1.98 \\ \times 3.10 \\ \hline \end{array}$

Dividing Decimals

When dividing with decimals, the principles of dividing still apply, except that the dividing number is changed to a whole number by moving the decimal point to the right. The number being divided also changes by accepting the same number of decimal point moves.

EXAMPLE 1.13

$0.5\overline{)0.75}$

Step 1 Move decimal point one place to the right.

Step 2

$$\begin{array}{r} 1.5 \\ 5\overline{)7.5} \\ \underline{5} \\ 2\,5 \\ \underline{2\,5} \\ 0 \end{array}$$

1.5

Exercise 1.6 **Dividing Decimals**
(See pages 23–24 for answers)

Practice dividing the following decimals and rounding the answers to the tenth.

1. $3.4\overline{)9.6}$

2. $0.25\overline{)12.50}$

3. $0.56\overline{)18.65}$

(Exercise continues on page 14)

4. $0.3\overline{)0.192}$

5. $0.4\overline{)12.43}$

6. $0.5\overline{)12.50}$

7. $0.125\overline{)0.25}$

8. $0.08\overline{)0.085}$

CONVERTING FRACTIONS TO DECIMALS

When problem solving with dimensional analysis, medication dosage-calculation problems may frequently contain both fractions and decimals. Some of you may have fraction phobia and prefer to convert fractions to decimals when solving problems. To convert a fraction to a decimal, divide the numerator portion of the fraction by the denominator portion of the fraction.

When dividing fractions, remember to add a decimal point and a zero if the numerator cannot be divided by the denominator.

EXAMPLE 1.14

$$\frac{1}{2} \text{ or } \frac{1\ (\text{numerator})}{2\ (\text{denominator})} = 2\overline{)1.0} \quad \begin{array}{r} 0.5 \\ \hline 1.0 \\ \underline{1\ 0} \end{array} = 0.5$$

EXAMPLE 1.15

$$\frac{3}{4} \text{ or } \frac{3\ (\text{numerator})}{4\ (\text{denominator})} = 4\overline{)3.00} \quad \begin{array}{r} 0.75 \\ \hline 3.00 \\ \underline{2\ 8\ } \\ 20 \\ \underline{20} \end{array} = 0.75$$

Exercise 1.7 **Converting Fractions to Decimals**
(See page 24 for answers)

To decrease fraction phobia, practice converting the following fractions to decimals.

1. $\frac{1}{8} =$

2. $\frac{1}{4} =$

3. $\frac{2}{5}$ =

4. $\frac{3}{5}$ =

5. $\frac{2}{3}$ =

6. $\frac{6}{8}$ =

7. $\frac{3}{8}$ =

8. $\frac{1}{3}$ =

9. $\frac{3}{6}$ =

10. $\frac{2}{10}$ =

SUMMARY

This chapter has reviewed basic arithmetic that will assist you to successfully implement dimensional analysis as a problem-solving method for medication dosage calculations. To assess your understanding and retention, complete the following practice problems.

Practice Problems for Chapter 1 Arithmetic Review

(See pages 25–26 for answers)

Change the following Arabic numbers to Roman numerals.

1. 2 =
2. 4 =
3. 5 =
4. 14 =
5. 19 =

Change the following Roman numerals to Arabic numbers.

6. VI =
7. IX =

(Practice problems continue on page 16)

8. XII =

9. XVII =

10. XIX =

Multiply the following fractions and reduce the answer to the lowest fractional term.

11. $\frac{3}{4} \times \frac{2}{5} =$

12. $\frac{2}{3} \times \frac{5}{8} =$

13. $\frac{1}{2} \times \frac{2}{3} =$

14. $\frac{7}{8} \times \frac{1}{3} =$

15. $\frac{4}{5} \times \frac{2}{7} =$

Divide the following fractions and reduce the answer to the lowest fractional term.

16. $\frac{1}{2} \div \frac{3}{4} =$

17. $\frac{1}{3} \div \frac{7}{8} =$

18. $\frac{1}{5} \div \frac{1}{2} =$

19. $\frac{4}{8} \div \frac{2}{3} =$

20. $\frac{1}{3} \div \frac{2}{3} =$

Multiply the following decimals.

21. $\begin{array}{r} 6.45 \\ \times\underline{1.36} \end{array}$

22. $\begin{array}{r} 3.14 \\ \times\underline{2.20} \end{array}$

23. $\begin{array}{r} 16.286 \\ \times\ 0.125 \\ \hline \end{array}$

24. $\begin{array}{r} 1.2 \\ \times 0.5 \\ \hline \end{array}$

25. $\begin{array}{r} 7.68 \\ \times 0.05 \\ \hline \end{array}$

Divide the following decimals.

26. $0.5\overline{)1.25}$

27. $0.20\overline{)40.80}$

28. $0.125\overline{)0.25}$

29. $0.75\overline{)0.125}$

30. $0.5\overline{)7.30}$

Convert the following fractions to decimals and round to the tenth.

31. $\frac{1}{2} =$

32. $\frac{1}{3} =$

33. $\frac{3}{4} =$

34. $\frac{2}{3} =$

35. $\frac{1}{8} =$

POST-TEST FOR CHAPTER 1: ARITHMETIC REVIEW

Name ______________________________ **Date** ____________

Converting Between Arabic Numbers and Roman Numerals

1. 4 = ______

2. IX = ______

Multiplying and Dividing Fractions

3. $\frac{1}{8} \times \frac{1}{8} =$ ______

4. $\frac{2}{4} \times \frac{1}{2} =$ ______

5. $\frac{1}{6} \div \frac{1}{3} =$ ______

6. $\frac{3}{4} \div \frac{7}{8} =$ ______

Converting Fractions to Decimals

7. $\frac{1}{2} =$ ______

8. $\frac{3}{4} =$ ______

Multiplying and Dividing Decimals

9. $0.25 \times 1.25 =$ ______

10. $0.125 \div 0.25 =$ ______

ANSWER KEY FOR CHAPTER 1: ARITHMETIC REVIEW

Exercise 1.1 Arabic Numbers and Roman Numerals

1. 1 = I
2. 1 + 1 = II
3. 1 + 1 + 1 = III
4. 5 − 1 = IV
5. 5 = V
6. 5 + 1 = VI
7. 5 + 1 + 1 = VII
8. 5 + 1 + 1 + 1 = VIII
9. 10 − 1 = IX
10. 10 = X
11. 10 + 1 = XI
12. 10 + 1 + 1 = XII
13. 10 + 1 + 1 + 1 = XIII
14. 10 + 5 − 1 = XIV
15. 10 + 5 = XV
16. 10 + 5 + 1 = XVI
17. 10 + 5 + 1 + 1 = XVII
18. 10 + 5 + 1 + 1 + 1 = XVIII
19. 10 + 10 − 1 = XIX
20. 10 + 10 = XX
21. 50 − 10 + 1 + 1 + 1 = XLIII
22. 10 + 10 + 5 − 1 = XXIV
23. 50 + 5 = LV
24. 10 + 10 + 10 + 1 + 1 = XXXII
25. 100 + 1 + 1 = CII
26. 100 + 50 = CL
27. 50 + 10 + 10 + 5 = LXXV
28. 100 − 10 + 1 + 1 = XCII
29. 50 + 10 + 5 − 1 = LXIV
30. 50 + 10 + 10 − 1 = LXIX
31. 1 + 1 = 2
32. 5 − 1 = 4
33. 5 + 1 = 6
34. 10 = 10
35. 5 + 1 + 1 + 1 = 8
36. 10 − 1 + 10 = 19
37. 10 + 10 = 20
38. 10 + 5 + 1 + 1 + 1 = 18
39. 1 = 1
40. 10 + 5 = 15
41. 1 + 1 + 1 = 3
42. 5 = 5
43. 10 − 1 = 9
44. 5 + 1 + 1 = 7
45. 10 + 1 = 11
46. 10 + 5 − 1 = 14
47. 10 + 5 + 1 = 16
48. 10 + 1 + 1 = 12
49. 10 + 5 + 1 + 1 = 17
50. 10 + 1 + 1 + 1 = 13
51. 19 = XIX
52. XII = 12
53. 7 = VII
54. IX = 9
55. IV = 4
56. 11 = XI
57. VIII = 8
58. 16 = XVI
59. XX = 20
60. 5 = V
61. I = 1
62. 18 = XVIII
63. VI = 6
64. 2 = II
65. III = 3
66. 10 = X
67. XIII = 13
68. 14 = XIV
69. XV = 15
70. 17 = XVII

Exercise 1.2 Multiplying Fractions

1. $\frac{3}{4} \times \frac{5}{8} = \frac{3 \times 5 = 15}{4 \times 8 = 32} = \frac{15}{32}$

2. $\frac{1}{3} \times \frac{4}{9} = \frac{1 \times 4 = 4}{3 \times 9 = 27} = \frac{4}{27}$

3. $\frac{2}{3} \times \frac{4}{5} = \frac{2 \times 4 = 8}{3 \times 5 = 15} = \frac{8}{15}$

4. $\frac{3}{4} \times \frac{1}{2} = \frac{3 \times 1 = 3}{4 \times 2 = 8} = \frac{3}{8}$

5. $\frac{1}{8} \times \frac{4}{5} = \frac{1 \times 4 = 4(4) = 1}{8 \times 5 = 40(4) = 10} = \frac{1}{10}$

6. $\frac{2}{3} \times \frac{5}{8} = \frac{2 \times 5 = 10(2) = 5}{3 \times 8 = 24(2) = 12} = \frac{5}{12}$

7. $\frac{3}{8} \times \frac{2}{3} = \frac{3 \times 2 = 6(6) = 1}{8 \times 3 = 24(6) = 4} = \frac{1}{4}$

8. $\frac{4}{7} \times \frac{2}{4} = \frac{4 \times 2 = 8(4) = 2}{7 \times 4 = 28(4) = 7} = \frac{2}{7}$

9. $\frac{4}{5} \times \frac{1}{2} = \frac{4 \times 1 = 4(2) = 2}{5 \times 2 = 10(2) = 5} = \frac{2}{5}$

10. $\frac{1}{4} \times \frac{1}{8} = \frac{1 \times 1 = 1}{4 \times 8 = 32} = \frac{1}{32}$

Exercise 1.3 Dividing Fractions

1. $\frac{3}{4} \div \frac{2}{3} = \frac{3}{4} \times \frac{3}{2}$ or $\frac{3 \times 3 = 9}{4 \times 2 = 8} = \begin{array}{r} 1\frac{1}{8} \\ 8\overline{)9} \\ \underline{8} \\ 1 \end{array} = 1\frac{1}{8}$

2. $\frac{1}{9} \div \frac{3}{9} = \frac{1}{9} \times \frac{9}{3}$ or $\frac{1 \times 9 = 9(9) = 1}{9 \times 3 = 27(9) = 3} = \frac{1}{3}$

3. $\frac{2}{3} \div \frac{1}{6} = \frac{2}{3} \times \frac{6}{1}$ or $\frac{2 \times 6 = 12}{3 \times 1 = 3} = \begin{array}{r} 4 \\ 3\overline{)12} \\ \underline{12} \end{array} = 4$

4. $\frac{1}{5} \div \frac{4}{5} = \frac{1}{5} \times \frac{5}{4}$ or $\frac{1 \times 5 = 5(5) = 1}{5 \times 4 = 20(5) = 4} = \frac{1}{4}$

5. $\frac{3}{6} \div \frac{4}{8} = \frac{3}{6} \times \frac{8}{4}$ or $\frac{3 \times 8 = 24}{6 \times 4 = 24} = \begin{array}{r} 1 \\ 24\overline{)24} \end{array} = 1$

6. $\frac{5}{8} \div \frac{5}{8} = \frac{5}{8} \times \frac{8}{5}$ or $\frac{5 \times 8 = 40}{8 \times 5 = 40} = \begin{array}{r} 1 \\ 40\overline{)40} \end{array} = 1$

7. $\frac{1}{8} \div \frac{2}{3} = \frac{1}{8} \times \frac{3}{2}$ or $\frac{1 \times 3 = 3}{8 \times 2 = 16} = \frac{3}{16}$

8. $\frac{1}{5} \div \frac{1}{2} = \frac{1}{5} \times \frac{2}{1}$ or $\frac{1 \times 2 = 2}{5 \times 1 = 5} = \frac{2}{5}$

Exercise 1.4 Rounding Decimals

1. 0.75 = 0.8
2. 0.88 = 0.9
3. 0.44 = 0.4
4. 0.23 = 0.2
5. 0.67 = 0.7
6. 0.27 = 0.3
7. 0.98 = 1.0
8. 0.92 = 0.9

Exercise 1.5 Multiplying Decimals

1. 2.5 (1 decimal point)
×4.6 (1 decimal point)
150
1000
1150
11.50 (2 decimal points from the right to left)

2. 1.45 (2 decimal points)
×0.25 (2 decimal points)
725
2900
0000
3625
0.3625 (4 decimal points from the right to left)

3. 3.9 (1 decimal point)
×0.8 (1 decimal point)
312
000
312
3.12 (2 decimal points from the right to left)

4. 2.56 (2 decimal points)
×0.45 (2 decimal points)
1280
10240
00000
11520
1.1520 (4 decimal points from the right to left)

5. 10.65 (2 decimal points)
×0.05 (2 decimal points)
5325
0000
5325
0.5325 (4 decimal points from the right to left)

6. 1.98 (2 decimal points)
×3.10 (2 decimal points)
000
1980
59400
61380
6.1380 (4 decimal points from the right to left)

Exercise 1.6 Dividing Decimals

1. $3.4\overline{)9.6}$

(Move decimal points one place to the right)

Answer: 2.82 = 2.8

$$
\begin{array}{r}
2.82 \\
34\overline{)96.00} \\
\underline{68} \\
28\ 0 \\
\underline{27\ 2} \\
80 \\
\underline{68} \\
12
\end{array}
$$

2. $0.25\overline{)12.50}$

(Move decimal points two places to the right)

Answer: 50. = 50

$$
\begin{array}{r}
50. \\
25\overline{)1250.} \\
\underline{125} \\
00
\end{array}
$$

3. $0.56\overline{)18.65}$

(Move decimal points two places to the right)

Answer: 33.30 = 33.3

$$
\begin{array}{r}
33.30 \\
56\overline{)1865.00} \\
\underline{168} \\
185 \\
\underline{168} \\
17\ 0 \\
\underline{16\ 8} \\
20
\end{array}
$$

4. $0.3\overline{)0.192}$

(Move decimal points one place to the right)

Answer: 0.64 = 0.6

$$
\begin{array}{r}
.64 \\
3\overline{)01.92} \\
\underline{1\ 8} \\
12 \\
\underline{12} \\
0
\end{array}
$$

5. $0.4\overline{)12.43}$

(Move decimal points one place to the right)

Answer: 31.075 = 31.1

$$
\begin{array}{r}
31.075 \\
4\overline{)124.300} \\
\underline{12} \\
04 \\
\underline{4} \\
0\ 30 \\
\underline{28} \\
20 \\
\underline{20} \\
0
\end{array}
$$

6. $0.5\overline{)12.50}$

(Move decimal points one place to the right)

Answer: 25.0 = 25

$$
\begin{array}{r}
25.0 \\
5\overline{)125.0} \\
\underline{10} \\
25 \\
\underline{25} \\
0
\end{array}
$$

7. $0.125\overline{)0.25}$

(Move decimal points three places to the right)

Answer: 2. = 2

$$
\begin{array}{r}
2 \\
125\overline{)250} \\
\underline{250} \\
0
\end{array}
$$

8. $0.08\overline{)0.085}$

(Move decimal points two places to the right)

Answer: 1.0625 = 1.1

```
   1.0625
8)8.5000
  8
   50
   48
    20
    16
    40
    40
     0
```

Exercise 1.7 Converting Fractions to Decimals

1. $\frac{1}{8} = 0.125$

Answer = 0.125

```
  0.125
8)1.000
   8
   20
   16
    40
    40
     0
```

2. $\frac{1}{4} = 0.25$

Answer = 0.25

```
   .25
4)1.00
   8
   20
   20
    0
```

3. $\frac{2}{5} = 0.4$

Answer = 0.4

```
  0.4
5)2.0
  2 0
    0
```

4. $\frac{3}{5} = 0.6$

Answer = 0.6

```
  0.6
5)3.0
  3 0
    0
```

5. $\frac{2}{3} = 0.66$

Answer = 0.66

```
  0.66
3)2.00
  1 8
   20
   18
    2
```

6. $\frac{6}{8} = 0.75$

Answer = 0.75

```
  0.75
8)6.00
  5 6
   40
   40
    0
```

7. $\frac{3}{8} = 0.375$

Answer = 0.375

```
   .375
8)3.00
  2 4
   60
   56
    40
    40
     0
```

8. $\frac{1}{3} = 0.33$

Answer = 0.33

$$3\overline{)1.00}$$ quotient 0.33; 9; 10; 9; 1

9. $\frac{3}{6} = 0.5$

Answer = 0.5

$$6\overline{)3.0}$$ quotient 0.5; 3 0; 0

10. $\frac{2}{10} = 0.2$

Answer = 0.2

$$10\overline{)2.0}$$ quotient 0.2; 2 0; 0

Practice Problems

1. II
2. IV
3. V
4. XIV
5. XIX
6. 6
7. 9
8. 12
9. 17
10. 19
11. $\frac{3 \times 2 = 6(2) = 3}{4 \times 5 = 20(2) = 10} = \frac{3}{10}$
12. $\frac{2 \times 5 = 10(2) = 5}{3 \times 8 = 24(2) = 12} = \frac{5}{12}$
13. $\frac{1 \times 2 = 2(2) = 1}{2 \times 3 = 6(2) = 3} = \frac{1}{3}$
14. $\frac{7 \times 1 = 7}{8 \times 3 = 24} = \frac{7}{24}$
15. $\frac{4 \times 2 = 8}{5 \times 7 = 35} = \frac{8}{35}$
16. $\frac{1}{2} \div \frac{3}{4} = \frac{1 \times 4 = 4(2) = 2}{2 \times 3 = 6(2) = 3} = \frac{2}{3}$
17. $\frac{1}{3} \div \frac{7}{8} = \frac{1 \times 8 = 8}{3 \times 7 = 21} = \frac{8}{21}$
18. $\frac{1}{5} \div \frac{1}{2} = \frac{1 \times 2 = 2}{5 \times 1 = 5} = \frac{2}{5}$
19. $\frac{4}{8} \div \frac{2}{3} = \frac{4 \times 3 = 12(4) = 3}{8 \times 2 = 16(4) = 4} = \frac{3}{4}$
20. $\frac{1}{3} \div \frac{2}{3} = \frac{1 \times 3 = 3(3) = 1}{3 \times 2 = 6(3) = 2} = \frac{1}{2}$
21. 6.45 (2 decimal points)
    ×1.36 (2 decimal points)
    3870
    19350
    64500
    87720
    8.7720 (4 decimal points from right to left)
22. 3.14 (2 decimal points)
    ×2.20 (2 decimal points)
    000
    6280
    62800
    69080
    6.9080 (4 decimal points from right to left)
23. 16.286 (3 decimal points)
    ×0.125 (3 decimal points)
    81430
    325720
    1628600
    2035750
    2.035750 (6 decimal points from right to left)
24. 1.2 (1 decimal point)
    ×0.5 (1 decimal point)
    60
    000
    060
    0.60 (2 decimal points from right to left)

25.
```
   7.68 (2 decimal points)
 ×0.05 (2 decimal points)
  3840
  0000
 00000
 03840
 0.3840 (4 decimal points from right to left)
```

26. $0.5\overline{)1.25}$

(Move decimal points one place to the right)

Answer: 2.5 = 2.5

```
   2.5
 5)12.5
   10
    25
    25
     0
```

27. $0.20\overline{)40.80}$

(Move decimal points two places to the right)

Answer: 204. = 204

```
    204
 20)4080
    40
     080
      80
       0
```

28. $0.125\overline{)0.25}$

(Move decimal points three places to the right)

Answer: 2. = 2

```
       2
 125)250
     250
       0
```

29. $0.75\overline{)0.125}$

(Move decimal points two places to the right)

Answer: 0.166 = 0.2

```
      .166
 75)12.500
     7 5
     5 00
     4 50
       50
```

30. $0.5\overline{)7.30}$

(Move decimal point one place to the right)

Answer: 14.6 = 14.6

```
   14.6
 5)73.0
   5
   23
   20
    30
    30
     0
```

31. 0.5
32. 0.33 = 0.3
33. 0.75 = 0.8
34. 0.66 = 0.7
35. 0.125 = 0.1

Medication calculation need not be difficult if you have a problem-solving method that is easy to understand and implement. In addition, you need to understand common equivalents and units of measurement to visualize all parts of a medication dosage calculation problem.

This chapter will help you to understand the measurement systems used for medication administration. This knowledge is necessary to accurately implement the problem-solving method of dimensional analysis.

2

SYSTEMS OF MEASUREMENT AND COMMON EQUIVALENTS

Outline

Objectives

After completing this chapter, you will be able to:

1. Identify measurements included in the metric, apothecary, and household systems.
2. Understand abbreviations used in the metric, apothecary, and household systems.

There are three systems of measurement used for medication dosage administration: the metric system, the apothecary system, and the household system. To be able to accurately administer medication, it is necessary to understand all three of these systems.

THE METRIC SYSTEM

The **metric system** is a decimal system of weights and measures based on units of ten in which gram, meter, and liter are the basic units of measurement. However, gram and liter are the only measurements from the metric system that are used in medication administration. The meter is a unit of distance, the gram (abbreviated g or gm) is a unit of weight, and the liter (abbreviated L) is a unit of volume. Frequently used metric units are displayed in Figure 2.1.

Weight: Basic unit is gram (g)

Equivalents:
- Kilogram (kg) 1 kg = 1,000 g
- Milligram (mg) 1 mg = 1/1,000 g
- Microgram (mcg) 1 mcg = 1/1,000 mg = 1/1,000,000 g

Volume: Basic unit is liter (L)

Equivalents:
- Milliliter (mL) 1 mL = 1/1,000 L
- Cubic centimeter (cc) 1 cc = 1 mL = 1/1,000 L

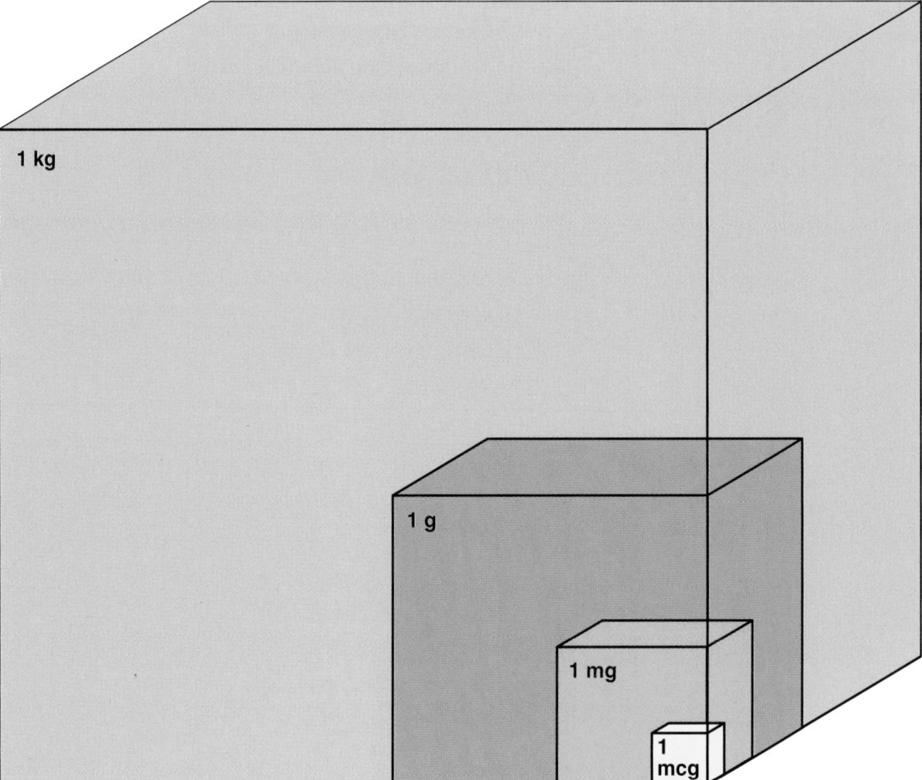

Figure 2-1. Metric units frequently used for drug administration. Another way to understand metric equivalents is to visualize the relationships between equivalent measurements. Please note that the figure is not drawn to scale.

THE APOTHECARY SYSTEM

The **apothecary system** is a system of measuring and weighing drugs and solutions in which fractions are used to identify parts of the unit of measure. The basic units of measurement in the apothecary system include weights and liquid volume. Although this may be replaced by the metric system, it is still necessary to understand it because some physicians continue to order medications using this system, and they also may include Roman numerals in the medication order.

The most frequently used measurements and equivalents within the apothecary system are summarized in Figure 2.2.

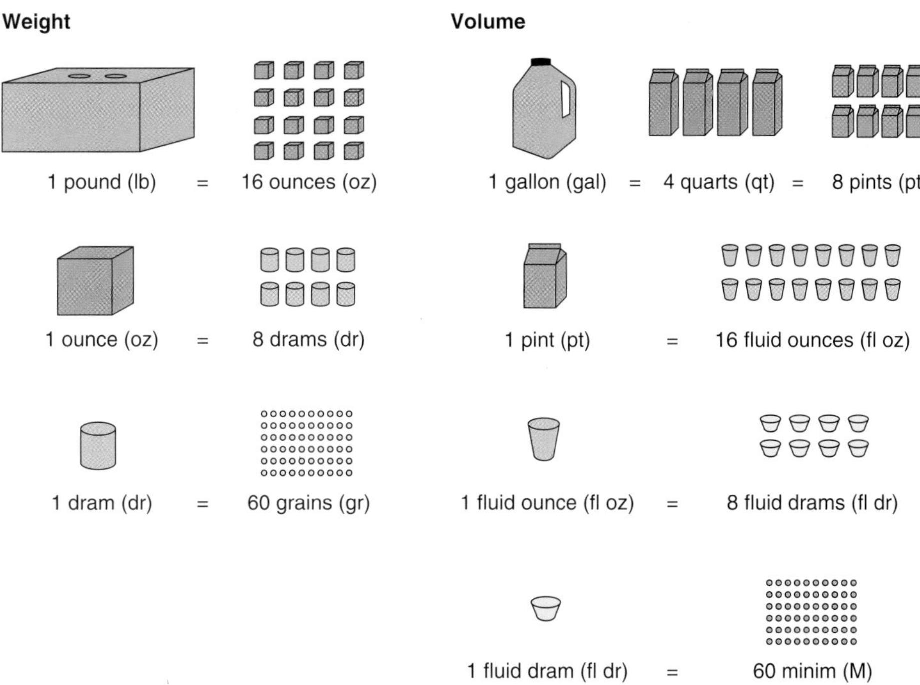

Figure 2-2. Apothecary system of equivalents for weight and volume. Please note that the figures are not shown to scale.

HOUSEHOLD MEASUREMENTS

The use of household measurements is considered inaccurate because of the varying sizes of cups, glasses, and eating utensils, and this system generally has been replaced with the metric system. However, as patient care moves away from hospitals, which use the metric system, and into the community, it is once again necessary for the nurse to have an understanding of the household measurement system to be able to use and teach it to clients and families.

The most frequently used measurements and equivalents within the household measurement system are summarized in Figure 2.3.

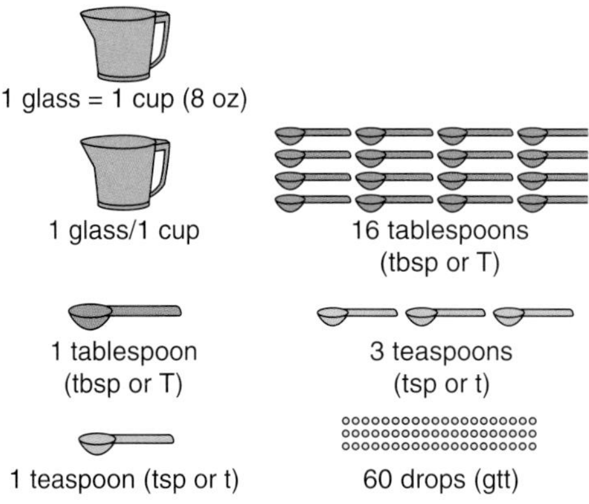

Figure 2-3. Household measurement system and equivalents for volume. Please note that the figures are not shown to scale.

COMMON EQUIVALENTS

Sometimes it is necessary to convert from one system to another to accurately administer medication. See Table 2.1 for approximate equivalents for weight and Table 2.2 for approximate equivalents for volume.

● TABLE 2.1 Approximate Equivalents for Weight

METRIC	APOTHECARY
1 kg (1000 g)	2.2 lb
1 g (1000 mg)	15 gr
60 mg	1 gr

● TABLE 2.2 Approximate Equivalents for Volume

METRIC	APOTHECARY	HOUSEHOLD
4000 mL	1 gal (4 qt)	
1 L (1000 mL)	1 qt (2 pt)	
500 mL	1 pt (16 fl oz)	
240 mL	8 oz	1 cup (1 glass)
30 mL	1 oz (8 dr)	2 tbsp
15 mL	½ oz (4 dr)	1 tbsp (3 tsp)
5 mL	1 dr (60 M)	1 tsp (60 gtt)
1 mL (1 cc)	15 M	15 gtt
	1 M	1 gtt

SUMMARY

This chapter has reviewed the metric, apothecary, and household systems of measurement. To assess your understanding and retention of the systems of measurement, complete the following practice problems.

Practice Problems for Chapter 2 Systems of Measurement and Common Equivalents

(See page 37 for answers)

Write the correct abbreviation symbols for the following measurements from the metric system:

1. kilogram =
2. gram =
3. milligram =
4. microgram =
5. liter =
6. milliliter =
7. cubic centimeter =

Write the correct abbreviation symbols for the following measurements from the apothecary system:

8. pound =
9. ounce =
10. dram =
11. grain =
12. gallon =
13. quart =
14. pint =
15. fluid ounce =
16. fluid dram =
17. minim =

Write the correct abbreviation symbols for the following measurements from the household system:

18. tablespoon =
19. teaspoon =
20. drop =

Identify the correct numerical values for the following measurements:

21. 1 kg = ____ lb
22. 1 kg = ____ g
23. 1 g = ____ mg
24. 1 mg = ____ mcg
25. 1 g = ____ gr

(Practice problems continue on page 34)

26. 1 gr = ____ mg
27. 1000 mg = ____ g
28. 1000 mL = ____ L = ____ qt
29. 500 mL = ____ pt
30. 240 mL = ____ oz
31. 30 mL = ____ oz = ____ tbsp
32. 15 mL = ____ oz = ____ tsp
33. 5 mL = ____ tsp
34. 1 mL = ____ M = ____ gtt
35. 1 mL = ____ cc

POST-TEST FOR CHAPTER 2: SYSTEMS OF MEASUREMENTS AND COMMON EQUIVALENTS

Name ______________________ **Date** __________

1. 2.2 lb = ____ kg
2. 16 fl oz = ____ pt
3. 1 tsp = ____ mL
4. 15 gr = ____ g
5. 1 oz = ____ mL
6. 1000 mcg = ____ mg
7. 60 mg = ____ gr
8. 1 pt = ____ mL
9. 1 cc = ____ mL
10. 1000 mg = ____ g
11. 1 L = ____ mL
12. 4 qt = ____ gal
13. 1 tbsp = ____ tsp
14. 1 glass = ____ oz
15. 8 oz = ____ mL
16. 3 tsp = ____ mL
17. 15 gtt = ____ M
18. 1 dr = ____ cc
19. 15 M = ____ mL
20. 1000 g = ____ kg

ANSWER KEY FOR CHAPTER 2: SYSTEMS OF MEASUREMENT AND COMMON EQUIVALENTS

Practice Problems

1. kilogram = kg
2. gram = g
3. milligram = mg
4. microgram = mcg
5. liter = L
6. milliliter = mL
7. cubic centimeter = cc
8. pound = lb
9. ounce = oz
10. dram = dr
11. grain = gr
12. gallon = gal
13. quart = qt
14. pint = pt
15. fluid ounce = fl oz
16. fluid dram = fl dr
17. minim = M
18. tablespoon = tbsp
19. teaspoon = tsp
20. drop = gtt
21. 1 kg = 2.2 lb
22. 1 kg = 1000 g
23. 1 g = 1000 mg
24. 1 mg = 1000 mcg
25. 1 g = 15 gr
26. 1 gr = 60 mg
27. 1000 mg = 1 g
28. 1000 mL = 1 L = 1 qt
29. 500 mL = 1 pt
30. 240 mL = 8 oz
31. 30 mL = 1 oz = 2 tbsp
32. 15 mL = $\frac{1}{2}$ oz = 3 tsp
33. 5 mL = 1 tsp
34. 1 mL = 15 M = 15 gtt
35. 1 mL = 1 cc

Dimensional analysis provides a systematic, straightforward way to set up problems and to organize and evaluate data. It is not only easy to learn, but also can reduce errors when mathematical conversion is required. This system allows conceptualization of a problem through visualization of all its parts using critical thinking.

This chapter introduces you to dimensional analysis with a step-by-step explanation of this problem-solving method. The chapter also provides the opportunity to practice solving problems that involve common equivalents.

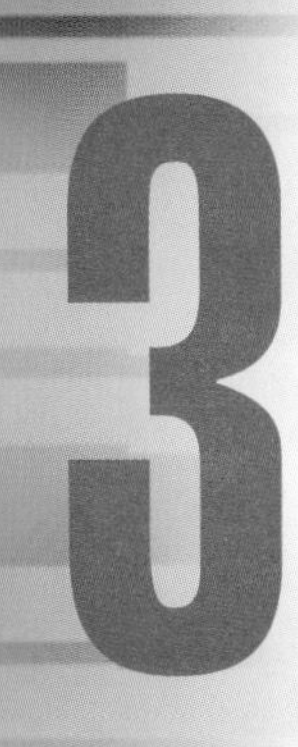

SOLVING PROBLEMS USING DIMENSIONAL ANALYSIS

Outline

Objectives

After completing this chapter, you will be able to:

1. Define the terms used in dimensional analysis.
2. Explain the step-by-step problem-solving method of dimensional analysis.
3. Solve problems involving common equivalents using dimensional analysis as a problem-solving method.

TERMS USED IN DIMENSIONAL ANALYSIS

Dimensional analysis is a problem-solving method that can be used whenever two quantities are directly proportional to each other and one quantity must be converted to the other by using a common equivalent, conversion factor, or conversion relation. All medication dosage calculation problems can be solved by dimensional analysis.

It is important to understand the following four terms that provide the basis for dimensional analysis.

- **Given quantity:** the beginning point of the problem
- **Wanted quantity:** the answer to the problem
- **Unit path:** the series of conversions necessary to achieve the answer to the problem
- **Conversion factors:** equivalents necessary to convert between systems of measurement and to allow unwanted units to be canceled from the problem

  Each conversion factor is a ratio of units that equals 1.

Dimensional analysis also uses the same terms as fractions: numerators and denominators.

- *The numerator* = the top portion of the problem
- *The denominator* = the bottom portion of the problem

Some problems will have a given quantity and a wanted quantity that contain only numerators. Other problems will have a given quantity and a wanted quantity that contain both a numerator and a denominator. This chapter contains only problems with numerators as the given quantity and the wanted quantity.

Once the beginning point in the problem is identified, then a series of conversions necessary to achieve the answer is established that leads to the problem's solution.

Below is an example of the problem-solving method, showing the placement of basic terms used in dimensional analysis.

Unit Path

Given Quantity	Conversion Factor for Given Quantity	Conversion Factor for Wanted Quantity	Conversion Computation		Wanted Quantity
1 liter (L)	1000 mL	1 oz	1 × 1000 × 1	1000	= 33.3 oz
	1 liter (L)	30 mL	1 × 30	30	

THE FIVE STEPS OF DIMENSIONAL ANALYSIS

Once the given quantity is identified, the unit path leading to the wanted quantity is established. The problem-solving method of dimensional analysis uses the following five steps.

1. Identify the *given quantity* in the problem.
2. Identify the *wanted quantity* in the problem.
3. Establish the *unit path* from the given quantity to the wanted quantity using equivalents as *conversion factors*.

4. Set up the conversion factors to permit cancellation of unwanted units. Carefully choose each conversion factor and ensure that it is correctly placed in the numerator or denominator portion of the problem to allow the unwanted units to be canceled from the problem.
5. Multiply the numerators, multiply the denominators, and divide the product of the numerators by the product of the denominators to provide the numerical value of the wanted quantity.

The following examples use the five steps to solve problems using dimensional analysis.

EXAMPLE 3.1

1 liter (L) equals how many ounces (oz)?

Step 1 Identify the *given quantity* in the problem.

The given quantity is *1 L*.

Unit Path

Given Quantity	Conversion Factor for Given Quantity	Conversion Factor for Wanted Quantity	Conversion Computation		Wanted Quantity
1 liter (L)					=

Step 2 Identify the *wanted quantity* in the problem.

The wanted quantity is the number of *ounces* (oz) in 1 L.

Unit Path

Given Quantity	Conversion Factor for Given Quantity	Conversion Factor for Wanted Quantity	Conversion Computation		Wanted Quantity
1 liter (L)					= oz

Step 3 Establish the *unit path* from the given quantity to the wanted quantity. You must determine what conversion factors are needed to convert the given quantity to the wanted quantity.

Given quantity: 1 L = 1000 mL
Wanted quantity: 1 oz = 30 mL

(Example continues on page 42)

Step 4 Write the unit path for the problem so that each unit cancels out the preceding unit until all unwanted units are canceled from the problem except the wanted quantity.

The wanted quantity must be within the numerator portion of the problem to identify that the problem is set up correctly.

Unit Path

Given Quantity	Conversion Factor for Given Quantity	Conversion Factor for Wanted Quantity	Conversion Computation		Wanted Quantity
1 liter (L)	1000 mL	1 oz			= oz
	1 liter (L)	30 mL			

Unit Path

Given Quantity	Conversion Factor for Given Quantity	Conversion Factor for Wanted Quantity	Conversion Computation		Wanted Quantity
1 ~~liter (L)~~	1000 ~~mL~~	1 (oz)			= oz
	1 ~~liter (L)~~	30 ~~mL~~			

Step 5 After the unwanted units are canceled from the problem, only the numerical values remain. Multiply the numerators, multiply the denominators, and divide the product of the numerators by the product of the denominators to provide the numerical value for the wanted quantity.

One (1) times (×) any number equals that number, therefore 1s may be automatically canceled from the problem. Other factors that can be canceled from the problem include like numerical values in the numerator and denominator portion of the problem and the same number of zeroes in the numerator and denominator portion of the problem.

Unit Path

Given Quantity	Conversion Factor for Given Quantity	Conversion Factor for Wanted Quantity	Conversion Computation		Wanted Quantity
1 ~~liter (L)~~	1000 ~~mL~~	1 (oz)	1000 × 1	1000	= 33.3 oz
	1 ~~liter (L)~~	30 ~~mL~~	1 × 30	30	

33.3 oz is the wanted quantity and the answer to the problem.

EXAMPLE 3.2

One gallon (gal) equals how many milliliters?

Step 1 Identify the given quantity in the problem.

The given quantity is 1 gal.

1 gal		=

Step 2 Identify the wanted quantity in the problem.

The wanted quantity is the number of *milliliters* (mL) in 1 gal.

1 gal	

= mL

Step 3 Establish the unit path from the given quantity to the wanted quantity by selecting the equivalents that will be used as conversion factors.

Given quantity: 1 gal = 4 quarts (qt); 1 qt = 1 L
Wanted quantity: 1 L = 1000 mL

Step 4 Write the unit path for the problem so that each unit cancels out the preceding unit until all unwanted units are canceled from the problem except the wanted quantity.

~~1 gal~~	4 ~~qt~~	1 ~~L~~	1000 (mL)
	1 ~~gal~~	1 ~~qt~~	1 ~~L~~

= mL

Step 5 After the unwanted units are canceled from the problem, only the numerical values remain. Multiply the numerators, multiply the denominators, and divide the product of the numerators by the product of the denominators to provide the numerical value for the wanted quantity.

~~1 gal~~	4 ~~qt~~	~~1 L~~	1000 (mL)	4 × 1000
	~~1 gal~~	~~1 qt~~	1 ~~L~~	1

= 4000 mL

Exercise 3.1 Dimensional Analysis

(See page 51 for answers)

Use dimensional analysis to change the following units of measurement.

1. Problem: 4 mg = How many g?

   Given quantity =

   Wanted quantity =

4 mg	

   = g

2. Problem: 5000 g = How many kg?

   Given quantity =

   Wanted quantity =

5000 g	

   = kg

(Exercise continues on page 44)

3. Problem: 0.3 L = How many cc?

Given quantity =

Wanted quantity =

0.3 L		= cc

4. Problem: 10 cc = How many mL?

Given quantity =

Wanted quantity =

10 cc		= mL

5. Problem: 120 lb = How many kg?

Given quantity =

Wanted quantity =

120 lb		= kg

6. Problem: 5 gr = How many mg?

Given quantity =

Wanted quantity =

5 gr		= mg

7. Problem: 2 g = How many gr?

Given quantity =

Wanted quantity =

2 g		= gr

8. Problem: 5 fl dr = How many mL?

Given quantity =

Wanted quantity =

5 fl dr		= mL

9. Problem: 8 fl dr = How many fl oz?

Given quantity =

Wanted quantity =

8 fl dr | = fl oz

10. Problem: 10 M = How many fl dr?

Given quantity =

Wanted quantity =

10 M | = fl dr

11. Problem: 35 kg = How many lb?

Given quantity =

Wanted quantity =

35 kg | = lb

12. Problem: 10 mL = How many tsp?

Given quantity =

Wanted quantity =

10 mL | = tsp

13. Problem: 30 mL = How many tbsp?

Given quantity =

Wanted quantity =

30 mL | = tbsp

14. Problem: 0.25 g = How many mg?

Given quantity =

Wanted quantity =

0.25 g | = mg

(Exercise continues on page 46)

15. Problem: 350 mcg = How many mg?

Given quantity =

Wanted quantity =

350 mcg | = mg

16. Problem: 0.75 L = How many mL?

Given quantity =

Wanted quantity =

0.75 L | = mL

17. Problem: 3 hr = How many minutes?

Given quantity =

Wanted quantity =

3 hr | = min

18. Problem: 3.5 mL = How many M?

Given quantity =

Wanted quantity =

3.5 mL | = M

19. Problem: 500 mcg = How many mg?

Given quantity =

Wanted quantity =

500 mcg | = mg

20. Problem: 225 M = How many tsp?

Given quantity =

Wanted quantity =

225 M | = tsp

SUMMARY

This chapter has introduced you to dimensional analysis with a step-by-step explanation and an opportunity to practice solving problems involving common equivalents. To demonstrate your understanding of dimensional analysis and conversions between systems of measurement, complete the following practice problems.

Practice Problems for Chapter 3 — Solving Problems Using Dimensional Analysis

(See page 53 for answers)

1. Problem: $\frac{3}{4}$ mL = How many M?
2. Problem: gtt XV = How many M?
3. Problem: $\frac{5}{6}$ gr = How many mg?
4. Problem: How many mL in 3 oz?
5. Problem: 0.5 mg = How many mcg?
6. Problem: 35 gtt = How many mL?
7. Problem: How many cc in 3 qt?
8. Problem: 4 gal = How many qt?
9. Problem: 1.5 cup = How many cc?
10. Problem: 24 oz = How many glasses?

POST-TEST FOR CHAPTER 3: SOLVING PROBLEMS USING DIMENSIONAL ANALYSIS

Name ______________________________ **Date** ______________

Use dimensional analysis to solve the following conversion problems:

1. 2045 g = How many lb?
2. 1/150 gr = How many mg?
3. 0.004 g = How many mcg?
4. 6 tsp = How many dr?
5. 0.5 L = How many pt?
6. How many L in 250 oz?
7. How many tbsp in 30 cc?
8. How many minims in 60 cc?
9. How many g in 45 gr?
10. How many oz in 1800 g?

ANSWER KEY FOR CHAPTER 3: SOLVING PROBLEMS USING DIMENSIONAL ANALYSIS

Exercise 3.1 Dimensional Analysis

1. Problem: 4 mg = How many g?
   Given quantity = 4 mg
   Wanted quantity = g
   Conversion factor = 1 g = 1000 mg

4 ~~mg~~	1 g	4 × 1	4 = 0.004 g
	1000 ~~mg~~	1000	1000

2. Problem: 5000 g = How many kg?
   Given quantity = 5000 g
   Wanted quantity = kg
   Conversion factor = 1 kg = 1000 g

~~5000 g~~	1 kg	5 × 1	5 = 5 kg
	~~1000 g~~	1	1

3. Problem: 0.3 L = How many cc?
   Given quantity = 0.3 L
   Wanted quantity = cc
   Conversion factor = 1 L = 1000 cc

0.3 ~~L~~	1000 cc	0.3 × 1000	300 = 300 cc
	1 ~~L~~	1	1

4. Problem: 10 cc = How many mL?
   Given quantity = 10 cc
   Wanted quantity = mL
   Conversion factor = 1 cc = 1 mL

10 ~~cc~~	1 mL	10 × 1	10 = 10 mL
	1 ~~cc~~	1	1

5. Problem: 120 lb = How many kg?
   Given quantity = 120 lb
   Wanted quantity = kg
   Conversion factor = 2.2 lb = 1 kg

120 ~~lb~~	1 kg	120 × 1	120 = 54.5 kg
	2.2 ~~lb~~	2.2	2.2

6. Problem: 5 gr = How many mg?
   Given quantity = 5 gr
   Wanted quantity = mg
   Conversion factor = 1 gr = 60 mg

5 ~~gr~~	60 mg	5 × 60	300 = 300 mg
	1 ~~gr~~	1	1

7. Problem: 2 g = How many gr?
   Given quantity = 2 g
   Wanted quantity = gr
   Conversion factor = 1 g = 15 gr

2 ~~g~~	15 gr	2 × 15	30 = 30 gr
	1 ~~g~~	1	1

8. Problem: 5 fl dr = How many mL?
   Given quantity = 5 fl dr
   Wanted quantity = mL
   Conversion factor = 1 fl dr = 5 mL

5 ~~fl dr~~	5 mL	5 × 5	25 = 25 mL
	1 ~~fl dr~~	1	1

9. Problem: 8 fl dr = How many fl oz?
   Given quantity = 8 fl dr
   Wanted quantity = fl oz
   Conversion factor = 1 fl dr = 5 mL
   Conversion factor = 1 fl oz = 30 mL

8 ~~fl dr~~	5 ~~mL~~	1 fl oz	8 × 5 × 1	40 = 1.3 fl oz
	1 ~~fl dr~~	30 ~~mL~~	1 × 30	30

10. Problem: 10 M = How many fl dr?
    Given quantity = M
    Wanted quantity = fl dr
    Conversion factor = 1 mL = 15 M
    Conversion factor = 1 fl dr = 5 mL

10 ~~M~~	1 ~~mL~~	1 fl dr	10 × 1 × 1	10 = 0.13 fl dr
	15 ~~M~~	5 ~~mL~~	15 × 5	75

11. Problem: 35 kg = How many lb?
Given quantity = 35 kg
Wanted quantity = lb
Conversion factor = 1 kg = 2.2 lb

35 ~~kg~~	2.2 (lb)	35 × 2.2	77 = 77 lb
	1 ~~kg~~	1	1

12. Problem: 10 mL = How many tsp?
Given quantity = 10 mL
Wanted quantity = tsp
Conversion factor = 1 tsp = 5 mL

10 ~~mL~~	1 (tsp)	10 × 1	10 = 2 tsp
	5 ~~mL~~	5	5

13. Problem: 30 mL = How many tbsp?
Given quantity = 30 mL
Wanted quantity = tbsp
Conversion factor = 1 tbsp = 15 mL

30 ~~mL~~	1 (tbsp)	30 × 1	30 = 2 tbsp
	15 ~~mL~~	15	15

14. Problem: 0.25 g = How many mg?
Given quantity = 0.25 g
Wanted quantity = mg
Conversion factor = 1 g = 1000 mg

0.25 ~~g~~	1000 (mg)	0.25 × 1000	250 = 250 mg
	1 ~~g~~	1	1

15. Problem: 350 mcg = How many mg?
Given quantity = 350 mcg
Wanted quantity = mg
Conversion factor = 1 mg = 1000 mcg

350 ~~mcg~~	1 (mg)	350 × 1	350 = 0.35 mg
	1000 ~~mcg~~	1000	1000

16. Problem: 0.75 L = How many mL?
Given quantity = 0.75 L
Wanted quantity = mL
Conversion factor = 1 L = 1000 mL

0.75 ~~L~~	1000 (mL)	0.75 × 1000	750 = 750 mL
	1 ~~L~~	1	1

17. Problem: 3 hr = How many minutes?
Given quantity = 3 hr
Wanted quantity = minutes
Conversion factor = 1 hr = 60 min

3 ~~hr~~	60 (min)	3 × 60	180 = 180 min
	1 ~~hr~~	1	1

18. Problem: 3.5 mL = How many M?
Given quantity = 3.5 mL
Wanted quantity = M
Conversion factor = 1 mL = 15 M

3.5 ~~mL~~	15 (M)	3.5 × 15	52.5 = 52.5 M
	1 ~~mL~~	1	1

19. Problem: 500 mcg = How many mg?
Given quantity = 500 mcg
Wanted quantity = mg
Conversion factor = 1 mg = 1000 mcg

500 ~~mcg~~	1 (mg)	500 × 1	500 = 0.5 mg
	1000 ~~mcg~~	1000	1000

20. Problem: 225 M = How many tsp?
Given quantity = 225 M
Wanted quantity = tsp
Conversion factor = 1 mL = 15 M
Conversion factor = 1 tsp = 5 mL

225 ~~M~~	1 ~~mL~~	1 (tsp)	225 × 1 × 1	225 = 3 tsp
	15 ~~M~~	5 ~~mL~~	15 × 5	75

Practice Problems

1. Problem: $\frac{3}{4}$ mL = How many M?
   Given quantity = $\frac{3}{4}$ mL
   Wanted quantity = M
   Conversion factor = 1 mL = 15 M

$\frac{3}{4}$ ~~mL~~	15 (M)	$\frac{3}{4} \times 15$	$\frac{3}{4} \times \frac{15}{1}$	$\frac{45}{4}$ = 11.25 M
	1 ~~mL~~	1	1	1

2. Problem: gtt XV = How many M?
   Given quantity = 15 gtt
   Wanted quantity = M
   Conversion factor = 1 gtt = 1 M

15 ~~gtt~~	~~1~~ (M)	15 = 15 M
	~~1~~ ~~gtt~~	

3. Problem: $\frac{5}{6}$ gr = How many mg?
   Given quantity = $\frac{5}{6}$ gr
   Wanted quantity = mg
   Conversion factor = 1 gr = 60 mg

$\frac{5}{6}$ ~~gr~~	60 (mg)	$\frac{5}{6} \times 60$	$\frac{5}{6} \times \frac{60}{1}$	$\frac{300}{6}$	50 = 50 mg
	1 ~~gr~~	1	1	1	1

4. Problem: How many mL in 3 oz?
   Given quantity = 3 oz
   Wanted quantity = mL
   Conversion factor = 1 oz = 30 mL

3 ~~oz~~	30 (mL)	3×30	90 = 90 mL
	1 ~~oz~~	1	1

5. Problem: 0.5 mg = How many mcg?
   Given quantity = 0.5 mg
   Wanted quantity = mcg
   Conversion factor = 1 mg = 1000 mcg

0.5 ~~mg~~	1000 (mcg)	0.5×1000	500 = 500 mcg
	1 ~~mg~~	1	1

6. Problem: 35 gtt = How many mL?
   Given quantity = 35 gtt
   Wanted quantity = mL
   Conversion factor = 1 gtt = 1 M
   Conversion factor = 15 M = 1 mL

35 ~~gtt~~	1 ~~M~~	1 (mL)	$35 \times 1 \times 1$	35 = 2.3 mL
	1 ~~gtt~~	15 ~~M~~	1×15	15

7. Problem: How many cc in 3 qt?
   Given quantity = 3 qt
   Wanted quantity = cc
   Conversion factor = 1 qt = 1000 mL
   Conversion factor = 1 cc = 1 mL

3 ~~qt~~	1000 ~~mL~~	1 (cc)	$3 \times 1000 \times 1$	3000 = 3000 cc
	1 ~~qt~~	1 ~~mL~~	1×1	1

8. Problem: 4 gal = How many qt?
   Given quantity = 4 gal
   Wanted quantity = qt
   Conversion factor = 1 gal = 4 qt

4 ~~gal~~	4 (qt)	4×4	16 = 16 qt
	1 ~~gal~~	1	1

9. Problem: 1.5 cup = How many cc?
   Given quantity = 1.5 cup
   Wanted quantity = cc
   Conversion factor = 1 cup = 240 cc

1.5 ~~cup~~	240 (cc)	1.5×240	360 = 360 cc
	1 ~~cup~~	1	1

10. Problem: 24 oz = How many glasses?
    Given quantity = 24 oz
    Wanted quantity = glasses
    Conversion factor = 1 glass = 8 oz

24 ~~oz~~	1 (glass)	24×1	24 = 3 glasses
	8 ~~oz~~	8	8

For accurate administration of medication, the "five rights of medication administration" form the foundation of communication between the physician and the nurse. The physician writes a medication order using the five rights, and the nurse administers the medication to the patient based on the five rights. There may be a slight variation in the way each physician writes a medication order, but information pertaining to the five rights should be included in the medication order to ensure safe administration by the nurse.

To calculate the change from a one-factor–given quantity to a one-factor–wanted quantity by dimensional analysis, it is necessary to have a clear understanding of the five rights. This chapter teaches you to interpret medication orders correctly and to calculate medication problems accurately using dimensional analysis.

4

ONE-FACTOR MEDICATION PROBLEMS

Outline

Objectives

After completing this chapter, you will be able to:

1. Interpret medication orders correctly, based on the five rights of medication administration.
2. Identify components from a drug label that are needed for accurate medication administration.
3. Describe the different routes of medication administration: tablets and capsules, liquids given by medicine cup or syringe, and parenteral injections using different types of syringes.
4. Calculate medication problems accurately from the one-factor–given quantity to the one-factor–wanted quantity using the sequential or random method of dimensional analysis.

INTERPRETATION OF MEDICATION ORDERS

Physicians order medications using the five rights of medication administration, which are:

1. Right **patient** (person receiving the medication)
2. Right **drug** (name of the medication)
3. Right **dosage** (amount of medication to be given)
4. Right **route** (how the medication is to be given)
5. Right **time** (when and how often the medication is to be given)

Once you are able to interpret the important components of an order for medication, you can perform accurate calculations for the correct drug dosage by using dimensional analysis.

Exercise 4.1 Interpretation of Medication Orders

(See page 93 for answers)

In the following medication orders, identify the five rights of medication administration.

1. Give gr 10 aspirin to Mrs. C. Clark orally every 4 hours, as needed for fever.

   a. Right patient ______________________

   b. Right drug ______________________

   c. Right dosage ______________________

   d. Right route ______________________

   e. Right time ______________________

2. Administer PO to Mr. S. Smith, Advil (ibuprofen) 400 mg every 6 hours for arthritis.

   a. Right patient ______________________

   b. Right drug ______________________

   c. Right dosage ______________________

   d. Right route ______________________

   e. Right time ______________________

3. Tylenol (acetaminophen) gr 10 PO every 4 hours for Mr. J. Jones prn for headache.

   a. Right patient ______________________

   b. Right drug ______________________

   c. Right dosage ______________________

   d. Right route ______________________

   e. Right time ______________________

ONE-FACTOR MEDICATION PROBLEMS

Medication problems can be easily solved using the five steps of dimensional analysis:

- The first step in interpreting any physician's order for medication is to identify the **given quantity** or the exact dosage that the physician ordered.
- The second step is to identify the **wanted quantity** or the answer to the medication problem.
- The third step is to establish the **unit path** from the given quantity to the wanted quantity, using equivalents as **conversion factors** to complete the problem. Identification of the available dosage of medicine (dose on hand) is considered part of the unit path.
- The fourth step is to set up the problem to cancel out unwanted units.
- The fifth step is to multiply the numerators, multiply the denominators, and divide the product of the numerators by the product of the denominators to provide the numerical value of the **wanted quantity** or answer to the problem.

You may choose to implement either the **sequential method** or the **random method** of dimensional analysis.

Below is an example of a one-factor problem showing the placement of components used in dimensional analysis.

Unit Path

Given Quantity	Conversion Factor for Given Quantity	Conversion Computation		Wanted Quantity
10 gr	tablets	10	=	2 tablets
	5 gr	5		
	Conversion Factor for Wanted Quantity			

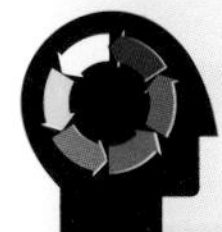

THINKING IT THROUGH

Both *10 gr* and *tablets* are numerators without denominators. This is called a **one-factor** medication problem because the given quantity and the wanted quantity contain only numerators.

The dose on hand (5 gr/tablets) is an equivalent that is used as a conversion factor and is factored into the unit path.

The unwanted units (gr) can be canceled from the problem leaving the wanted quantity (tablets) in the numerator.

(Thinking It Through continues on page 58)

EXAMPLE 4.1

The physician orders gr 10 aspirin orally every 4 hours, as needed for fever. The unit dose of medication on hand is gr 5 per tablet (5 gr/tab).

How many tablets will you administer?

Given quantity = 10 gr
Wanted quantity = tablets
Dose on hand = 5 gr/tab

Step 1 Identify the *given quantity* (the physician's order).

Unit Path

Given Quantity	Conversion Factor for Given Quantity	Conversion Computation		Wanted Quantity
10 gr			=	
	Conversion Factor for Wanted Quantity			

(Example continues on page 58)

The **sequential method** of dimensional analysis has been used to factor in the dose on hand, which allows the previous unit (given quantity) to be canceled. When using the sequential method, the conversion factor that is factored in always cancels out the preceding unit.

Step 2 Identify the *wanted quantity* (the answer to the problem).

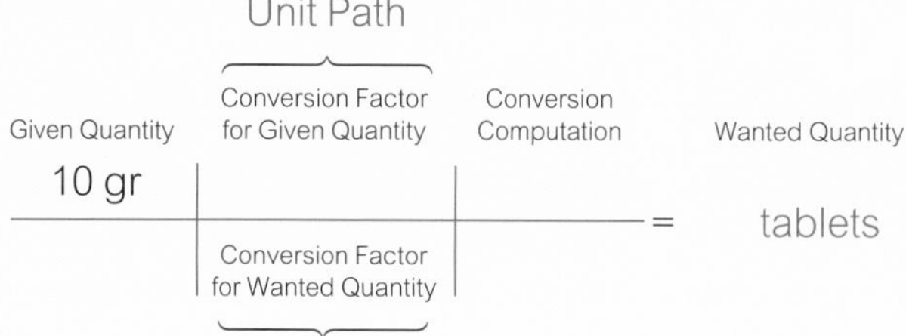

Step 3 Establish the unit path from the given quantity to the wanted quantity using equivalents as conversion factors.

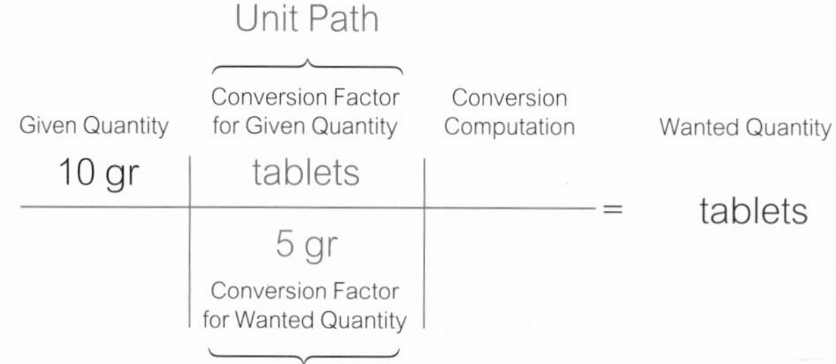

Step 4 Set up the problem to allow cancellation of unwanted units and circle the wanted quantity within the unit path to demonstrate correct placement.

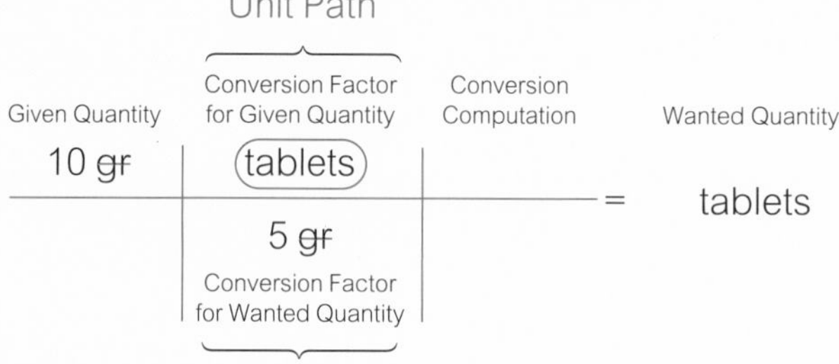

Step 5 Multiply the numerators, multiply the denominators, and divide the product of the numerators by the product of the denominators to provide the numerical value for the wanted quantity.

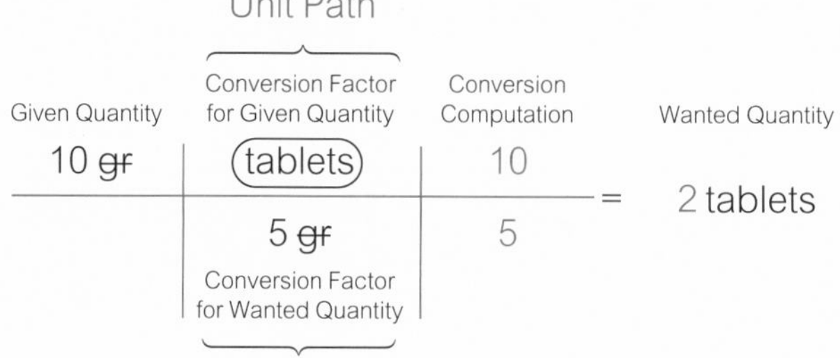

2 tablets is the wanted quantity and the answer to the problem.

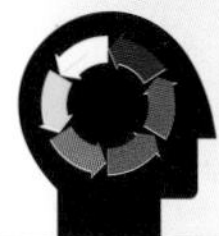

EXAMPLE 4.2

Administer PO Advil (ibuprofen) 400 mg every 6 hours for arthritis. The dosage on hand is 200 mg/tablet.

How many tablets will you give?

Given quantity = 400 mg
Wanted quantity = tablets
Dose on hand = 200 mg/tablet

▶ **Step 1** Identify the *given quantity.*

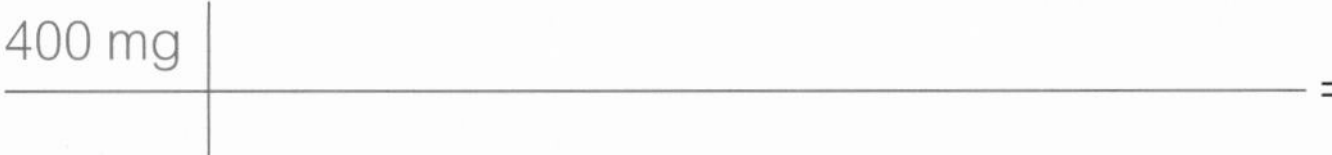

$$\frac{400\text{ mg}}{\quad} =$$

▶ **Step 2** Identify the *wanted quantity.*

$$\frac{400\text{ mg}}{\quad} = \text{tablets}$$

▶ **Step 3** Establish the unit path from the given quantity to the wanted quantity using equivalents as conversion factors.

$$\frac{400\text{ mg}}{\quad} \bigg| \frac{\text{tablet}}{200\text{ mg}} = \text{tablets}$$

▶ **Step 4** Set up the problem to allow cancellation of unwanted units and circle the wanted quantity within the unit path to demonstrate correct placement.

$$\frac{400\text{ }\cancel{\text{mg}}}{\quad} \bigg| \frac{\boxed{\text{tablet}}}{200\text{ }\cancel{\text{mg}}} = \text{tablets}$$

▶ **Step 5** Multiply the numerators, multiply the denominators, and divide the product of the numerators by the product of the denominators to provide the numerical value of the wanted quantity.

$$\frac{\cancel{400}\text{ }\cancel{\text{mg}}}{\quad} \bigg| \frac{\boxed{\text{tablet}}}{\cancel{200}\text{ }\cancel{\text{mg}}} \bigg| \frac{4}{2} = 2 \text{ tablets}$$

2 tablets is the wanted quantity and the answer to the problem.

THINKING IT THROUGH

The **sequential method** of dimensional analysis has been used to set up the problem. The unwanted units (mg) have been canceled from the unit path by correctly factoring in the dose on hand (200 mg/tablet). The same number of zeroes has also been canceled from the numerator and denominator.

If an answer does not result in a whole number, but instead a decimal in the tenths (4.7) or hundredths (4.75), the answer must be rounded up or down to allow for administration of the medication.

If the tablets are scored, a half of the tablet can be administered. If a tablet is not scored, a decision must be made by the nurse whether to give one or two tablets. If a liquid medication to be administered involves decimals, then the nurse must make a decision regarding the amount of medication to be given.

If the number following the decimal is 5 or greater, then the number is rounded up.
Example in the tenths: 4.7 → 5
Example in the hundredths: 4.75 → 4.8

If the number following the decimal is less than 5, then the number is rounded down.
Example in the tenths: 4.4 → 4
Example in the hundredths: 4.42 → 4.4

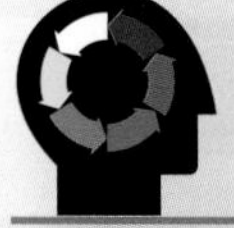

THINKING IT THROUGH

The **sequential method** of dimensional analysis has been used. The unwanted unit (gr) has been canceled by factoring in a conversion factor (1 gr = 60 mg).

The dose on hand (325 mg/caplet) is factored into the unit path, which allows the unwanted unit (mg) to be canceled.

The remaining unit (caplet) is in the numerator and correctly correlates with the wanted quantity in the numerator.

EXAMPLE 4.3

Tylenol (acetaminophen) gr 10 PO every 4 hours for headache. The unit dose of medication on hand is 325 mg per caplet.

How many caplets will you give?

Given quantity = 10 gr
Wanted quantity = caplets
Dose on hand = 325 mg/caplet

Step 1 Identify the *given quantity.*

10 gr		=

Step 2 Identify the *wanted quantity.*

10 gr		= caplets

Step 3 Establish the *unit path* from the given quantity to the wanted quantity using equivalents as conversion factors.

10 gr	60 mg	caplet	= caplets
	1 gr	325 mg	

▶ **Step 4** Set up the problem to allow cancellation of unwanted units and circle the wanted quantity within the unit path to demonstrate correct placement.

10 ~~gr~~	60 ~~mg~~	(caplet)	= caplets
	1 ~~gr~~	325 ~~mg~~	

▶ **Step 5** Multiply the numerators, multiply the denominators, and divide the product of the numerators by the product of the denominators to provide the numerical value of the wanted quantity.

10 ~~gr~~	60 ~~mg~~	(caplet)	10 × 60	600	= 1.8 caplets
	1 ~~gr~~	325 ~~mg~~	1 × 325	325	

> 1.8 caplets is the wanted quantity and the answer to the problem, but, by using the rounding rule, 2 caplets would be given.

Dimensional analysis is a problem-solving method that uses critical thinking, not a specific formula. Therefore, the important concept to remember is that *all* unwanted units must be canceled from the unit path. The **random method** of dimensional analysis can also be used when solving medication problems. When using the random method of dimensional analysis, the focus is on the correct placement of the conversion factor. It must correlate with the wanted quantity in the numerator portion of the unit path, without considering the preceding units.

EXAMPLE 4.4

The random method of dimensional analysis will be used to calculate the answer for Example 4.3.

▶ **Step 1** Identify the *given quantity.*

10 gr	=

▶ **Step 2** Identify the *wanted quantity.*

10 gr	= caplet

(Example continues on page 62)

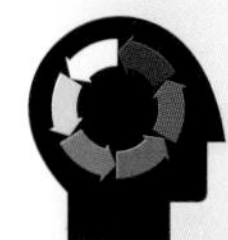

THINKING IT THROUGH

When using the random method, the focus is on the correct placement of the conversion factor to correspond with the wanted quantity. The problem is set up correctly as long as the dose on hand (caplet) correlates with the wanted quantity (caplet), both in the numerator.

A conversion factor (1 gr = 60 mg) is factored into the problem to cancel out the unwanted units (gr and mg). The remaining unit (caplet) correlates with the wanted quantity.

Step 3 Establish the *unit path* from the given quantity to the wanted quantity using equivalents as conversion factors.

10 gr	caplet	= caplet
	325 mg	

Step 4 Set up the problem to allow cancellation of unwanted units and circle the wanted quantity within the unit path to demonstrate correct placement.

10 ~~gr~~	(caplet)	60 ~~mg~~	= caplet
	325 ~~mg~~	1 ~~gr~~	

Step 5 Multiply the numerators, multiply the denominators, and divide the product of the numerators by the product of the denominators to provide the numerical value of the wanted quantity.

10 ~~gr~~	(caplet)	60 ~~mg~~	10×60	600	= 1.8 caplets
	325 ~~mg~~	1 ~~gr~~	325×1	325	

1.8 caplets is the wanted quantity and the answer to the problem, but, by using the rounding rule, 2 caplets would be given.

Exercise 4.2 One-Factor Medication Problems

(See page 93 for answers)

1. The physician orders Achromycin (tetracycline) 0.25 g PO every 12 hours for acne. The dosage of medication on hand is 250 mg per capsule.

   How many capsules will you give? ____________

2. Administer phenobarbital gr $\frac{1}{2}$ PO tid for sedation. The dosage on hand is 15 mg/tablet.

   How many tablets will you give? ____________

3. Give 0.5 g Diuril PO bid for hypertension. Unit dose is 500 mg per tablet.

   How many tablets will you give? ____________

4. Order: Restoril 0.03 g PO hs for sedation. Supply: Restoril 30-mg capsules.

   How many capsules will you give? ____________

5. Order: Thorazine gr $\frac{1}{2}$ PO tid for singultus. Supply: Thorazine 30-mg capsules.

How many capsules will you give? ________

COMPONENTS OF A DRUG LABEL

All medications (stock and unit dose) are labeled with a drug label that includes specific information to assist in the accurate administration of the medication.

Identifying the Components

Information on the drug label includes:

- Name of the drug, including the trade name (name given by the pharmaceutical company identified with a trademark symbol) and the generic name (chemical name given to the drug)
- Dosage of medication (the amount of medication in each tablet, capsule, or liquid)
- Form of medication (tablet, capsule, or liquid)
- Expiration date (how long the medication will remain stable and safe to administer)
- Lot number (the manufacturer's batch series that the medication came from)
- Manufacturer (the pharmaceutical company that produced the medication)

EXAMPLE 4.5

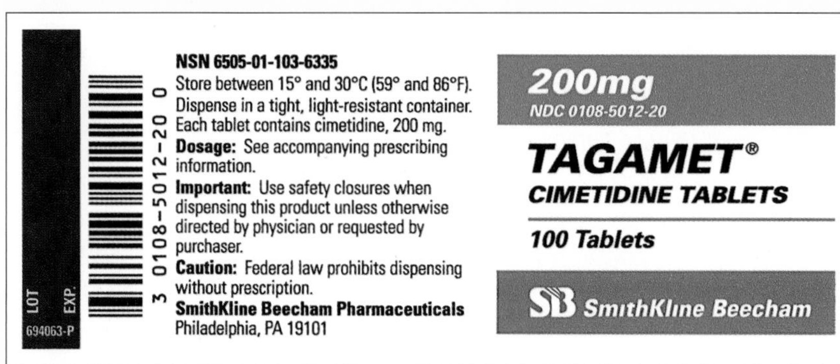

Courtesy of SmithKline Beecham Pharmaceuticals.

a. Trade name of the drug: Tagamet
b. Generic name of the drug: Cimetidine
c. Dosage of medication: 200 mg per tablet
d. Form of medication: 100 tablets
e. Expiration date:
f. Lot number:
g. Manufacturer: SmithKline Beecham Pharmaceuticals

Exercise 4.3 Identifying the Components of Drug Labels

(See pages 93–94 for answers)

1.

851310 NDC 0026-8513-51

CIPRO®

(ciprofloxacin hydrochloride)

Equivalent to

500 mg ciprofloxacin

100 Tablets

Caution: Federal (USA) law prohibits dispensing without a prescription.

Bayer

Bayer Corporation
Pharmaceutical Division
400 Morgan Lane
West Haven, CT 06516

DESCRIPTION: Each tablet contains ciprofloxacin hydrochloride equivalent to 500 mg of ciprofloxacin.
DOSAGE: See accompanying literature for complete information on dosage and administration.
RECOMMENDED STORAGE:
Store below 86°F (30°C).

Batch:
Expires:

3 0026-8513-51 0

PL500002 6505-01-333-4154 ©1995 Bayer Corporation 4743 Printed in USA

Courtesy of Bayer Corporation Pharmaceutical Division.

a. Trade name of the drug ________________

b. Generic name of the drug ________________

c. Dosage medication ________________

d. Form of medication ________________

e. Expiration date ________________

f. Batch number ________________

g. Manufacturer ________________

2.

Store at room temperature.
Container not for household use.
Dispense in a well-closed container.
Each capsule contains 100 mg trimethobenzamide hydrochloride.
Dosage: See accompanying prescribing information.
Important: Use safety closures when dispensing this product unless otherwise directed by physician or requested by purchaser.
Manufactured by King Pharmaceuticals, Inc., Bristol, TN 37620 for **SmithKline Beecham Pharmaceuticals**
Philadelphia, PA 19101

100mg

NDC 0029-4082-30

TIGAN®

TRIMETHO-BENZAMIDE HCl

100 Capsules

SB SmithKline Beecham

Caution: Federal law prohibits dispensing without prescription.

3 0029-4082-30 1

0938011 LOT EXP. 694040-B

Courtesy of SmithKline Beecham Pharmaceuticals.

a. Trade name of the drug ________________

b. Generic name of the drug ________________

c. Dosage medication ________________

d. Form of medication ________________

e. Expiration date ________________

f. Batch number ________________

g. Manufacturer ________________

3.

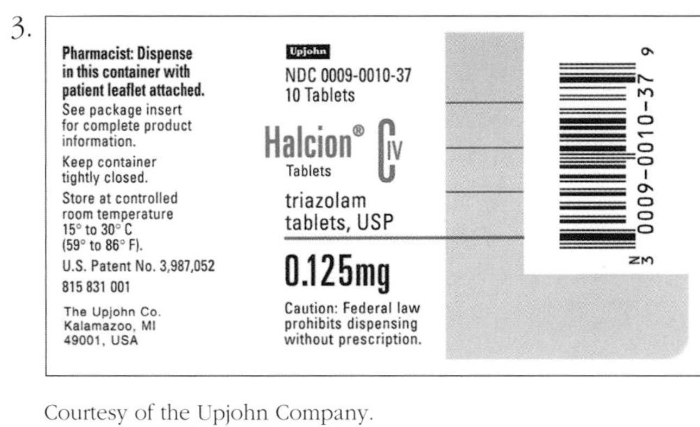

Courtesy of the Upjohn Company.

a. Trade name of the drug ________________

b. Generic name of the drug ________________

c. Dosage medication ________________

d. Form of medication ________________

e. Expiration date ________________

f. Batch number ________________

g. Manufacturer ________________

Solving Problems with Components of Drug Labels

Once you are able to identify the components of a drug label, you can use critical thinking to solve problems with dimensional analysis.

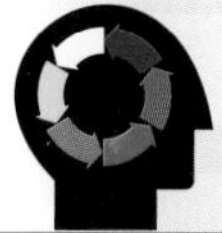

EXAMPLE 4.6

The physician orders Cipro 750 mg PO every 12 hours for a bacterial infection.

How many tablets will you give?

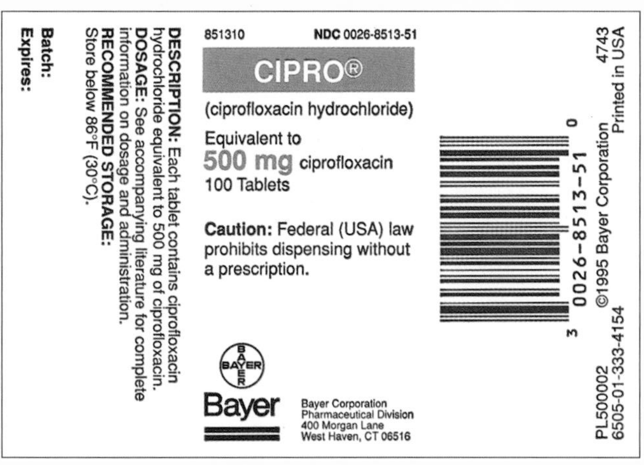

Courtesy of Bayer Corporation Pharmaceutical Division.

(Example continues on page 66)

THINKING IT THROUGH

The wanted quantity and the answer to the problem is 1.5 tablets. A scored tablet can be cut in half allowing the exact dosage to be administered.

Given quantity = 750 mg
Wanted quantity = tablets
Dose on hand = 500 mg/tablet

Sequential method:

75~~0~~ ~~mg~~	(tablet)	75	= 1.5 tablets
	50~~0~~ ~~mg~~	50	

1.5 tablets is the wanted quantity and the answer to the problem.

EXAMPLE 4.7

Administer Tigan 200 mg PO qid for nausea.

How many capsules will you give?

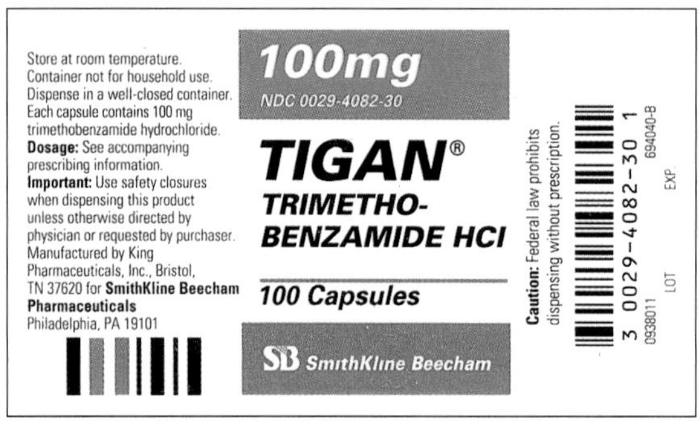

Courtesy of SmithKline Beecham Pharmaceuticals.

Given quantity = 200 mg
Wanted quantity = capsules
Dose on hand = 100 mg/capsules

Sequential method:

2~~00~~ ~~mg~~	(capsules)	2	= 2 capsules
	1~~00~~ ~~mg~~	1	

2 capsules is the wanted quantity and the answer to the problem.

EXAMPLE 4.8

Order: Halcion 0.25 mg PO hs prn.

How many tablets will you give?

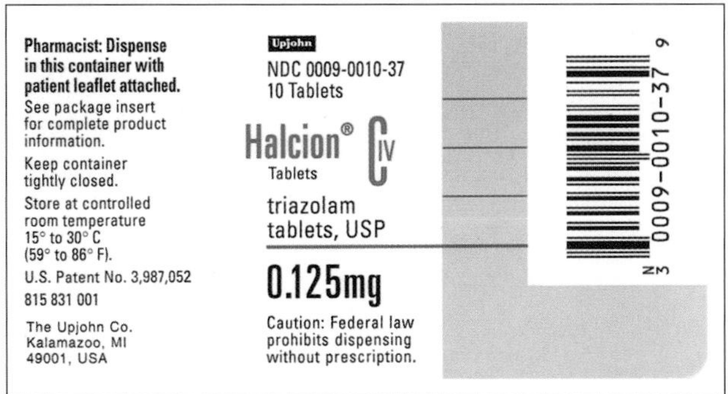

Courtesy of the Upjohn Company.

Given quantity = 0.25 mg
Wanted quantity = tablets
Dose on hand = 0.125 mg/tablet

Sequential method:

$$\frac{0.25\ \cancel{mg}}{} \bigg| \frac{\text{tablet}}{0.125\ \cancel{mg}} \bigg| \frac{0.25}{0.125} = 2\ \text{tablets}$$

2 tablets is the wanted quantity and the answer to the problem.

Exercise 4.4 Problems With Components of Drug Labels
(See page 94 for answers)

1. Order: methylphenidate 10 mg PO before breakfast and lunch for attention-deficit hyperactivity disorder (ADHD)

How many tablets will you give? ________

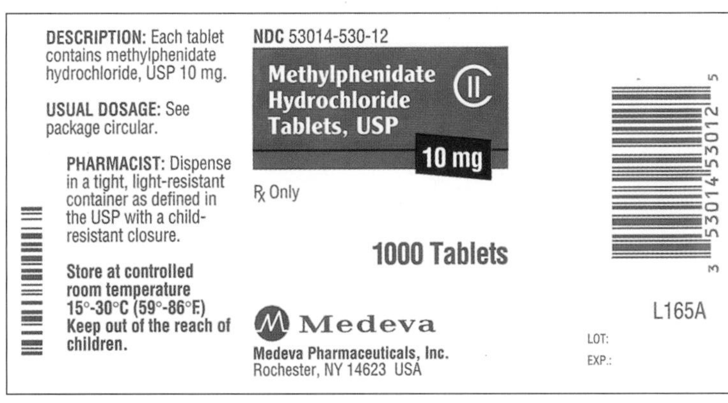

Courtesy of Medeva Pharmaceuticals.

(Exercise continues on page 68)

2. Order: Xanax 500 mcg PO bid for anxiety

How many tablets will you give? ____________

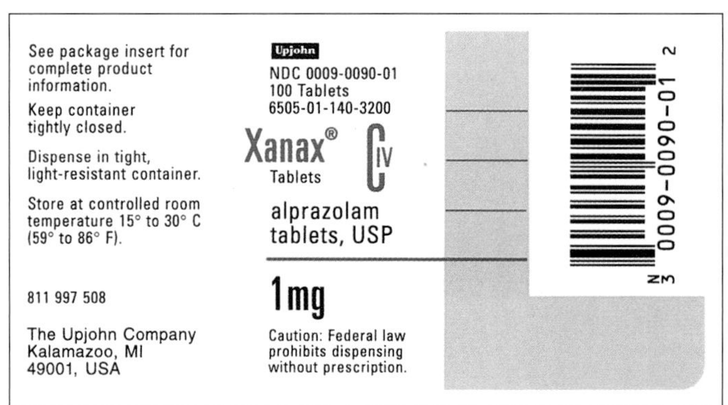

Courtesy of the Upjohn Company.

3. Order: Tolinase 375 mg PO every AM ac for type 2 diabetes mellitus

How many tablets will you give? ____________

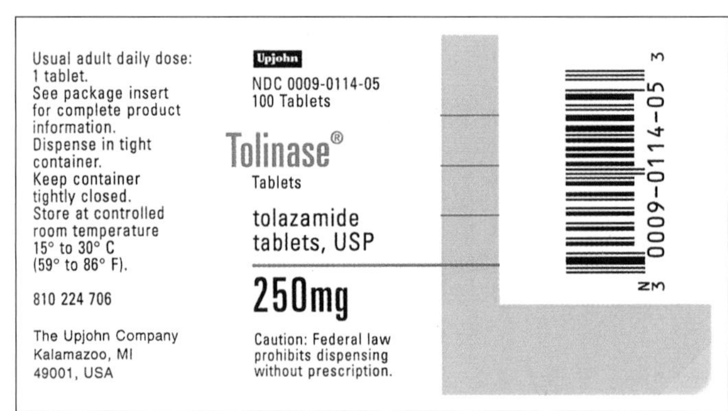

Courtesy of the Upjohn Company.

4. Order: vitamin B_{12} 2.5 mg daily as a daily vitamin supplement

How many tablets will you give? ____________

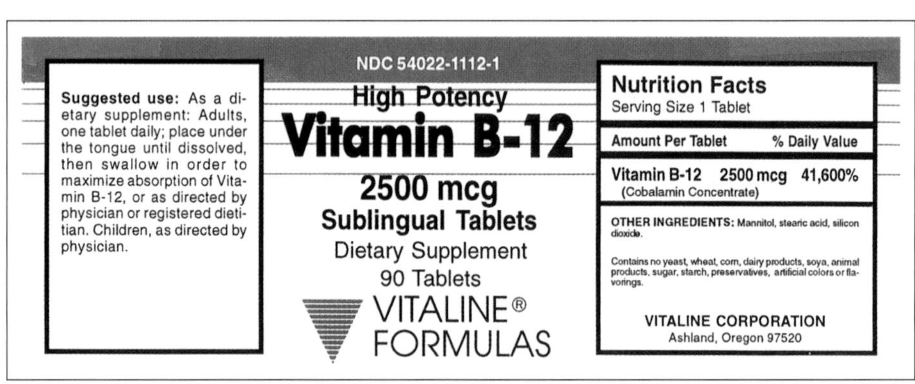

Courtesy of Vitaline Corporation.

5. Order: Tigan 250 mg PO qid prn for nausea

How many capsules will you give? ______________

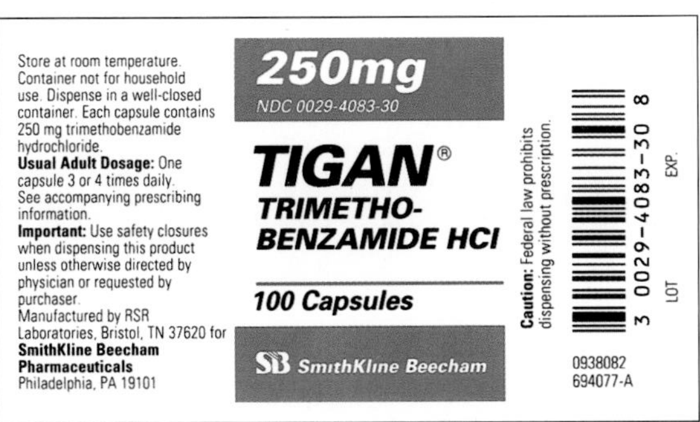

Courtesy of SmithKline Beecham Pharmaceuticals.

ADMINISTERING MEDICATION BY DIFFERENT ROUTES

Medication may be administered by various routes, including oral, parenteral, or intravenous, involving tablets, capsules, or liquid.

Enteral Medications

Oral (PO) medications are administered using tablets, caplets, capsules, or liquid. Tablets and caplets may be scored, which permits a more accurate administration when one fourth or one half of a tablet must be given.

Tablets and caplets may also be enteric coated, which allows the medication to bypass disintegration in the stomach to decrease irritation, and then later break down in the small intestine for absorption. Enteric-coated tablets and caplets should never be crushed, because such medications irritate the stomach.

Capsules are usually of the time-release type, and these should never be crushed or opened because the medication would be immediately released into the system, instead of being released slowly over time.

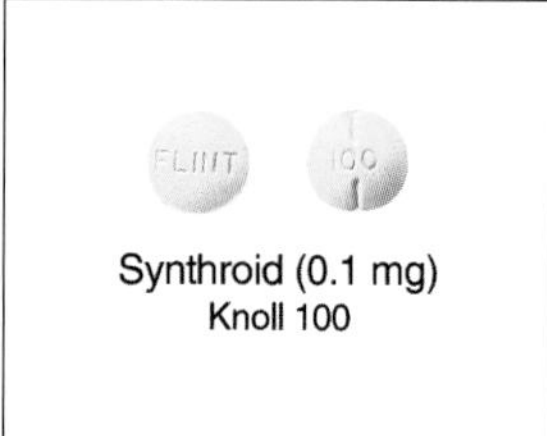

Tablets: note scored tablet on right.

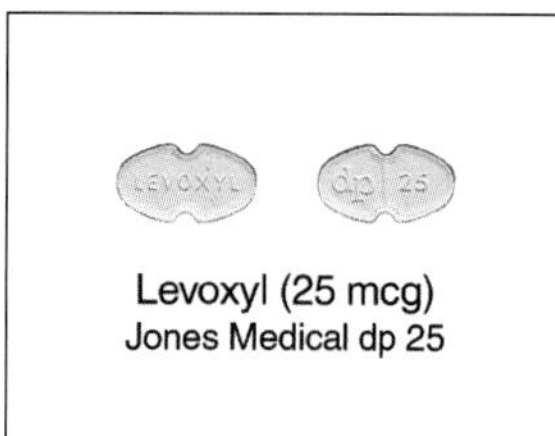

Caplets, note scored caplet on right.

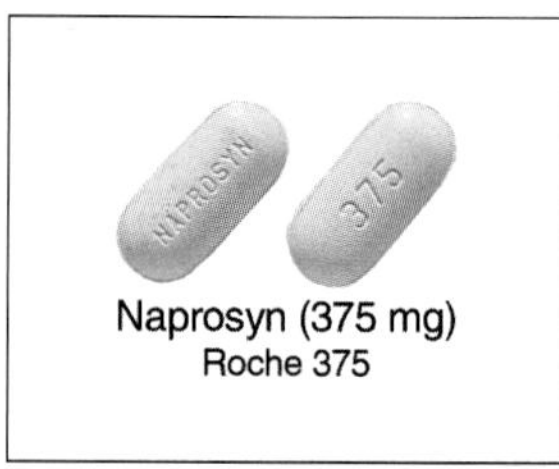

Enteric coated caplets.

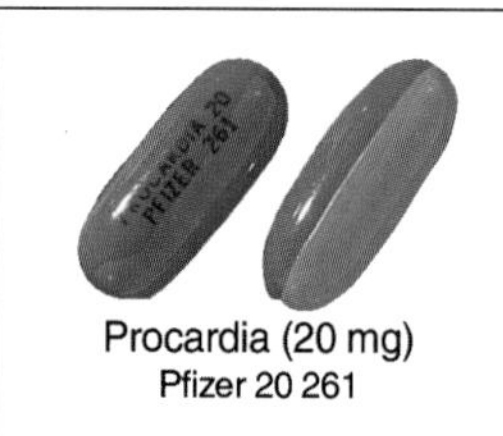

Capsules.

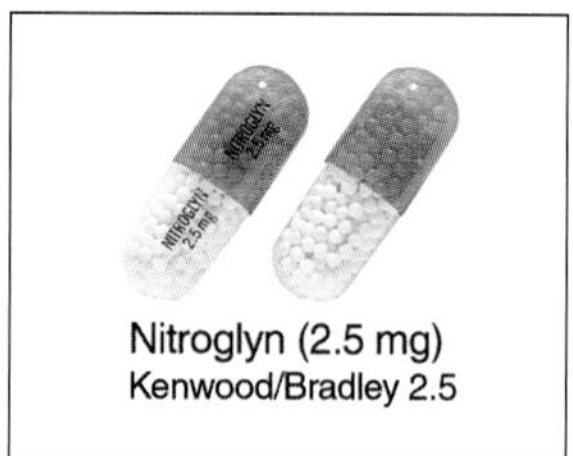

Control released capsules.

Liquid medication is accurately administered using a medication cup or medication syringe. The medication cup contains the common equivalents for the metric, apothecary, and household systems to permit adaptation of the medication's dosage for administration under various circumstances.

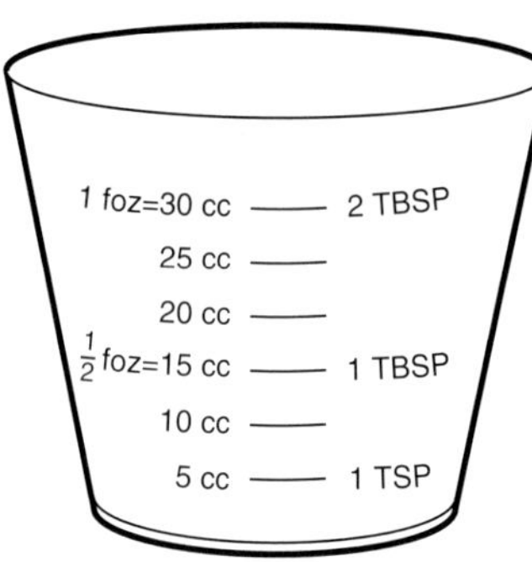

EXAMPLE 4.9

Order: Tagamet 600 mg PO bid for gastrointestinal (GI) bleeding.

How many tsp will you give?

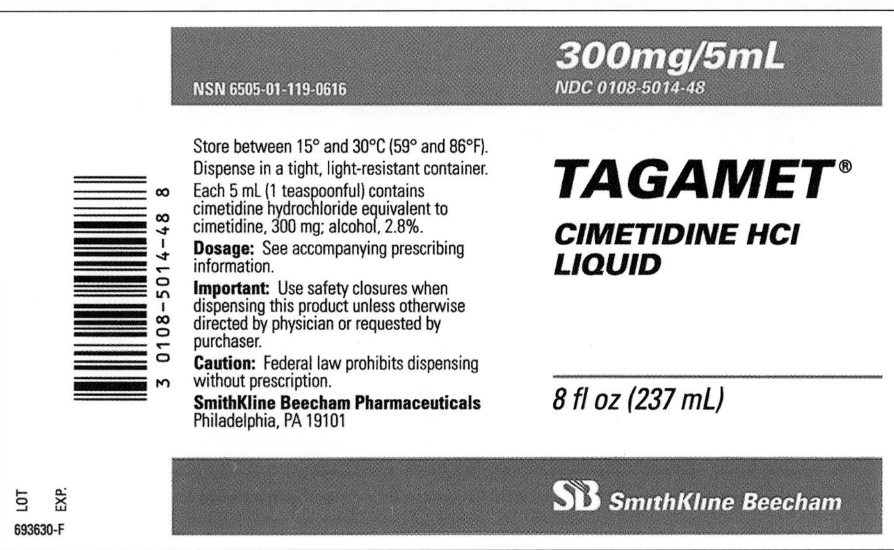

Courtesy of SmithKline Beecham Pharmaceuticals.

Given quantity = 600 mg
Wanted quantity = tsp
Dose on hand = 300 mg/5 mL

Sequential method:

6~~00 mg~~	5 ~~mL~~	(tsp)	6 × 5	30	= 2 tsp
	3~~00 mg~~	5 ~~mL~~	3 × 5	15	

2 tsp is the wanted quantity and the answer to the problem.

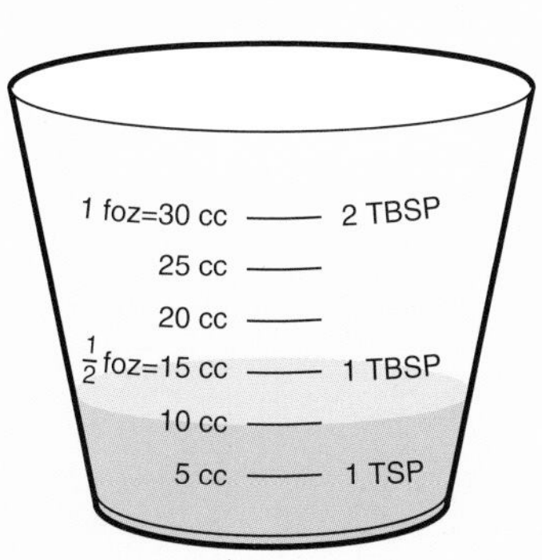

EXAMPLE 4.10

Order: Compazine 10 mg PO qid for psychomotor agitation.

How many mL will you give?

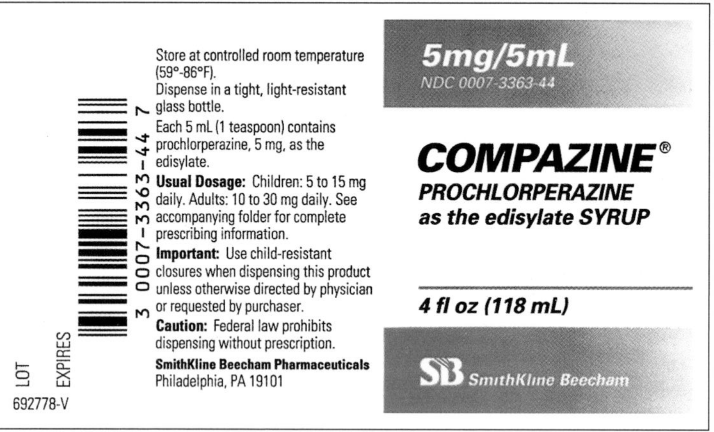

Courtesy of SmithKline Beecham Pharmaceuticals.

Given quantity = 10 mg
Wanted quantity = mL
Dose on hand = 5 mg/5 mL

Sequential method:

$$\frac{10\ \cancel{mg}}{} \bigg| \frac{5\ (mL)}{5\ \cancel{mg}} \bigg| \frac{10}{} = 10\ mL$$

10 mL is the wanted quantity and the answer to the problem.

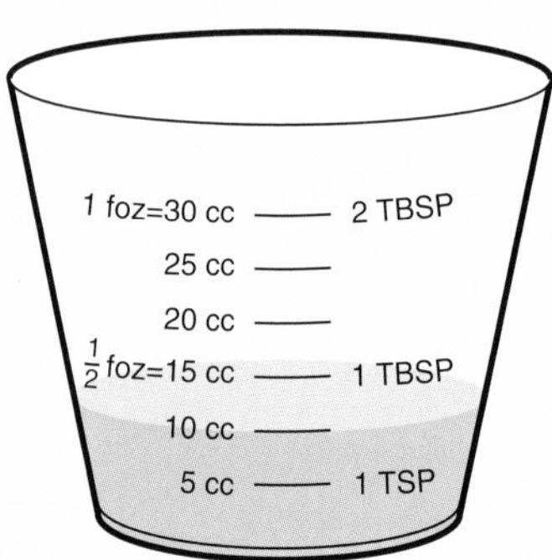

EXAMPLE 4.11

Order: Tegretol 100 mg PO qid for convulsions.

How many tsp will you give?

NDC 58887-019-76 FSC 1841
6505-01-302-4467

Tegretol®
carbamazepine USP
Suspension
100 mg/5 ml

EXP
LOT

450 ml

Dispense in tight, light-resistant container (USP).

Caution: Federal law prohibits dispensing without prescription.

BASEL Pharmaceuticals

Each 5 ml contains 100 mg carbamazepine USP.
Shake well before using.
Dosage: See package insert.
Do not store above 86°F (30°C).

BASEL Pharmaceuticals
Division of CIBA-GEIGY Corporation
Summit, New Jersey 07901

643754

N 3 58887-019-76 0

Courtesy of Basel Pharmaceuticals.

Given quantity = 100 mg
Wanted quantity = tsp
Dose on hand = 100 mg/5 mL

Random method:

~~100 mg~~	1 tsp	~~5 mL~~	1
	~~5 mL~~	~~100 mg~~	

= 1 tsp

1 tsp is the wanted quantity and the answer to the problem.

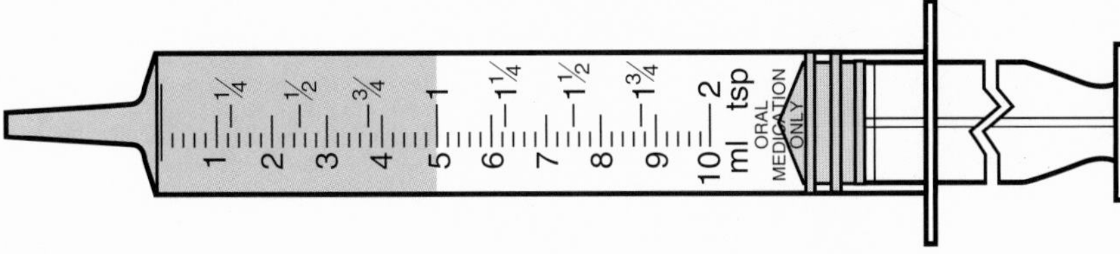

Exercise 4.5 Administering Enteral Medications

(See pages 94–95 for answers)

1. Order: phenobarbital gr $\frac{1}{2}$ PO daily for convulsions

   On hand: 20 mg/5 mL

   How many mL will you give? ____________

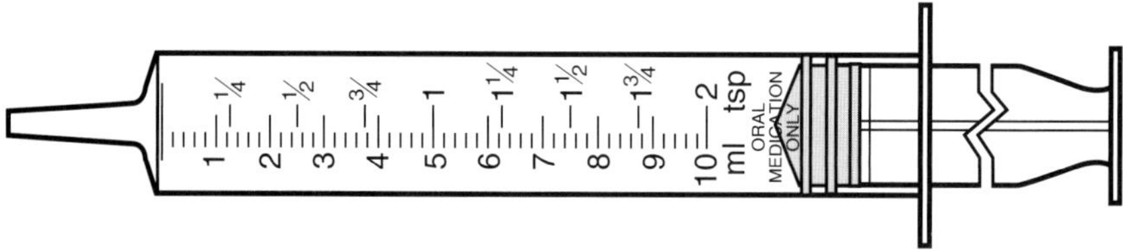

2. Order: Zantac 0.15 g PO bid for ulcers

   On hand: 15 mg/mL

   How many tsp will you give? ____________

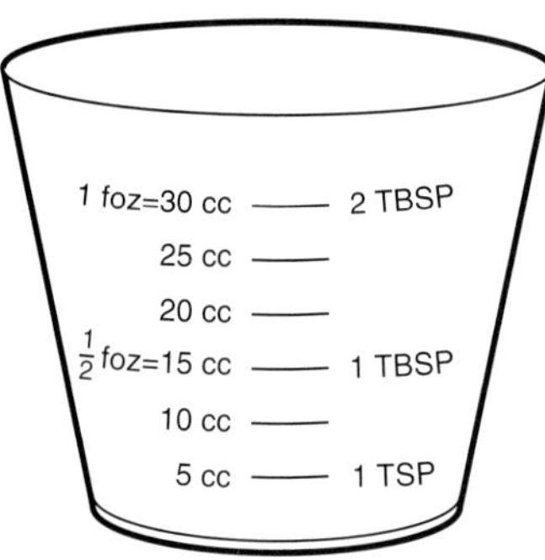

3. Order: Dilaudid 3 mg PO every 3 hour prn for pain

   On hand: Dilaudid Liquid 1 mg/mL

   How many mL will you give? ____________

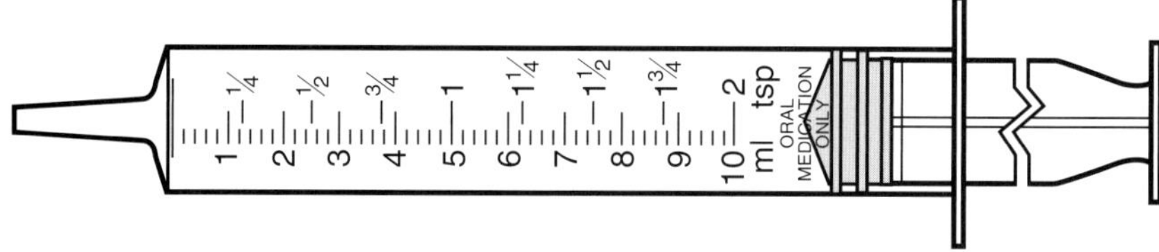

4. Order: lactulose 20 g PO tid for hepatic encephalopathy

On hand: lactulose 10 g/15 mL

How many oz will you give? ___________

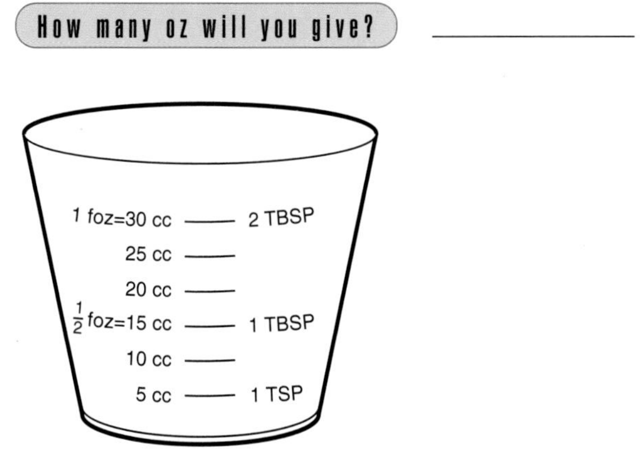

Parenteral Medications

Medications may also be ordered by the physician for the parenteral route of administration, including subcutaneous (SQ), intramuscular (IM), and intravenous (IV). Parenteral medications are sterile solutions obtained from vials or ampules and are administered using a syringe or prefilled syringes. The three syringes most often used are:

1. 3-cc syringe (used for a variety of medications requiring administration of doses from 0.2 to 3 cc).

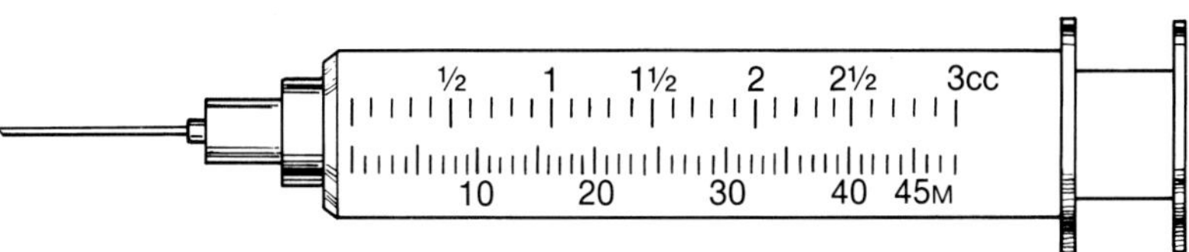

2. Insulin syringe (used specifically to administer insulin). Two types are illustrated below **A.** 0.5-mL (cc) low-dose syringe for U-100 insulin and **B.** 1-mL (cc) syringe for U-100 insulin.

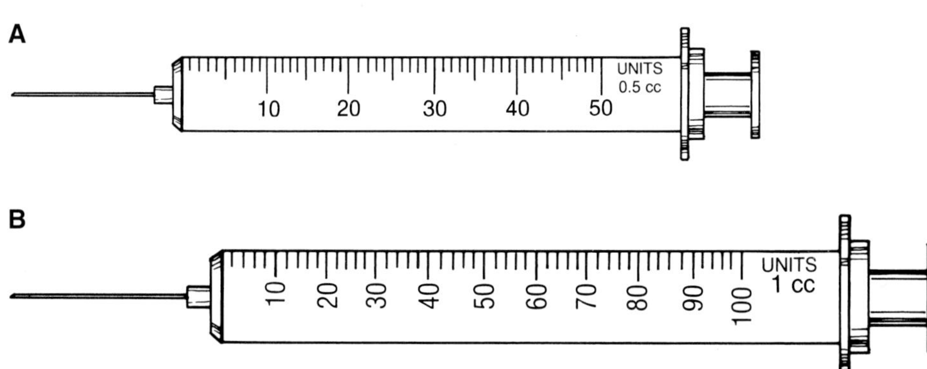

3. Tuberculin syringe (used for a variety of medications requiring administration of doses from 0.1 to 1 cc).

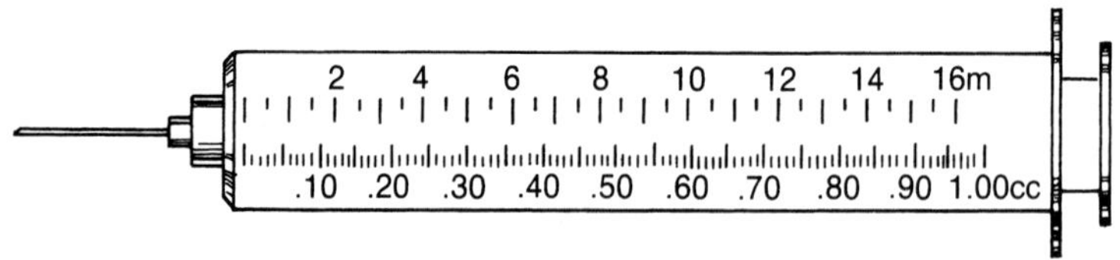

EXAMPLE 4.12

Order: Tigan 100 mg IM qid for nausea.

How many mL will you give?

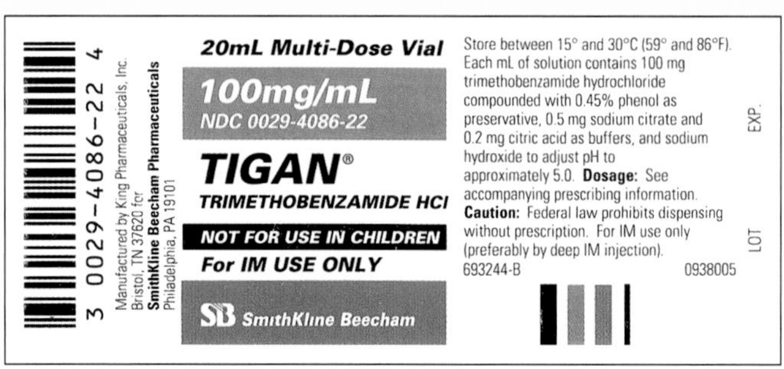

Courtesy of SmithKline Beecham Pharmaceuticals.

Given quantity = 100 mg
Wanted quantity = mL
Dose on hand = 100 mg/mL

Sequential method:

~~100 mg~~	(mL)	1	= 1 mL
	~~100 mg~~	1	

1 mL is the wanted quantity and the answer to the problem.

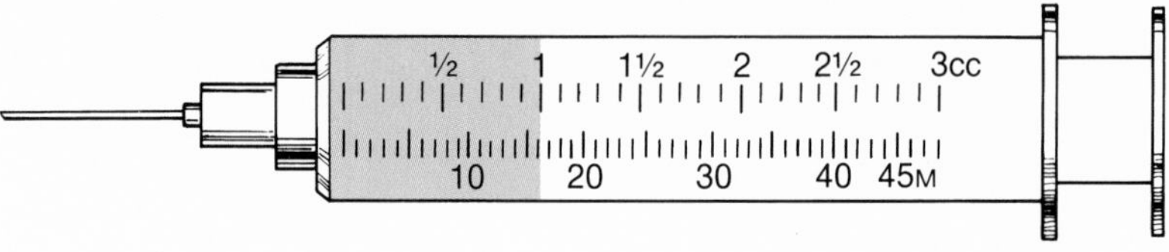

EXAMPLE 4.13

Order: Compazine 10 mg IM every 4 hour for psychoses.

How many mL will you give?

Store below 86°F. Do not freeze.
Protect from light. Discard if markedly discolored.
Each mL contains, in aqueous solution, prochlorperazine, 5 mg, as the edisylate; sodium biphosphate, 5 mg; sodium tartrate, 12 mg; sodium saccharin, 0.9 mg; benzyl alcohol, 0.75%, as preservative.
Dosage: For deep I.M. or I.V. injection.
See accompanying prescribing information.
Caution: Federal law prohibits dispensing without prescription.
SmithKline Beecham Pharmaceuticals
Philadelphia, PA 19101
LOT EXP. 693793-AD

10mL Multi-Dose Vial
5mg/mL
NDC 0007-3343-01
COMPAZINE®
PROCHLORPERAZINE
as the edisylate INJECTION
SB SmithKline Beecham

Courtesy of SmithKline Beecham Pharmaceuticals.

Given quantity = 10 mg
Wanted quantity = mL
Dose on hand = 5 mg/mL

Sequential method:

$$\frac{10\ \cancel{\text{mg}}}{} \left| \frac{\text{mL}}{5\ \cancel{\text{mg}}} \right| \frac{10}{5} = 2\ \text{mL}$$

2 mL is the wanted quantity and the answer to the problem.

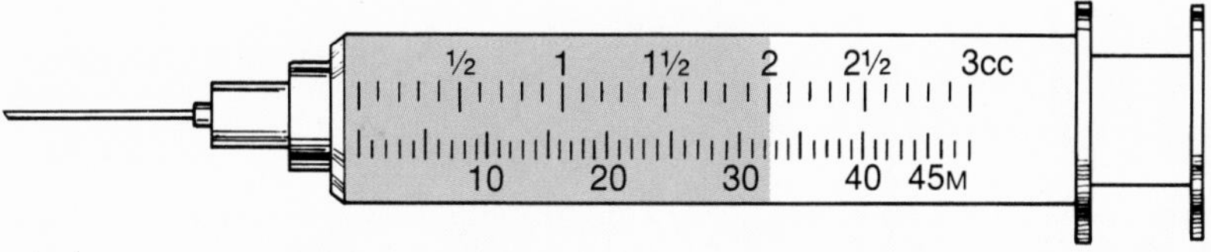

EXAMPLE 4.14

Order: morphine sulfate, $\frac{1}{4}$gr every 4 hour prn for pain.

How many mL will you give?

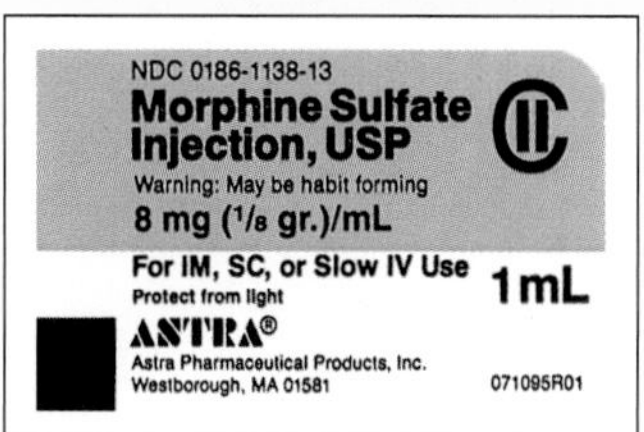

Courtesy of Astra Pharmaceutical Products.

(Example continues on page 78)

Given quantity $= \frac{1}{4}$ gr
Wanted quantity = mL
Dose on hand $= 8$ mg/mL or $\frac{1}{8}$ gr/mL

Random method:

$\frac{1}{4}$ ~~gr~~	(mL)	60 ~~mg~~	$\frac{1}{4} \times \frac{60}{1}$	$\frac{60}{4}$	15	= 1.87 mL or 1.9 mL
	8 ~~mg~~	1 ~~gr~~	8×1	8	8	

1.87 mL is the wanted quantity and the answer to the problem, but, by using the rounding rule, 1.9 mL would be given.

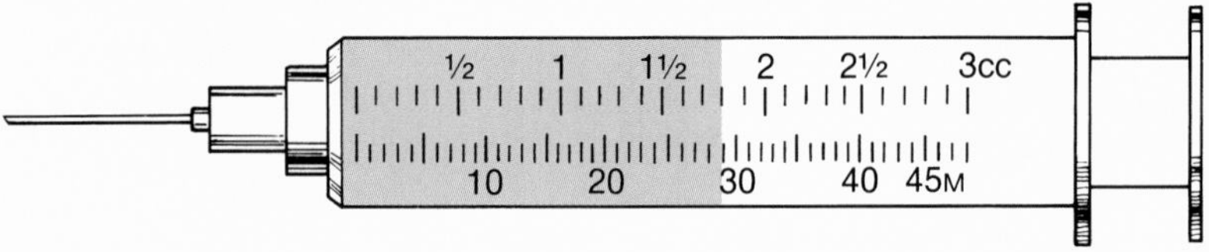

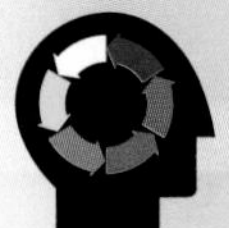

THINKING IT THROUGH

Insulin is given with an insulin syringe that requires no calculation. The number of units of insulin ordered by the physician equals the number of units that the nurse draws using the correct insulin syringe—low-dose or regular U-100.

EXAMPLE 4.15

Order: NPH human insulin 20 units SQ every AM for type 1 diabetes mellitus.

How many units will you give?

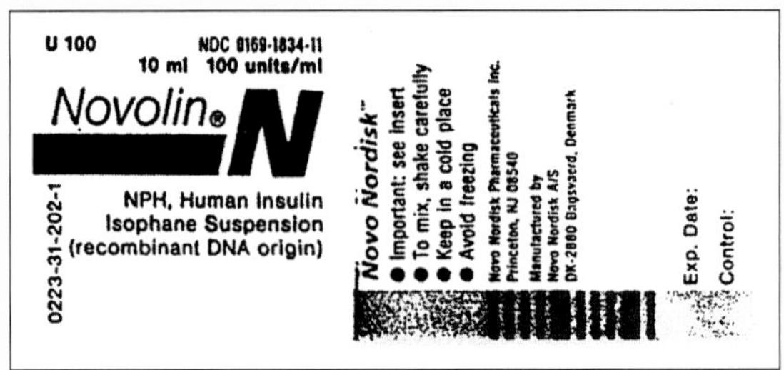

Courtesy of Novo Nordisk Pharmaceutical.

Sequential method:

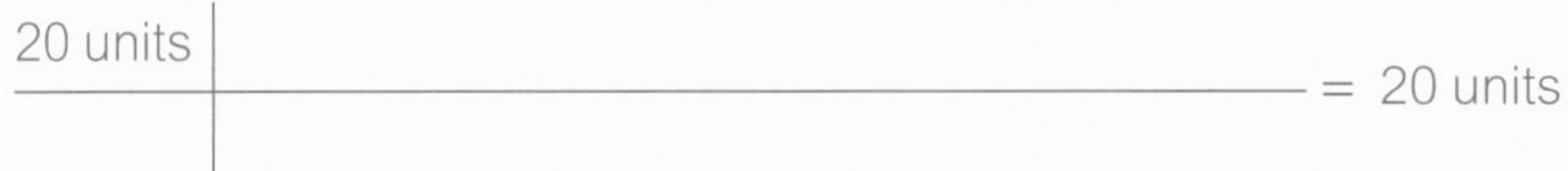

20 units		= 20 units

20 units is the wanted quantity and the answer to the problem.

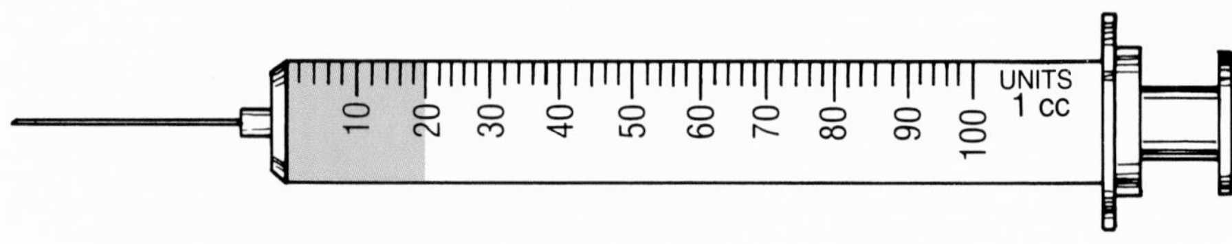

EXAMPLE 4.16

Order: Lente human insulin 45 units SQ every AM for type 1 diabetes mellitus.

How many units will you give?

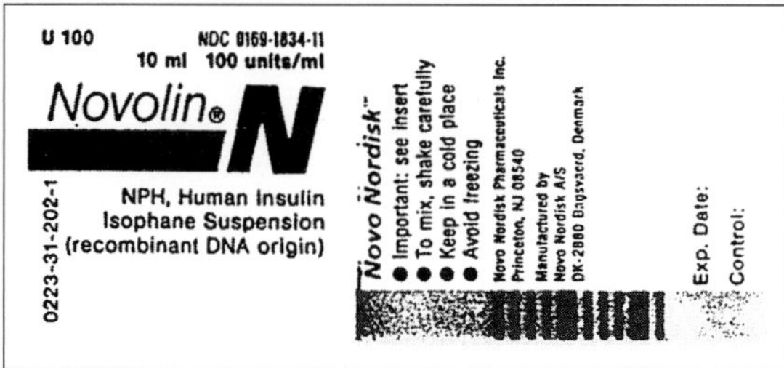

Courtesy of Novo Nordisk Pharmaceutical.

Sequential method:

45 units		= 45 units

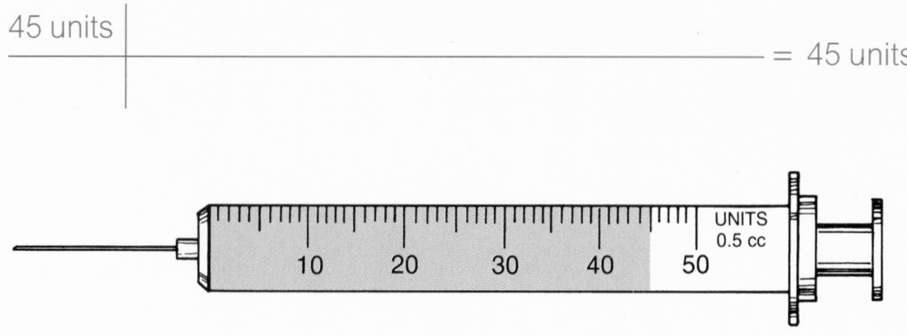

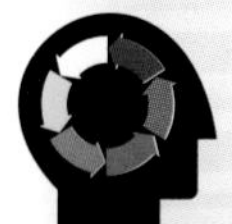

EXAMPLE 4.17

Order: heparin 5000 units SQ bid for prevention of thrombi. On hand: heparin 10,000 units/mL.

How many mL will you give?

Sequential method:

~~5000~~ ~~units~~	(mL)	5	= 0.5 mL
	10,~~000~~ ~~units~~	10	

0.5 mL is the wanted quantity and the answer to the problem.

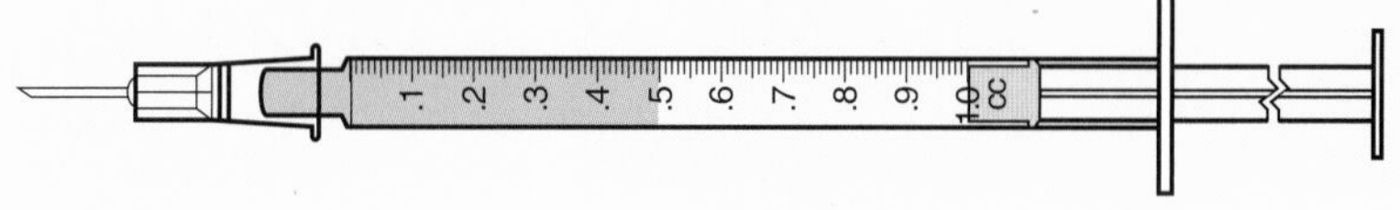

THINKING IT THROUGH

Heparin is administered using a tuberculin syringe, which is calibrated from 0.1 to 1 cc. This allows more accurate administration of medication dosages of less than 1 cc.

Exercise 4.6 Administering Parenteral Medications

(See page 95 for answers)

1. Order: atropine sulfate 300 mcg IM for preoperative medication.

How many mL will you give? ______________

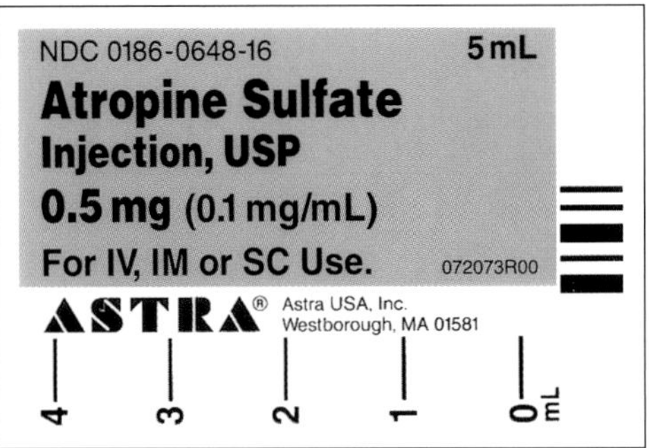

Courtesy of Astra Pharmaceutical Products.

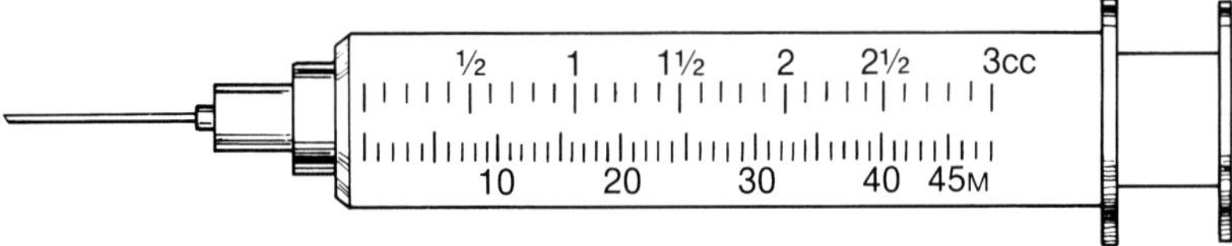

2. Order: hydromorphone 3 mg IM every 4 hours for pain.

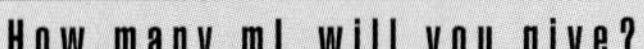

____

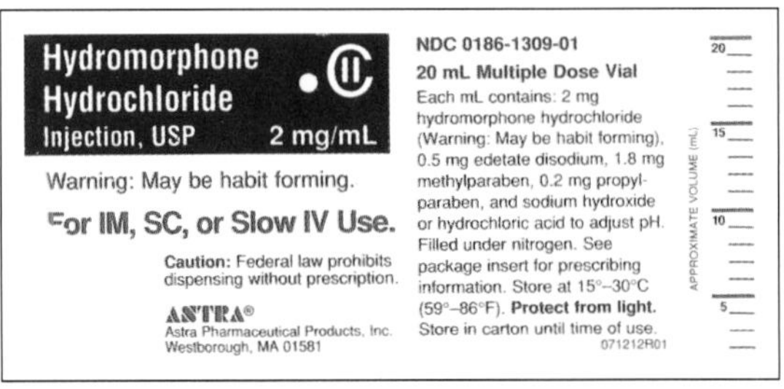

Courtesy of Astra Pharmaceutical Products.

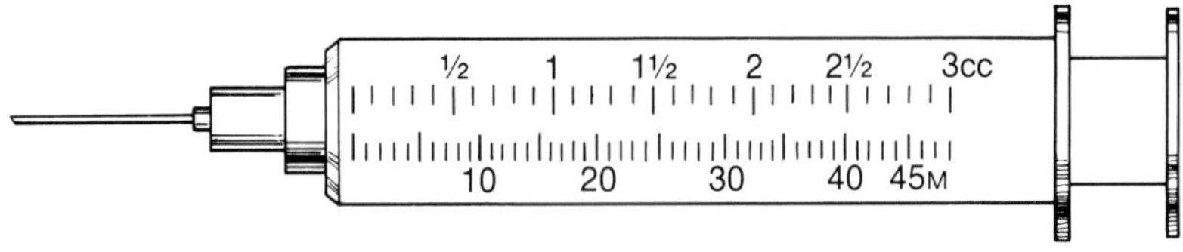

3. Order: meperidine 35 mg IV every hour for pain.

How many mL will you give? ____________

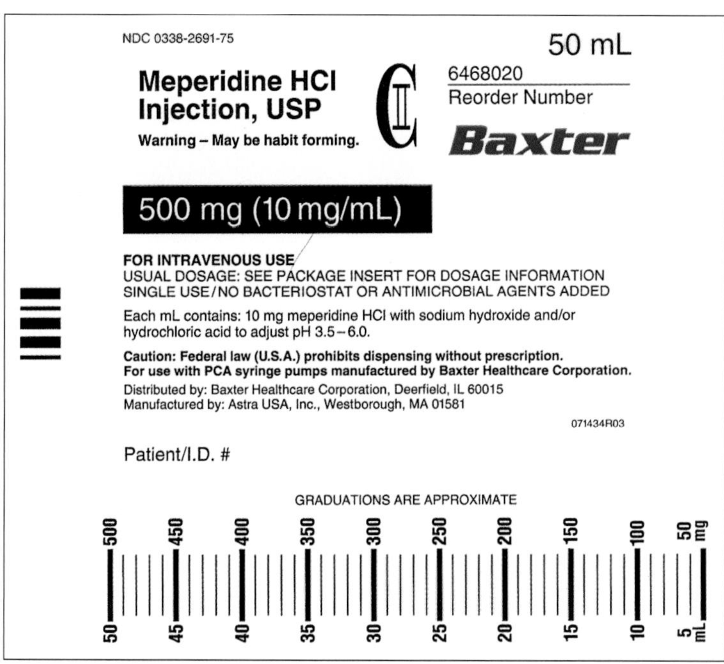

Courtesy of Baxter Pharmaceuticals.

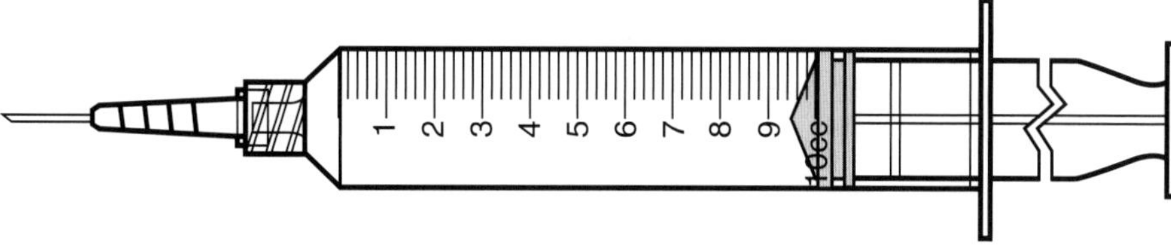

4. Order: regular insulin 10 units SQ every AM for type 1 diabetes mellitus.

On hand: regular insulin 100 units/mL.

How many units will you give? ____________

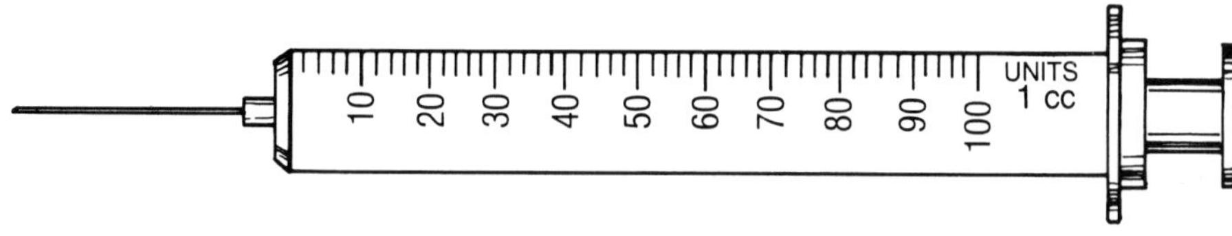

(Exercise continues on page 82)

5. Order: heparin 8000 units SQ bid for prevention of thrombi.

   On hand: heparin 10,000 units/mL.

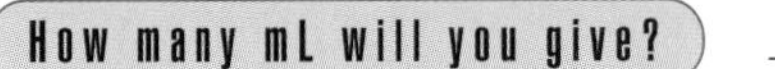

____

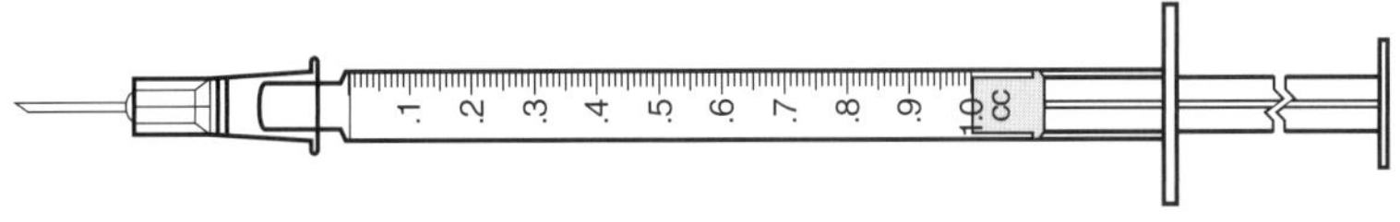

SUMMARY

This chapter has taught you to interpret medication orders and drug labels and to calculate one-factor medication problems using dimensional analysis. To demonstrate your ability to interpret correctly and calculate accurately, complete the following practice problems.

Practice Problems for Chapter 4 **One-Factor Medication Problems**

(See pages 95–96 for answers)

1. The physician orders Tigan 0.2 g IM qid for nausea. The dosage of medication on hand is a multiple-dose vial labeled 100 mg/mL.

   How many mL will you give? _______________

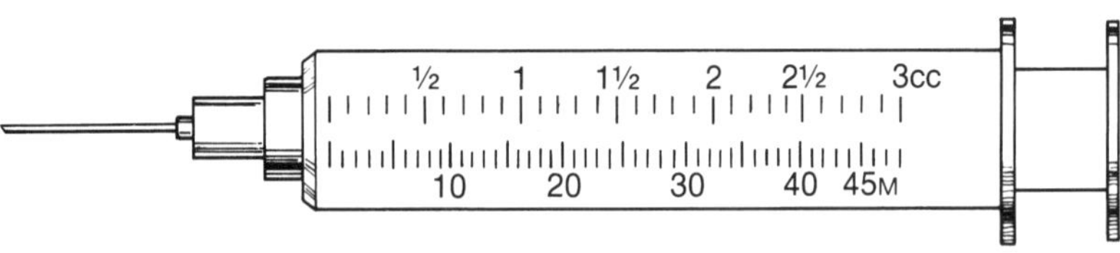

2. A physician orders Thorazine 50 mg tid prn for singultus. The dose on hand is Thorazine 25 mg tablets.

   How many tablets will you give? _______________

3. Order: Orinase 1 g PO bid for type 2 diabetes mellitus

How many tablets will you give? _______________

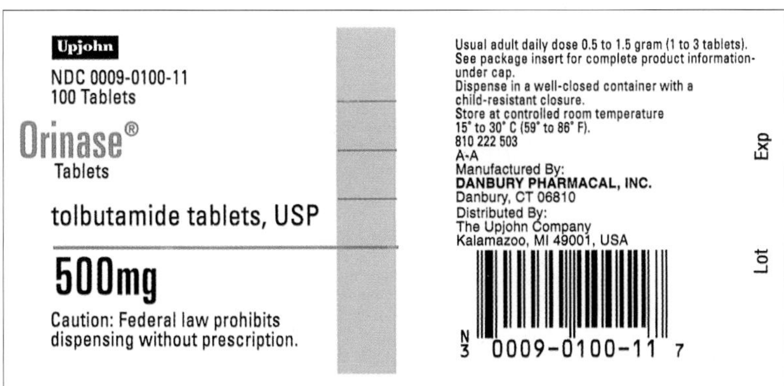

Courtesy of the Upjohn Company.

4. Order: Persantine 50 mg PO qid for prevention of thromboembolism

How many tablets will you give? _______________

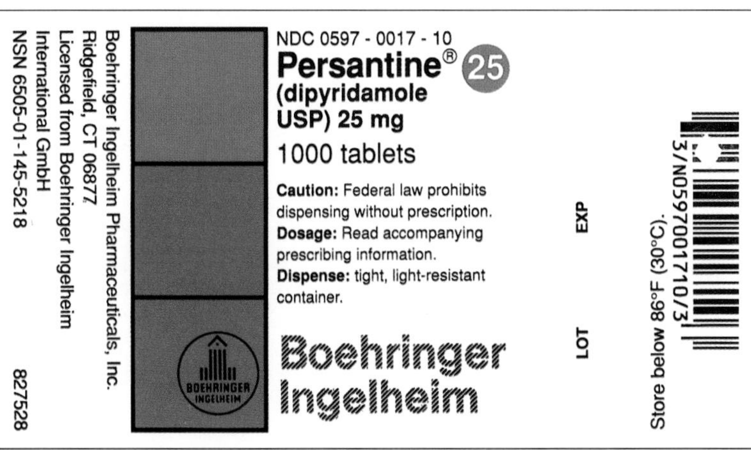

Courtesy of Boehringer Ingelheim Pharmaceuticals.

5. Order: NPH insulin 56 units SQ every AM for type 1 diabetes mellitus

On hand: NPH insulin 100 units/mL

How many units will you give? _______________

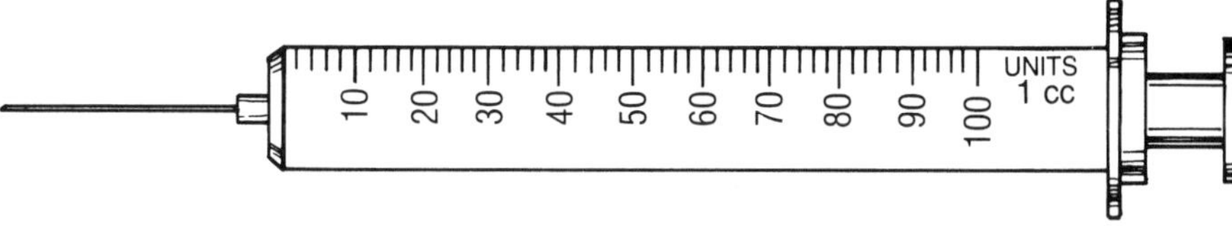

(Practice problems continue on page 84)

6. Order: heparin 7500 units SQ bid for prevention of thrombi

On hand: heparin 10,000 units/mL

How many mL will you give? ____________

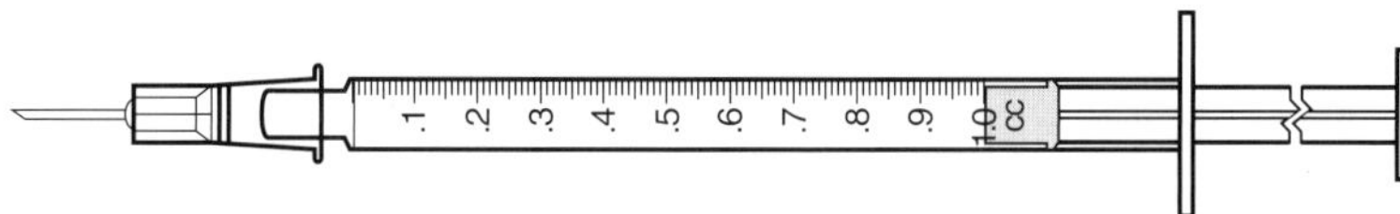

7. Order: Augmentin 500 mg PO every 8 hours for infection.

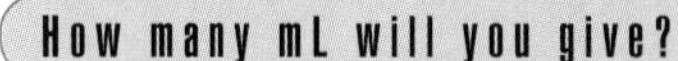

How many mL will you give? ____________

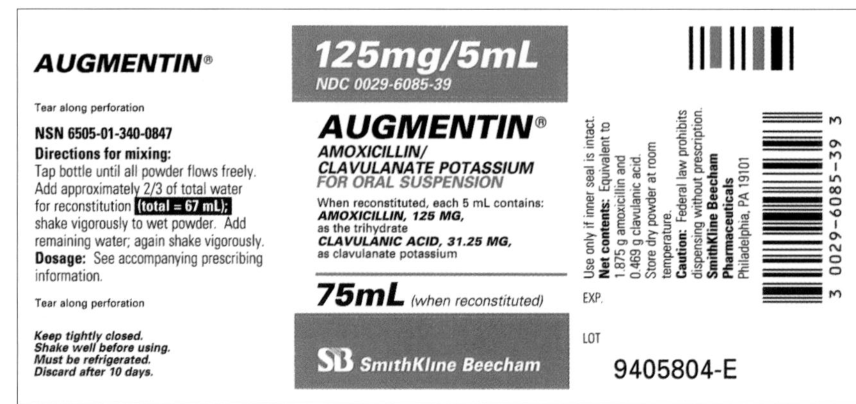

Courtesy of SmithKline Beecham Pharmaceuticals.

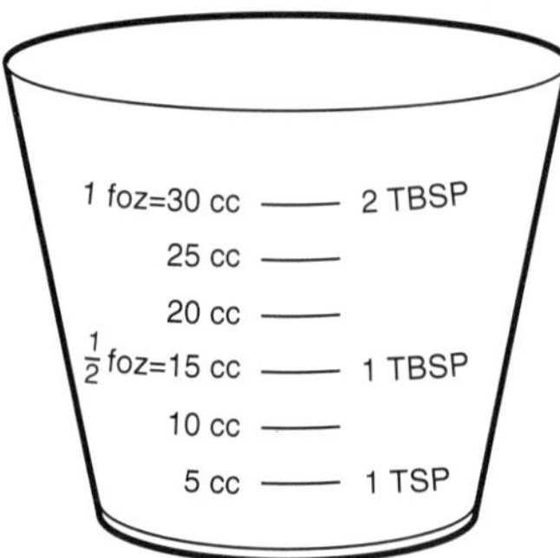

8. Order: Zaroxolyn 5 mg PO every AM for hypertension

How many tablets will you give? ____________

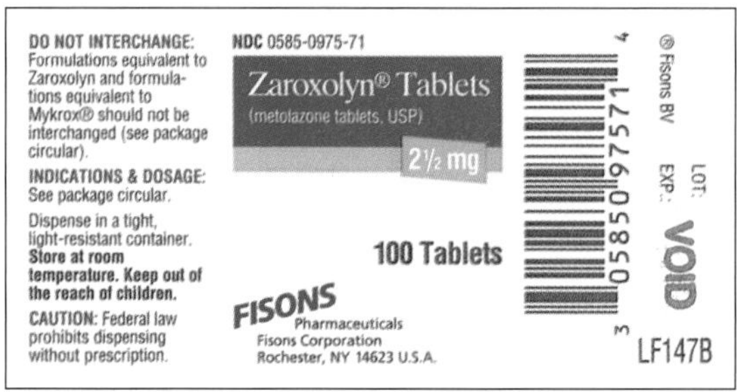

Courtesy of Fisons Pharmaceuticals.

9. Order: methylphenidate (Ritalin) 10 mg PO tid for attention-deficit hyperactivity disorder (ADHD)

How many tablets will you give? ____________

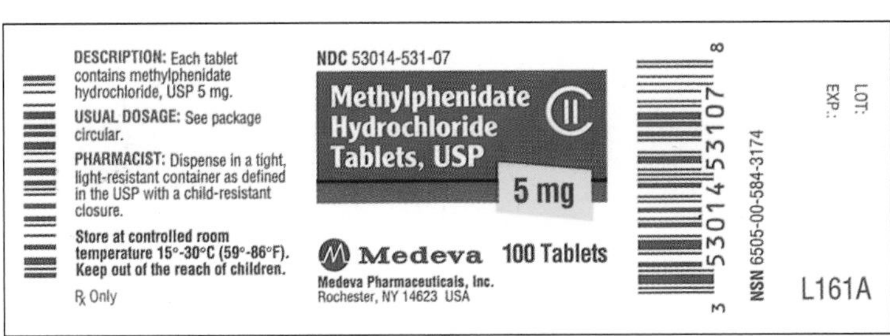

Courtesy of Medeva Pharmaceuticals.

10. Order: meperidine 50 mg IM every 3 hours prn for pain.

On hand: meperidine 100 mg/mL

How many mL will you give? ____________

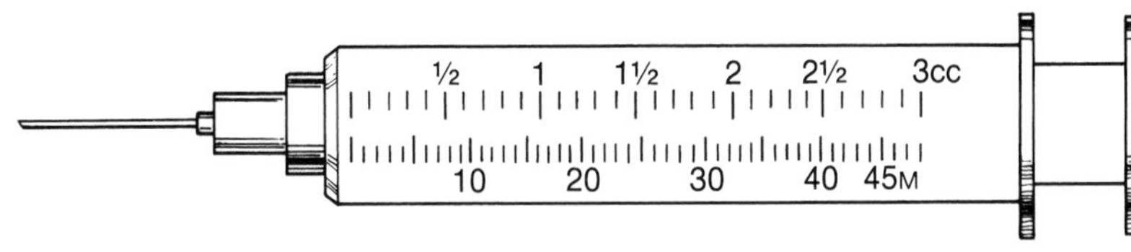

POST-TEST FOR CHAPTER 4: ONE-FACTOR MEDICATION PROBLEMS

Name ______________________ **Date** ____________

1. Order: Micronase 1.25 mg PO daily for non-insulin-dependent diabetes mellitus

   How many tablets will you give? ____________

See package insert for complete product information.
Dispense in tight, light-resistant container.
Keep container tightly closed.
Store at controlled room temperature 15° to 30° C (59° to 86° F).
812 372 405
The Upjohn Co.
Kalamazoo, MI
49001, USA

Upjohn
NDC 0009-0141-01
100 Tablets
6505-01-216-6289
Micronase®
Tablets
glyburide tablets
2.5mg
Caution: Federal law prohibits dispensing without prescription.

Courtesy of the Upjohn Company.

2. Order: Tegretol 50 mg PO qid for seizures

   How many tablets will you give? ____________

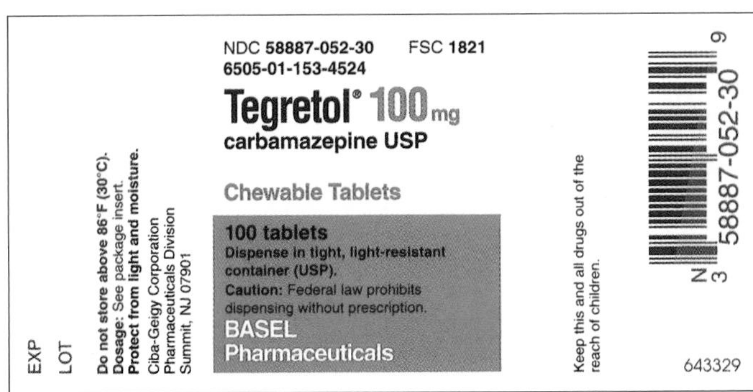

Courtesy of Basel Pharmaceuticals.

3. Order: acetaminophen 240 mg PO every 4 hours prn for moderate pain

How many milliliters will you give? ____________

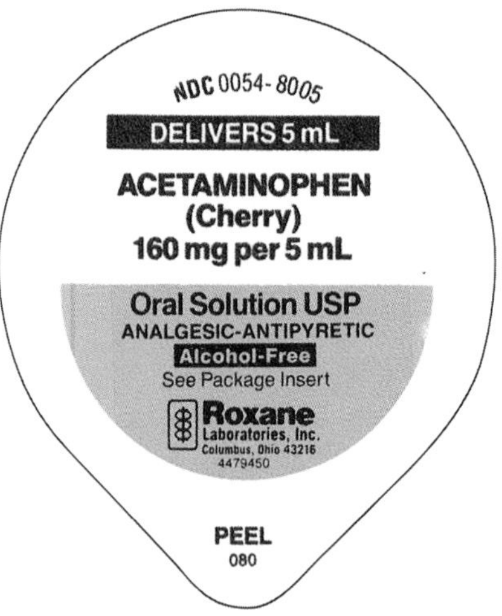

Courtesy of Roxane Laboratories, Inc.

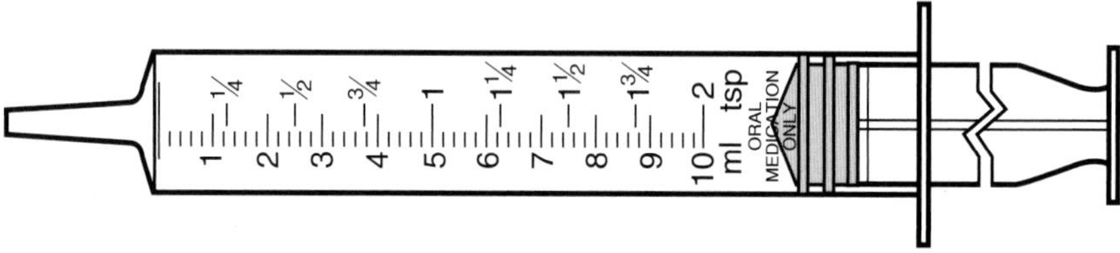

4. Order: lactulose 30 g PO qid for hepatic encephalopathy

How many milliliters will you give? ____________

NDC 0054-3486-68
1000 mL
LACTULOSE
Solution USP
10 g per 15 mL
Indication and Dosage:
For the treatment of constipation.
See insert labeling for full information.
Each 15 mL contains: 10 g lactulose (and less than 1.6 g galactose, less than 1.2 g lactose, 1.2 g or less of other sugars).
Usual Dosage: 1 to 2 tablespoonfuls (15 to 30 mL) daily. Since lactulose does not exert its effect until it reaches the colon, and since transit time through the colon may be slow, 24 to 48 hours may be required to produce a normal bowel movement.
Some patients have found that lactulose solution may be more acceptable when mixed with juice, water or milk.
Pharmacist: When ordering this product, include the NDC number in the description.
Dispense in tight, light-resistant container as defined in the USP/NF with a child-resistant closure.
Store at Controlled Room Temperature 15°-30°C (59°-86°F). DO NOT FREEZE.
Caution: Federal law prohibits dispensing without prescription.
0054-3486-68
LACTULOSE SOLUTION USP, 10 g per 15 mL
Store at Controlled Room Temperature 15°-30°C (59°-86°F)
LOT
EXP.
4120290
064
© RLI, 1994
Roxane
Laboratories, Inc.
Columbus, Ohio 43216
Product may darken slightly but therapeutic action is not affected. Do not use if extreme darkening or turbidity occurs. See accompanying information.

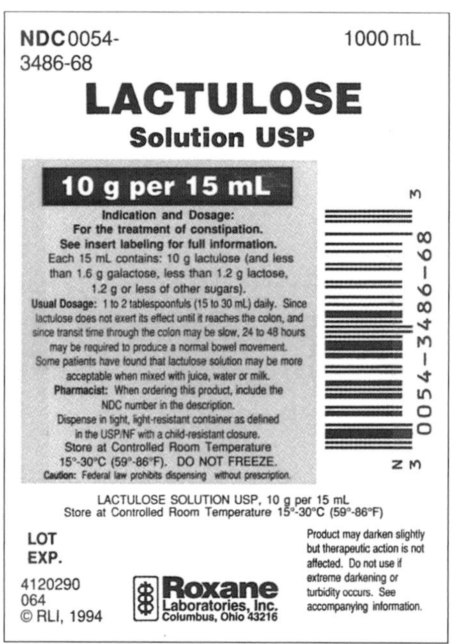

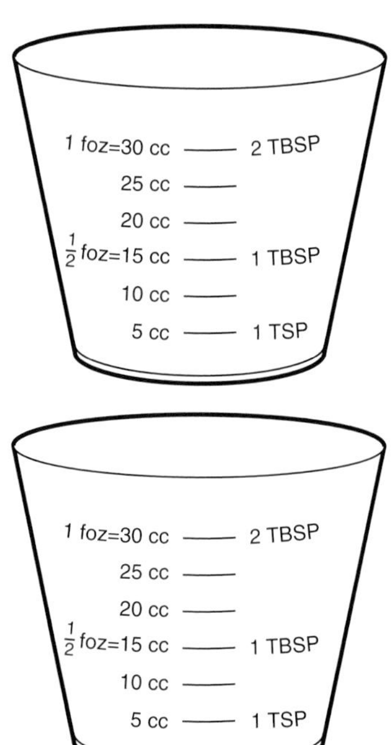

Courtesy of Roxane Laboratories, Inc.

5. Order: Tagamet 300 mg PO qid for short-term treatment of active ulcers

How many teaspoons will you give? ____________

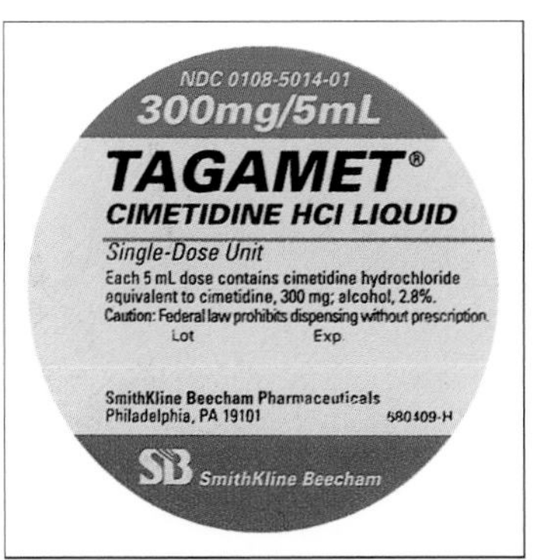

Courtesy of SmithKline Beecham Pharmaceuticals.

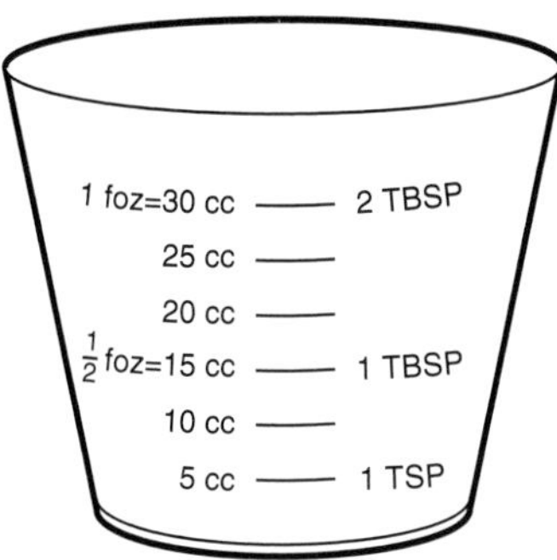

6. Order: Tigan 0.2 g IM tid prn for nausea

How many milliliters will you give? ____________

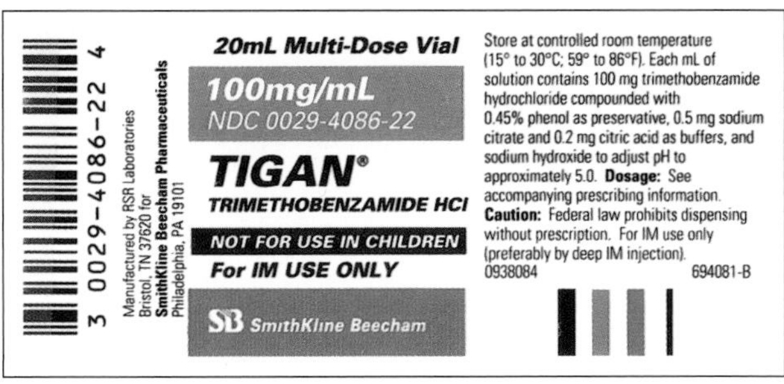

Courtesy of SmithKline Beecham Pharmaceuticals.

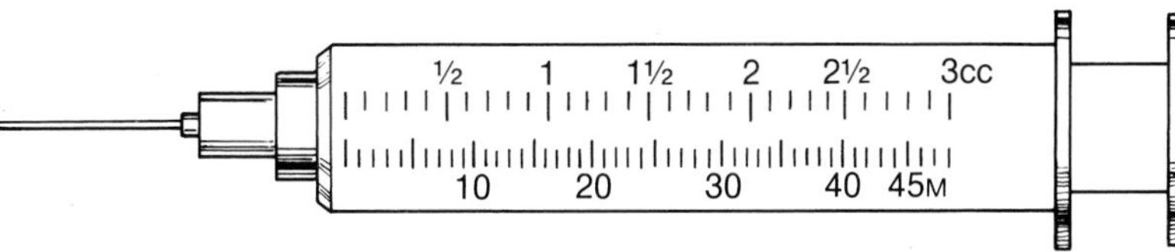

7. Order: hydromorphone 3 mg IM every 3 hours for pain

How many milliliters will you give? ______________

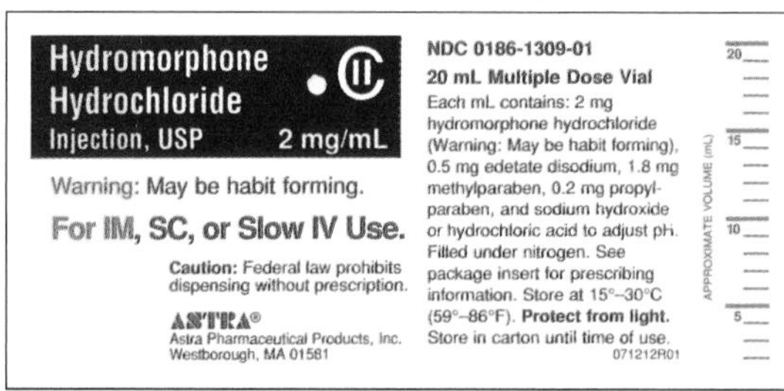

Courtesy of Astra Pharmaceutical Products.

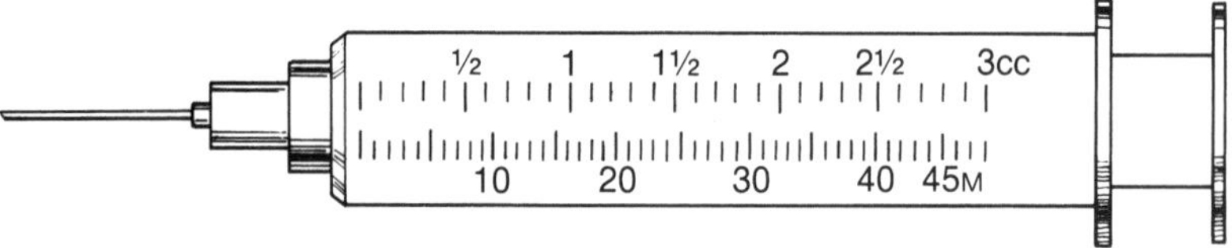

8. Order: magnesium sulfate 1000 mg IM in each buttock for hypomagnesemia

How many milliliters will you give? ______________

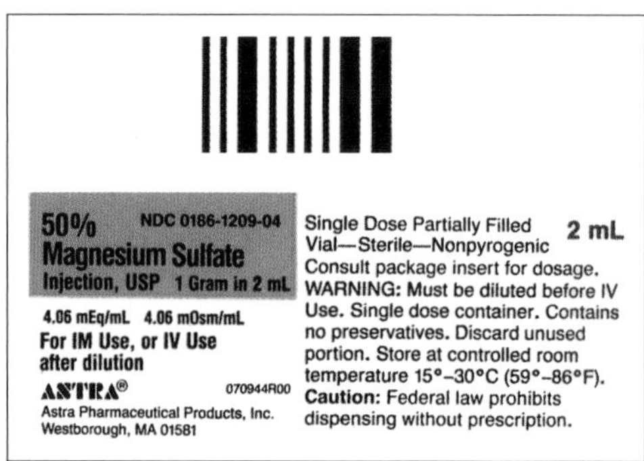

Courtesy of Astra Pharmaceutical Products.

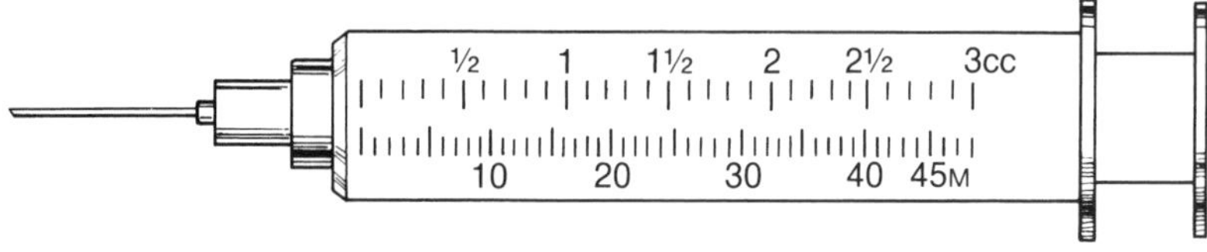

9. Order: naloxone HCl 200 mcg IV stat for respiratory depression

How many milliliters will you give? ______________

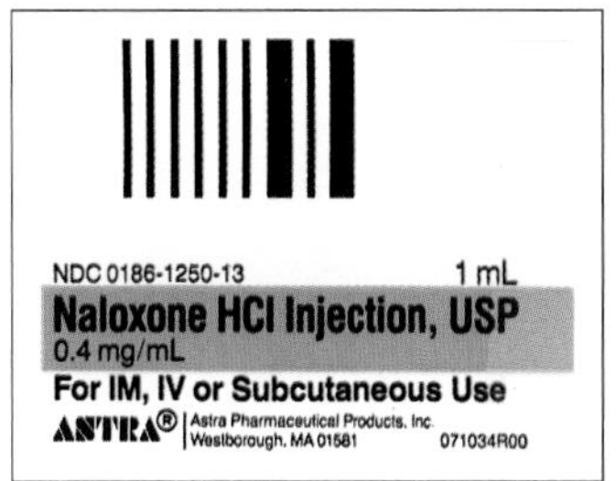

Courtesy of Astra Pharmaceutical Products.

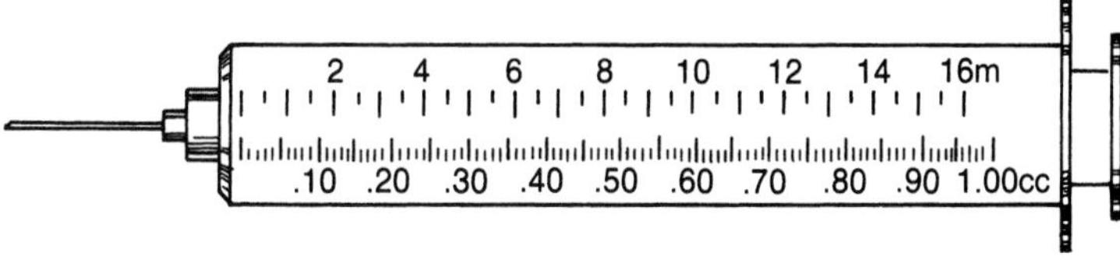

10. Order: Solu-Medrol 40 mg IM daily for autoimmune disorder

How many milliliters will you give? ______________

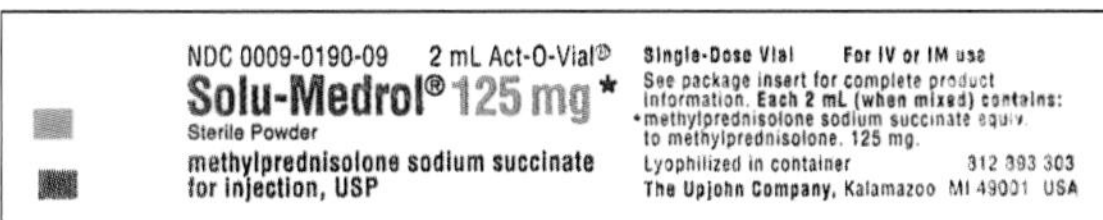

Courtesy of the Upjohn Company.

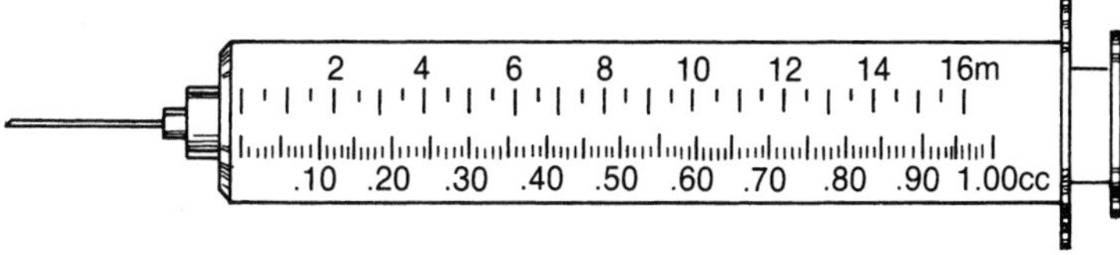

ANSWER KEY FOR CHAPTER 4: ONE-FACTOR MEDICATION PROBLEMS

Exercise 4.1 Interpretation of Medication Orders

1

a. Right patient Mrs. C. Clark
b. Right drug Aspirin for fever
c. Right dosage gr 10
d. Right route orally (PO)
e. Right time every 4 hr as needed (prn)

2

a. Right patient Mr. S. Smith
b. Right drug Advil (ibuprofen) for arthritis
c. Right dosage 400 mg
d. Right route PO (orally)
e. Right time every 6 hr

3

a. Right patient Mr. J. Jones
b. Right drug Tylenol (acetaminophen) for headache
c. Right dosage gr 10
d. Right route PO (orally)
e. Right time every 4 hr prn

Exercise 4.2 One-Factor Medication Problems

1. Sequential method:

$$\begin{array}{l|l|l|l|l} 0.25\ \cancel{\text{g}} & 100\cancel{0\ \text{mg}} & \text{(capsule)} & 0.25 \times 100 & 25 \\ \hline & 1\ \cancel{\text{g}} & 25\cancel{0\ \text{mg}} & 1 \times 25 & 25 \end{array} = 1 \text{ capsule}$$

Random method:

$$\begin{array}{l|l|l|l|l} 0.25\ \cancel{\text{g}} & \text{(capsule)} & 100\cancel{0\ \text{mg}} & 0.25 \times 100 & 25 \\ \hline & 25\cancel{0\ \text{mg}} & 1\ \cancel{\text{g}} & 25 \times 1 & 25 \end{array} = 1 \text{ capsule}$$

2. Sequential method:

$$\begin{array}{l|l|l|l|l|l} \frac{1}{2}\ \cancel{\text{gr}} & 60\ \cancel{\text{mg}} & \text{(tablet)} & \frac{1}{2} \times \frac{60}{1} & \frac{60}{2} & 30 \\ \hline & 1\ \cancel{\text{gr}} & 15\ \cancel{\text{mg}} & 1 \times 15 & 15 & 15 \end{array} = 2 \text{ tablets}$$

Random method:

$$\begin{array}{l|l|l|l|l|l} \frac{1}{2}\ \cancel{\text{gr}} & \text{(tablet)} & 60\ \cancel{\text{mg}} & \frac{1}{2} \times \frac{60}{1} & \frac{60}{2} & 30 \\ \hline & 15\ \cancel{\text{mg}} & 1\ \cancel{\text{gr}} & 15 \times 1 & 15 & 15 \end{array} = 2 \text{ tablets}$$

3. Sequential method:

$$\begin{array}{l|l|l|l|l} 0.5\ \cancel{\text{g}} & 10\cancel{00\ \text{mg}} & \text{(tablet)} & 0.5 \times 10 & 5 \\ \hline & 1\ \cancel{\text{g}} & 5\cancel{00\ \text{mg}} & 1 \times 5 & 5 \end{array} = 1 \text{ tablet}$$

Random method:

$$\begin{array}{l|l|l|l|l} 0.5\ \cancel{\text{g}} & \text{(tablet)} & 10\cancel{00\ \text{mg}} & 0.5 \times 10 & 5 \\ \hline & 5\cancel{00\ \text{mg}} & 1\ \cancel{\text{g}} & 5 \times 1 & 5 \end{array} = 1 \text{ tablet}$$

4. Sequential method:

$$\begin{array}{l|l|l|l|l} 0.03\ \cancel{\text{g}} & 100\cancel{0\ \text{mg}} & \text{(capsules)} & 0.03 \times 100 & 3 \\ \hline & 1\ \cancel{\text{g}} & 3\cancel{0\ \text{mg}} & 1 \times 3 & 3 \end{array} = 1 \text{ capsule}$$

Random method:

$$\begin{array}{l|l|l|l|l} 0.03\ \cancel{\text{g}} & \text{(capsules)} & 100\cancel{0\ \text{mg}} & 0.03 \times 100 & 3 \\ \hline & 3\cancel{0\ \text{mg}} & 1\ \cancel{\text{g}} & 3 \times 1 & 3 \end{array} = 1 \text{ capsule}$$

5. Sequential method:

$$\begin{array}{l|l|l|l|l|l} \frac{1}{2}\ \cancel{\text{gr}} & 60\ \cancel{\text{mg}} & \text{(capsules)} & \frac{1}{2} \times \frac{60}{1} & \frac{60}{2} & 30 \\ \hline & 1\ \cancel{\text{gr}} & 30\ \cancel{\text{mg}} & 1 \times 30 & 30 & 30 \end{array} = 1 \text{ capsule}$$

Random method:

$$\begin{array}{l|l|l|l|l|l} \frac{1}{2}\ \cancel{\text{gr}} & \text{(capsules)} & 60\ \cancel{\text{mg}} & \frac{1}{2} \times \frac{60}{1} & \frac{60}{2} & 30 \\ \hline & 30\ \cancel{\text{mg}} & 1\ \cancel{\text{gr}} & 30 \times 1 & 30 & 30 \end{array} = 1 \text{ capsule}$$

Exercise 4.3 Identifying the Components of Drug Labels

1

a. Cipro
b. Ciprofloxacin hydrochloride
c. 500 mg per tablet
d. 100 tablets
e. *Not listed on the label
f. *Not listed on the label
g. Bayer Corporation, Pharmaceutical Division

2

a. Tigan
b. Trimethobenzamide hydrochloride
c. 100 mg per capsule
d. 100 capsules

e. *Not listed on the label
f. *Not listed on the label
g. SmithKline Beecham Pharmaceuticals

3

a. Halcion
b. Triazolam
c. 0.125 mg per tablet
d. 10 tablets
e. *Not listed on the label
f. *Not listed on the label
g. The Upjohn Company

Exercise 4.4 Problems with Components of Drug Labels

1. Sequential method:

$$\begin{array}{c|c|c} 10\ \cancel{\text{mg}} & \text{tablet} & 10 \\ \hline & 10\ \cancel{\text{mg}} & 10 \end{array} = 1 \text{ tablet}$$

2. Random method:

$$\begin{array}{c|c|c|c} 5\cancel{00}\ \cancel{\text{mcg}} & \text{tablet} & \cancel{1}\ \cancel{\text{mg}} & 5 \\ \hline & \cancel{1}\ \cancel{\text{mg}} & 1\cancel{000}\ \cancel{\text{mcg}} & 10 \end{array} = \frac{1}{2} \text{ tablet}$$

3. Sequential method:

$$\begin{array}{c|c|c} 375\ \cancel{\text{mg}} & \text{tablet} & 375 \\ \hline & 250\ \cancel{\text{mg}} & 250 \end{array} = 1\frac{1}{2} \text{ tablets}$$

4. Random method:

$$\begin{array}{c|c|c|c|c} 2.5\ \cancel{\text{mg}} & \text{tablet} & 10\cancel{00}\ \cancel{\text{mcg}} & 2.5\times 10 & 25 \\ \hline & 25\cancel{00}\ \cancel{\text{mcg}} & 1\ \cancel{\text{mg}} & 25\times 1 & 25 \end{array} = 1 \text{ tablet}$$

5. Sequential method:

$$\begin{array}{c|c|c} 25\cancel{0}\ \cancel{\text{mg}} & \text{capsule} & 25 \\ \hline & 25\cancel{0}\ \cancel{\text{mg}} & 25 \end{array} = 1 \text{ capsule}$$

Exercise 4.5 Administering Enteral Medications

1. Random method:

$$\begin{array}{c|c|c|c|c|c} \frac{1}{2}\ \cancel{\text{gr}} & 5\ \text{mL} & 6\cancel{0}\ \cancel{\text{mg}} & \frac{1}{2}\times\frac{5}{1}\times\frac{6}{1} & \frac{30}{2} & 15 \\ \hline & 2\cancel{0}\ \cancel{\text{mg}} & 1\ \cancel{\text{gr}} & 2\times 1 & 2 & 2 \end{array} = 7.5 \text{ mL}$$

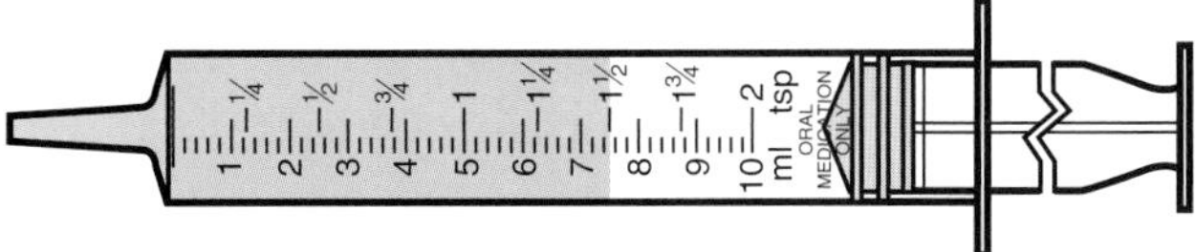

2. Sequential method:

$$\begin{array}{c|c|c|c|c|c} 0.15\ \cancel{\text{g}} & 1000\ \cancel{\text{mg}} & \cancel{\text{mL}} & \cancel{1}\ \text{tsp} & 0.15\times 1000 & 150 \\ \hline & \cancel{1}\ \cancel{\text{g}} & 15\ \cancel{\text{mg}} & 5\ \cancel{\text{mL}} & 15\times 5 & 75 \end{array} = 2 \text{ tsp}$$

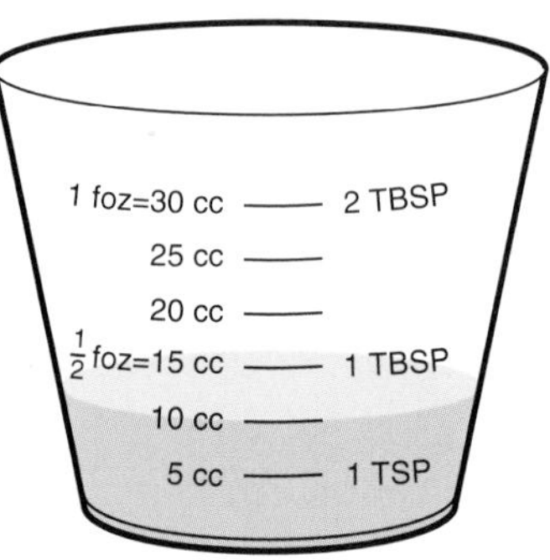

3. Sequential method:

$$\begin{array}{c|c|c} 3\ \cancel{\text{mg}} & \text{mL} & 3 \\ \hline & 1\ \cancel{\text{mg}} & 1 \end{array} = 3 \text{ mL}$$

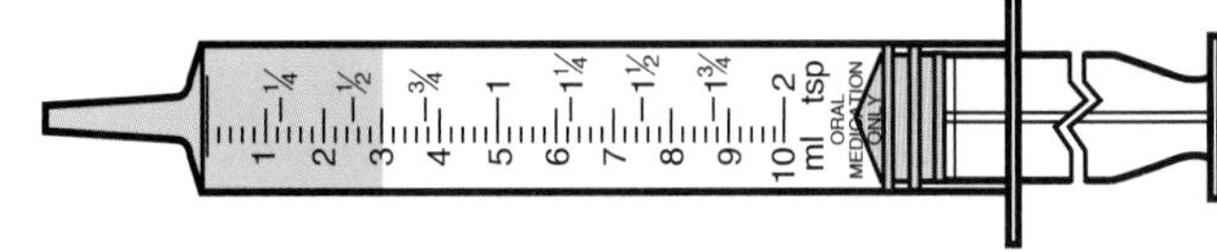

4. Sequential method:

$$\begin{array}{c|c|c|c|c} 2\cancel{0}\ \cancel{g} & 15\ \cancel{mL} & 1\ (oz) & 2\times15\times1 & 30 \\ \hline & 1\cancel{0}\ \cancel{g} & 30\ \cancel{mL} & 1\times30 & 30 \end{array} = 1\ oz$$

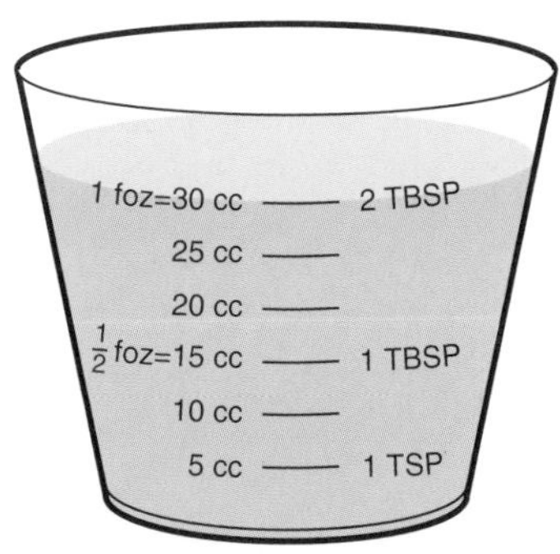

Exercise 4.6 Administering Parenteral Medications

1. Random method

$$\begin{array}{c|c|c|c|c} 3\cancel{00}\ \cancel{mcg} & (mL) & 1\ \cancel{mg} & 3\times1 & 3 \\ \hline & 0.1\ \cancel{mg} & 10\cancel{00}\ \cancel{mcg} & 0.1\times10 & 1 \end{array} = 3\ mL$$

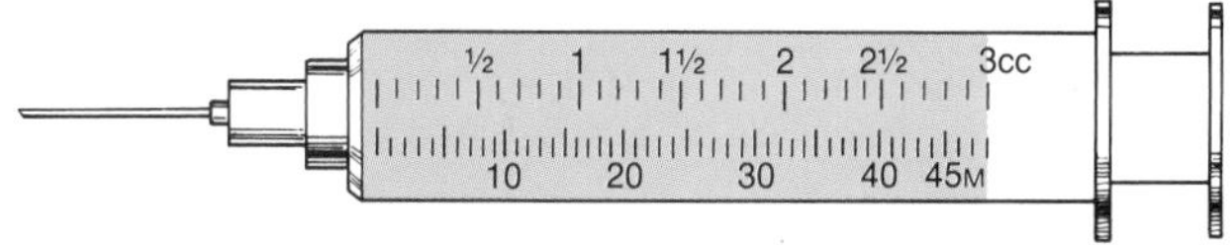

2. Sequential method:

$$\begin{array}{c|c|c} 3\ \cancel{mg} & (mL) & 3 \\ \hline & 2\ \cancel{mg} & 2 \end{array} = 1.5\ mL$$

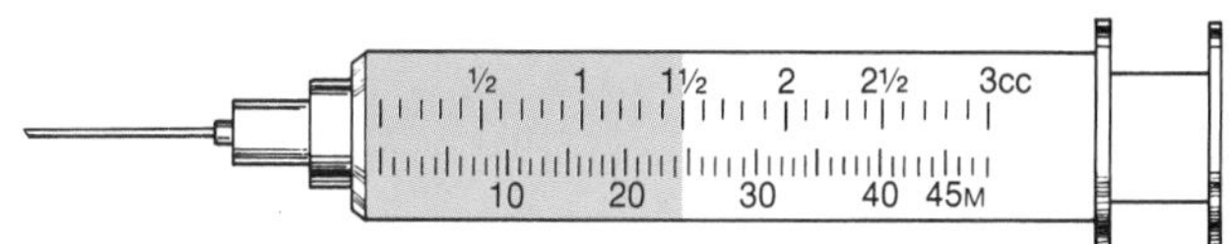

3. Sequential method:

$$\begin{array}{c|c|c} 35\ \cancel{mg} & (mL) & 35 \\ \hline & 10\ \cancel{mg} & 10 \end{array} = 3.5\ mL$$

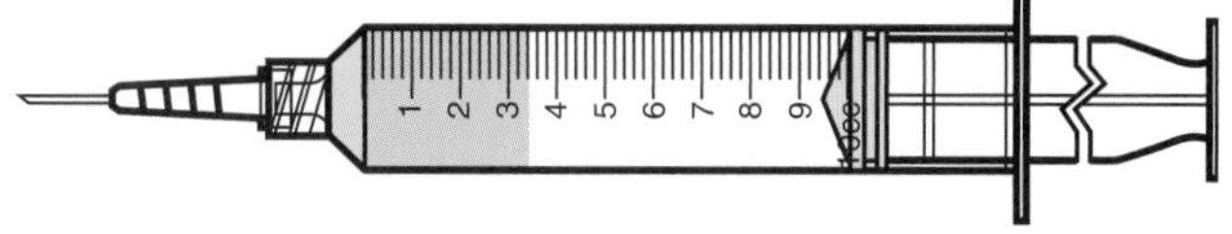

4. Sequential method:

$$\begin{array}{c|c} 10\ units & \\ \hline & \end{array} = 10\ units$$

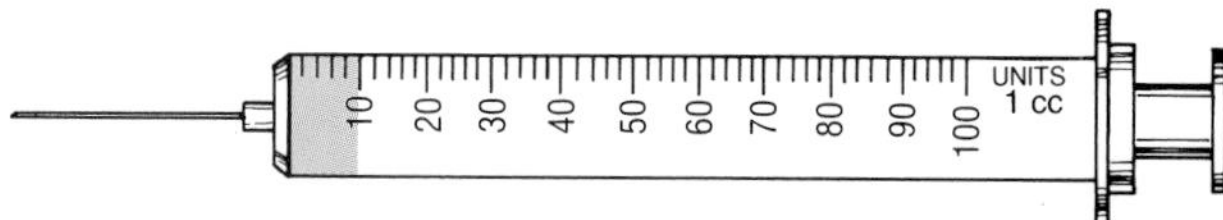

5. Sequential method:

$$\begin{array}{c|c|c} 8\cancel{000\ units} & (mL) & 8 \\ \hline & 10,\cancel{000\ units} & 10 \end{array} = 0.8\ mL$$

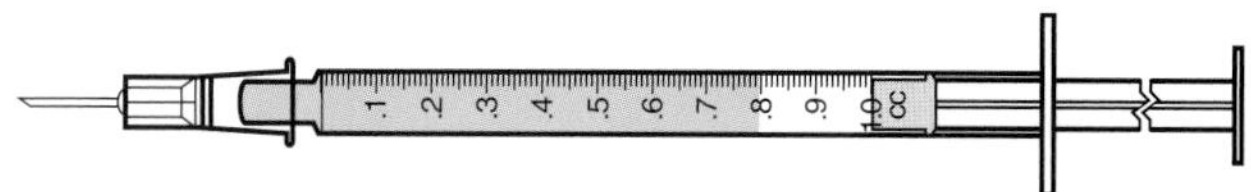

Practice Problems

1. Random method:

$$\begin{array}{c|c|c|c|c} 0.2\ \cancel{g} & (mL) & 10\cancel{00}\ \cancel{mg} & 0.2\times10 & 2 \\ \hline & 1\cancel{00}\ \cancel{mg} & 1\ \cancel{g} & 1\times1 & 1 \end{array} = 2\ mL$$

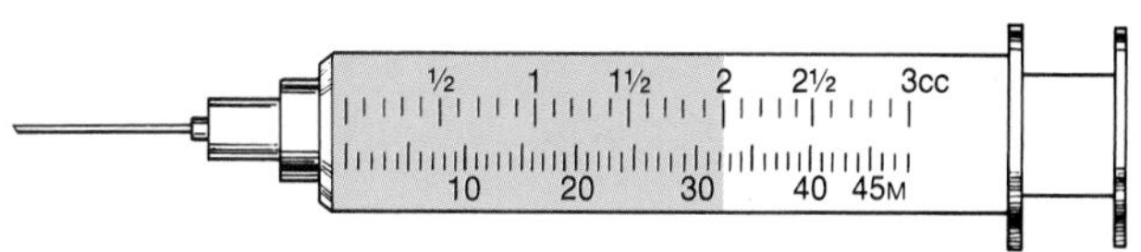

2. Sequential method:

$$\begin{array}{c|c|c} 50\ \cancel{mg} & (tablet) & 50 \\ \hline & 25\ \cancel{mg} & 25 \end{array} = 2\ tablets$$

3. Random method:

$$\begin{array}{c|c|c|c|c} 1\ \cancel{g} & (tablet) & 10\cancel{00}\ \cancel{mg} & 1\times10 & 10 \\ \hline & 5\cancel{00}\ \cancel{mg} & 1\ \cancel{g} & 5\times1 & 5 \end{array} = 2\ tablets$$

4. Random method:

$$\begin{array}{c|c|c} 50\ \cancel{mg} & (tablet) & 50 \\ \hline & 25\ \cancel{mg} & 25 \end{array} = 2\ tablets$$

5. Sequential method:

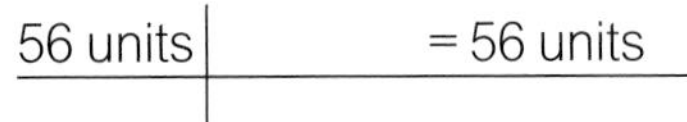

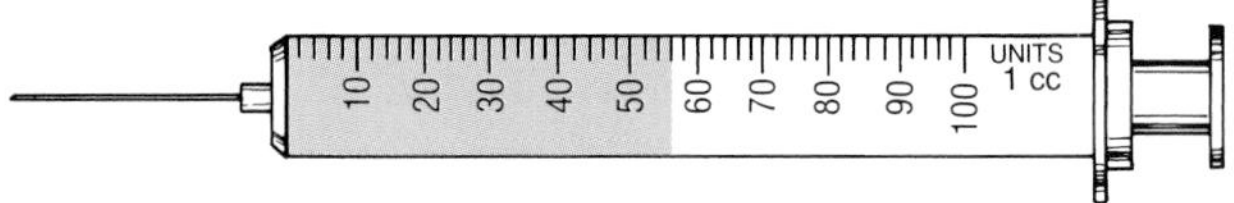

6. Sequential method:

$$\frac{75\cancel{00}\ \cancel{\text{units}}}{} \left| \frac{\text{(mL)}}{100\cancel{00}\ \cancel{\text{units}}} \right| \frac{75}{100} = 0.75\ \text{mL}$$

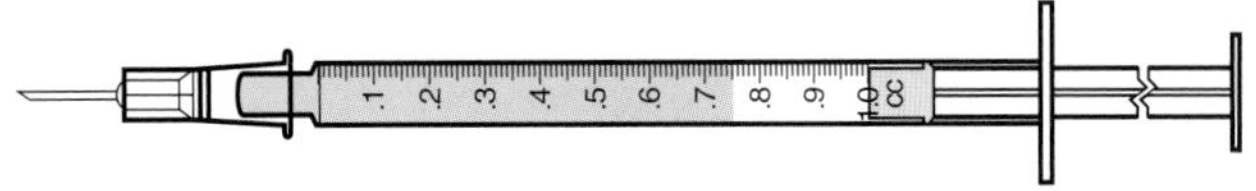

7. Sequential method:

$$\frac{500\ \cancel{\text{mg}}}{} \left| \frac{5\ \text{(mL)}}{125\ \cancel{\text{mg}}} \right| \frac{500 \times 5}{125} \left| \frac{2500}{125} \right. = 20\ \text{mL}$$

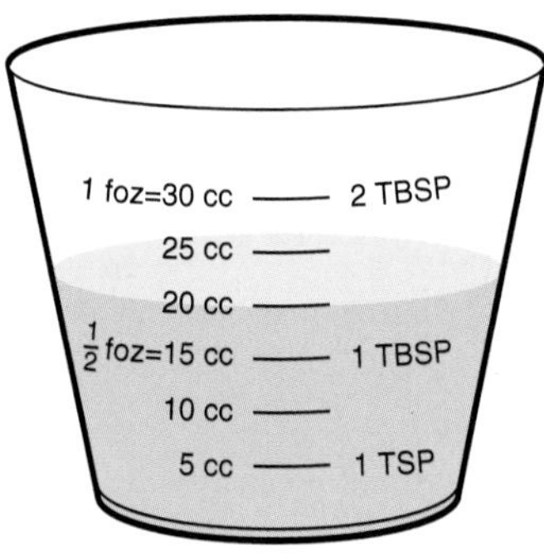

8. Sequential method:

$$\frac{5\ \cancel{\text{mg}}}{} \left| \frac{\text{(tablet)}}{2.5\ \cancel{\text{mg}}} \right| \frac{5}{2.5} = 2\ \text{tablets}$$

9. Sequential method:

$$\frac{10\ \cancel{\text{mg}}}{} \left| \frac{\text{(tablet)}}{5\ \cancel{\text{mg}}} \right| \frac{10}{5} = 2\ \text{tablets}$$

10. Sequential method:

$$\frac{5\cancel{0}\ \cancel{\text{mg}}}{} \left| \frac{\text{(mL)}}{100\ \cancel{\text{mg}}} \right| \frac{5}{10} = 0.5\ \text{mL}$$

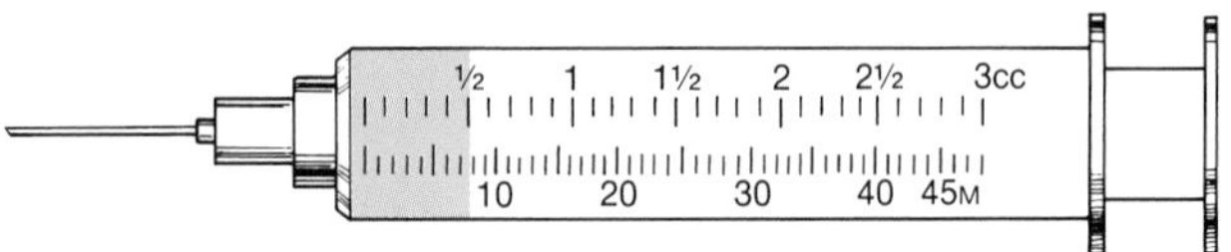

Although medications are ordered by physicians and administered by nurses using the "five rights of medication administration," other factors need to be considered when administering certain medications or intravenous fluids.

- The *weight* of the patient often must be factored into a medication problem when determining how much medication can safely be given to an infant or a child or the elderly.
- The dosage of medication available may be in a powdered form that needs *reconstitution* to a liquid form before parenteral or intravenous administration.
- Also, the length of *time* over which medications or intravenous fluids can be given plays an important role in the safe administration of intravenous therapy.

To be able to calculate a two-factor–given quantity to one-factor– or two-factor–wanted quantity medication problem, it is important to understand all factors that may need to be considered in some medication problems. With use of dimensional analysis, this chapter will teach you to calculate medication problems involving the weight of the patient, the reconstitution of medications from powder to liquid form, and the amount of time over which medications or intravenous fluids can be safely administered.

5

TWO-FACTOR MEDICATION PROBLEMS

Outline

Objectives

After completing this chapter, you will be able to:

1. Solve two-factor–given quantity to one-factor–wanted quantity medication problems involving a specific amount of medication ordered based on the weight of the patient.

2. Calculate medication problems requiring reconstitution of medications by using information from a nursing drug reference, label, or package insert.

3. Solve two-factor–given quantity to two-factor–wanted quantity medication problems involving a specific amount of fluid to be delivered over limited time using an intravenous pump delivering milliliters per hour (mL/hr).

4. Solve two-factor–given quantity to two-factor–wanted quantity medication problems involving a specific amount of fluid to be delivered over a limited time using different types of intravenous tubing that deliver drops per minute (gtt/min) based on a specific *drop factor*.

MEDICATION PROBLEMS INVOLVING WEIGHT

When solving problems with dimensional analysis, you can use either the *sequential method* or the *random method* to calculate two-factor–given quantity medication problems. The **given quantity** (the physician's order) contains two parts including a **numerator** (dosage of medication) and a **denominator** (the weight of the patient). This type of medication problem is called a *two-factor* medication problem because the *given quantity* now contains two parts (a numerator and a denominator) instead of just one part (a numerator).

Below is an example of the problem-solving method showing placement of basic terms used in dimensional analysis, applied to a two-factor medication problem involving weight.

Unit Path

Given Quantity	Conversion Factor for Given Quantity (Numerator)	Conversion Factor for Given Quantity (Denominator)		Conversion Computation		Wanted Quantity
2.5 mg	mL	1 kg	60 lb	2.5 × 1 × 6	15	= 1.7 mL
kg	40 mg	2.2 lb		4.22	8.8	

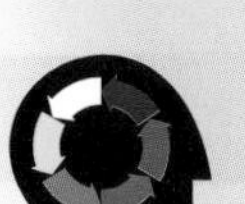

THINKING IT THROUGH

The two-factor–given quantity has been set up with a numerator (2.5 mg) and a denominator (kg) leading across the unit path to a one-factor–wanted quantity with only a numerator (mL).

The *dose on hand* (40 mg/mL) has been factored in to cancel out the preceding unwanted unit (mg). The wanted unit (mL) is in the numerator and corresponds with the one-factor–wanted quantity (mL).

A *conversion factor* (1 kg = 2.2 lb) is factored into the unit path to cancel out the preceding unwanted unit (kg).

The *weight* is finally factored in to cancel out the preceding unwanted unit (lb) in the denominator. All unwanted units are canceled and only the wanted unit (mL) remains and corresponds with the wanted quantity (mL). Multiply the numerators, multiply the denominators, and divide the product of the numerators by the product of the denominators to provide the numerical value.

EXAMPLE 5.1

The physician orders gentamicin 2.5 mg/kg IV (intravenous) every 8 hours for infection. The vial of medication is labeled 40 mg/mL. The child weighs 60 lb.

How many milliliters will you give?

Given quantity = 2.5 mg/kg
Wanted quantity = mL
Dose on hand = 40 mg/mL
Weight = 60 lb

Sequential method:

Step 1 Identify the two-factor–given quantity (the physician's order).

Unit Path

Given Quantity	Conversion Factor for Given Quantity (Numerator)	Conversion Factor for Given Quantity (Denominator)		Conversion Computation	Wanted Quantity
2.5 mg					= mL
kg					

Step 2

Unit Path

Given Quantity	Conversion Factor for Given Quantity (Numerator)	Conversion Factor for Given Quantity (Denominator)		Conversion Computation	Wanted Quantity
2.5 mg	(mL)				= mL
kg	40 mg				

Step 3

Unit Path

Given Quantity	Conversion Factor for Given Quantity (Numerator)	Conversion Factor for Given Quantity (Denominator)		Conversion Computation	Wanted Quantity
2.5 ~~mg~~	(mL)	1 ~~kg~~			= mL
~~kg~~	40 ~~mg~~	2.2 lb			

Step 4

Unit Path

Given Quantity	Conversion Factor for Given Quantity (Numerator)	Conversion Factor for Given Quantity (Denominator)		Conversion Computation	Wanted Quantity
2.5 ~~mg~~	(mL)	1 ~~kg~~	60 ~~lb~~		= mL
~~kg~~	40 ~~mg~~	2.2 ~~lb~~			

Step 5

Unit Path

Given Quantity	Conversion Factor for Given Quantity (Numerator)	Conversion Factor for Given Quantity (Denominator)		Conversion Computation	Wanted Quantity	
2.5 ~~mg~~	(mL)	1 ~~kg~~	60 ~~lb~~	2.5 × 1 × 6	15	= 1.7 mL
~~kg~~	~~40 mg~~	2.2 ~~lb~~		4 × 2.2	8.8	

1.7 mL is the wanted quantity and the answer to the problem.

Dimensional analysis is a problem-solving method that uses critical thinking. When implementing the *random method* of dimensional analysis, the medication problem can be set up in a number of different ways. The focus is on the correct placement of conversion factors to cancel out all unwanted units. The wanted unit is placed in the numerator to correctly correspond with the wanted quantity.

2.5 ~~mg~~	1 ~~kg~~	60 ~~lb~~	(mL)	2.5 × 1 × 6	15	= 1.7 mL
~~kg~~	2.2 ~~lb~~		~~40 mg~~	2.2 × 4	8.8	

Exercise 5.1 Medication Problems Involving Weight

(See page 129 for answers)

1. Order: furosemide 1 mg/kg IV bid for hypercalcemia. The child weighs 45 lb.

How many milliliters will you give? ______________

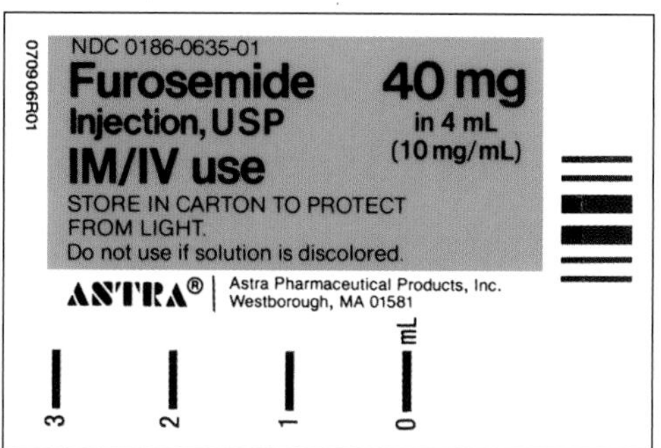

Courtesy of Astra Pharmaceutical Products.

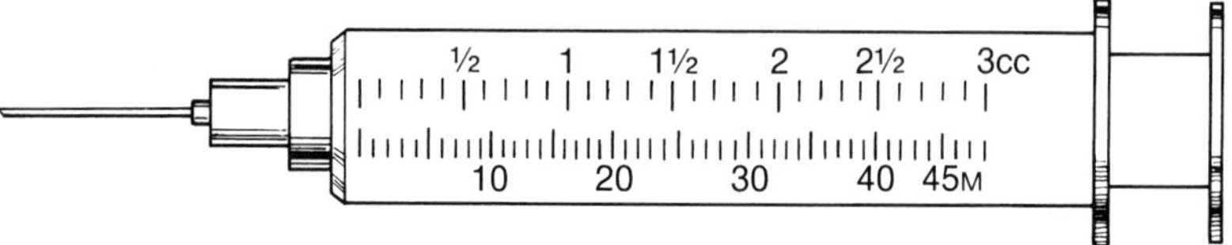

2. Order: atropine sulfate 0.01 mg/kg IV stat for bradycardia. The child weighs 20 lb.

How many milliliters will you give? ______________

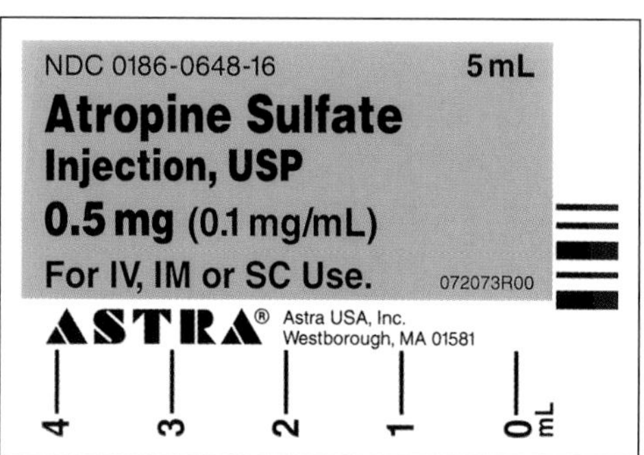

Courtesy of Astra Pharmaceutical Products.

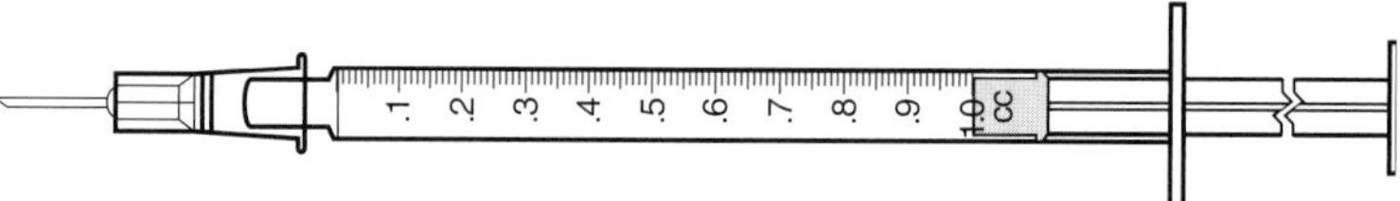

3. Order: phenergan 0.5 mg/kg IV every 4 hours prn for nausea. The dose on hand is 25 mg/mL. The child weighs 45 lb.

How many milliliters will you give? ______________

4. Order: morphine 50 mcg/kg IV every 4 hours prn for pain. The child weighs 75 lb.

How many milliliters will you give? ______________

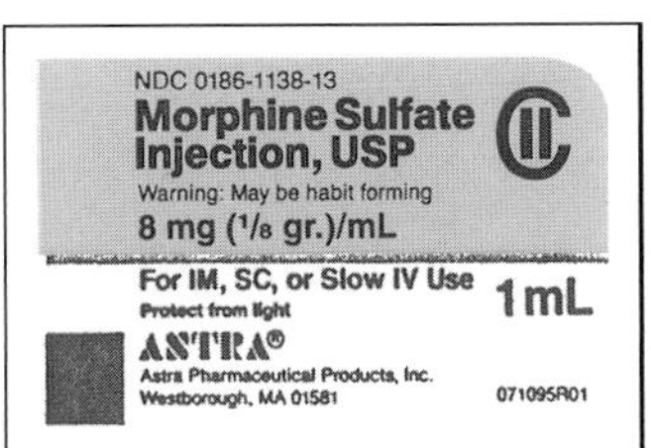

Courtesy of Astra Pharmaceutical Products.

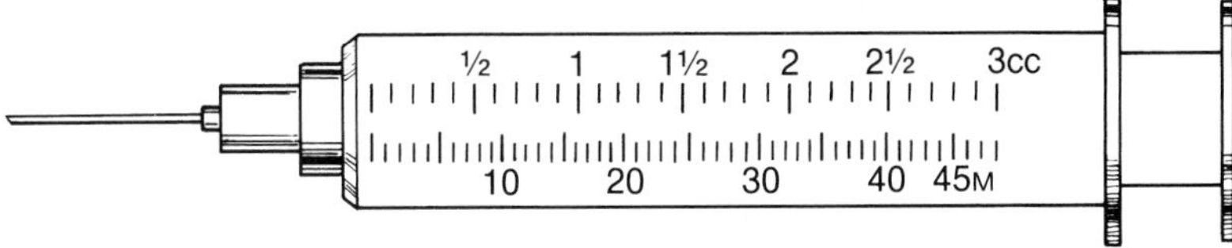

(Exercise continues on page 104)

5. Order: Tagamet 10 mg/kg PO qid for prophylaxis of duodenal ulcer. The dose on hand is 300 mg/5 mL. The child weighs 70 lb.

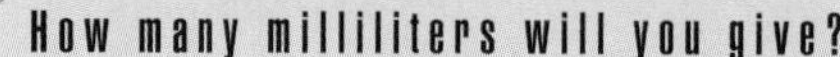

____

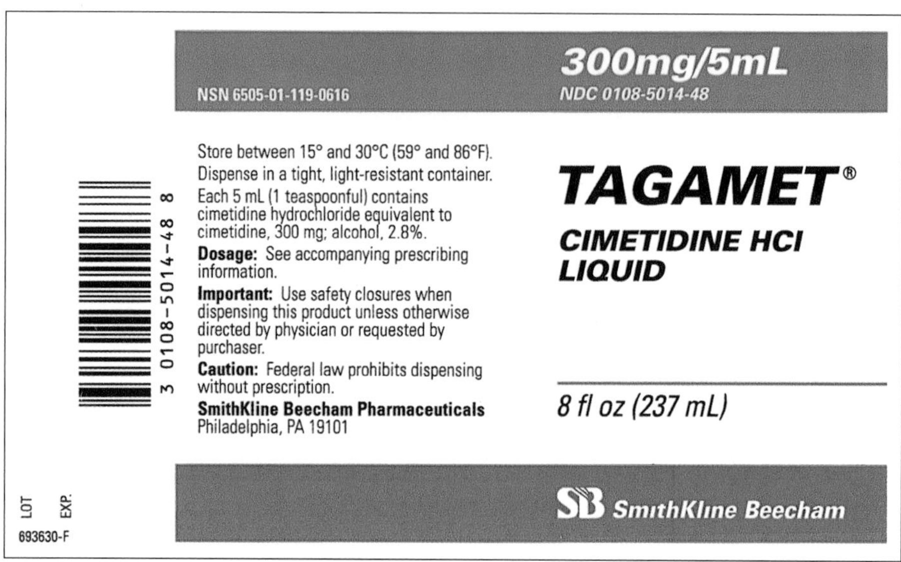

Courtesy of SmithKline Beecham Pharmaceuticals.

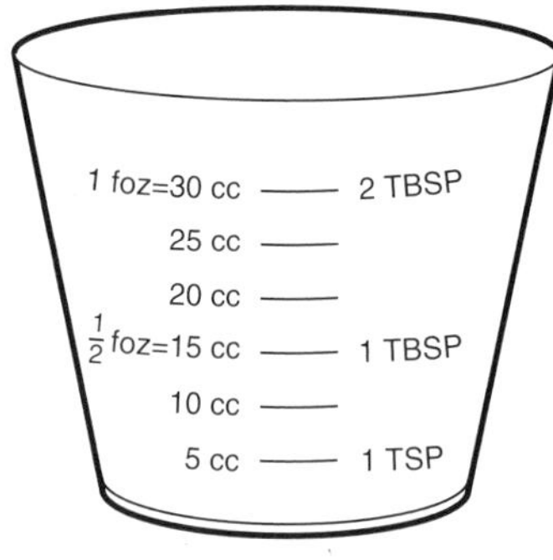

MEDICATION PROBLEMS INVOLVING RECONSTITUTION

Some medications in vials are in a powder form and need reconstitution before administration. **Reconstitution** involves adding a specific amount of sterile solution (also called **diluent**) to the vial to change the powder to a liquid form. Information on how much diluent to add to the vial and what dosage of medication per milliliter will result after reconstitution (also called **yield**) can be obtained from a nursing drug reference, label, or package insert.

EXAMPLE 5.2

The physician orders Mezlin (mezlocillin) 50 mg/kg every 4 hours IV for infection. The child weighs 60 lb. The pharmacy sends a vial of medication labeled Mezlin 1 g. The nursing drug reference provides information to reconstitute 1 g of medication with 10 mL of sterile water for injection, 0.9% NaCl, or D5W.

How many milliliters will you draw from the vial?

Given quantity = 50 mg/kg
Wanted quantity = mL
Dose on hand = 1 g/10 mL (yields 1 g/10 mL)
Weight = 60 lb

Random method:

Unit Path

Given Quantity	Conversion Factor for Given Quantity (Numerator)		Conversion Factor for Given Quantity (Denominator)		Conversion Computation		Wanted Quantity
~~50 mg~~	1 ~~kg~~	~~60 lb~~	~~10~~ (mL)	~~1 g~~	5 × 1 × 6 × 1	30	= 13.63 mL or 13.6 mL
~~kg~~	2.2 ~~lb~~		~~1 g~~	~~1000 mg~~	2.2	2.2	

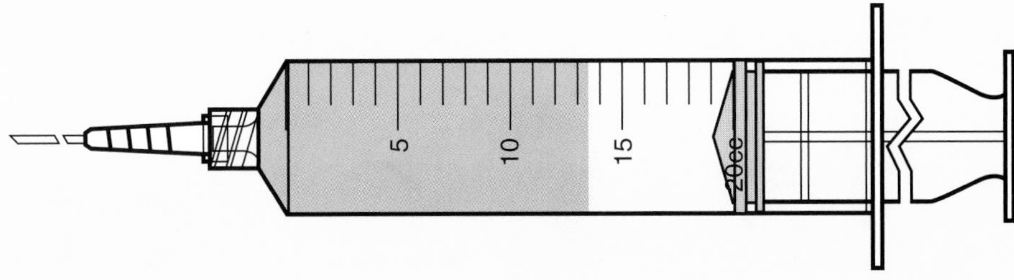

13.63 mL or 13.6 mL is the wanted quantity and the answer to the problem.

EXAMPLE 5.3

Order: Solu-Medrol 40 mg IV every 4 hours for inflammation.

How many milliliters will you draw from the vial?

Solu-Medrol®

Upjohn

brand of methylprednisolone sodium succinate sterile powder (methylprednisolone sodium succinate for injection, USP)

For Intravenous or Intramuscular Administration

125 mg Act-O-Vial System (Single-Dose Vial)—Each 2 mL (when mixed) contains methylprednisolone sodium succinate equivalent to 125 mg methylprednisolone; also 1.6 mg monobasic sodium phosphate anhydrous; 17.4 mg dibasic sodium phosphate dried; 17.6 mg benzyl alcohol added as preservative

DOSAGE AND ADMINISTRATION

When high dose therapy is desired, the recommended dose of SOLU-MEDROL Sterile Powder is 30 mg/kg administered intravenously over at least 30 minutes. This dose may be repeated every 4 to 6 hours for 48 hours.

In general, high dose corticosteroid therapy should be continued only until the patient's condition has stabilized; usually not beyond 48 to 72 hours.

Although adverse effects associated with high dose short-term corticoid therapy are uncommon, peptic ulceration may occur. Prophylactic antacid therapy may be indicated.

In other indications initial dosage will vary from 10 to 40 mg of methylprednisolone depending on the clinical problem being treated. The larger doses may be required for short-term management of severe, acute conditions. The initial dose usually should be given intravenously over a period of several minutes. Subsequent doses may be given intravenously or intramuscularly at intervals dictated by the patient's response and clinical condition. Corticoid therapy is an adjunct to, and not replacement for conventional therapy.

Dosage may be reduced for infants and children but should be governed more by the severity of the condition and response of the patient than by age or size. It should not be less than 0.5 mg per kg every 24 hours.

Dosage must be decreased or discontinued gradually when the drug has been administered for more than a few days. If a period of spontaneous remission occurs in a chronic condition, treatment should be discontinued. Routine laboratory studies, such as urinalysis, two-hour postprandial blood sugar, determination of blood pressure and body weight, and a chest X-ray should be made at regular intervals during prolonged therapy. Upper GI X-rays are desirable in patients with an ulcer history or significant dyspepsia.

SOLU-MEDROL may be administered by intravenous or intramuscular injection or by intravenous infusion, the preferred method for initial emergency use being intravenous injection. To administer by intravenous (or intramuscular) injection, prepare solution as directed. The desired dose may be administered intravenously over a period of several minutes. If desired, the medication may be administered in diluted solutions by adding Water for Injection or other suitable diluent (see below) to the **Act-O-Vial** and withdrawing the indicated dose.

To prepare solutions for intravenous infusion, first prepare the solution for injection as directed. This solution may then be added to indicated amounts of 5% dextrose in water, isotonic saline solution or 5% dextrose in isotonic saline solution.

Multiple Sclerosis

In treatment of acute exacerbations of multiple sclerosis, daily doses of 200 mg of prednisolone for a week followed by 80 mg every other day for 1 month have been shown to be effective (4 mg of methylprednisolone is equivalent to 5 mg of prednisolone).

DIRECTIONS FOR USING THE ACT-O-VIAL SYSTEM

1. Press down on plastic activator to force diluent into the lower compartment.
2. Gently agitate to effect solution.
3. Remove plastic tab covering center of stopper.
4. Sterilize top of stopper with a suitable germicide.
5. Insert needle **squarely through center** of stopper until tip is just visible. Invert vial and withdraw dose.

STORAGE CONDITIONS

Store unreconstituted product at controlled room temperature 15° to 30° C (59° to 86° F).
Store solution at controlled room temperature 15° to 30° C (59° to 86° F).
Use solution within 48 hours after mixing.

HOW SUPPLIED

SOLU-MEDROL Sterile Powder is available in the following packages:

40 mg Act-O-Vial System (Single-Dose Vial)
1 mL NDC 0009-0113-12
25—1 mL NDC 0009-0113-13
25—1 mL NDC 0009-0113-19

125 mg Act-O-Vial System (Single-Dose Vial)
2 mL NDC 0009-0190-09
25—2 mL NDC 0009-0190-10
25—2 mL NDC 0009-0190-16

500 mg Vial NDC 0009-0758-01
500 mg Vial with Diluent NDC 0009-0887-01
500 mg Act-O-Vial System (Single-Dose Vial)
4 mL NDC 0009-0765-02
1 gram Vial NDC 0009-0698-01
1 gram Act-O-Vial System (Single-Dose Vial)
8 mL NDC 0009-3389-01
2 gram Vial NDC 0009-0988-01
2 gram Vial with Diluent NDC 0009-0796-01

Courtesy of the Upjohn Company.

Given quantity = 40 mg
Wanted quantity = mL
Dose on hand = 125 mg/2 mL (yield from 2 mL Act-O-Vial)

Sequential method:

$$\frac{40\ \cancel{mg}}{} \bigg| \frac{2\ (mL)}{125\ \cancel{mg}} \bigg| \frac{40 \times 2}{125} \bigg| \frac{80}{125} = 0.64\ mL \text{ or } 0.6\ mL$$

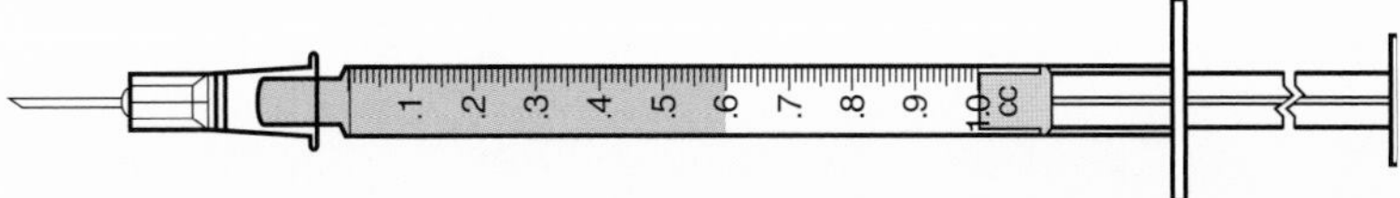

0.6 mL is the wanted quantity and the answer to the problem.

EXAMPLE 5.4

Order: Claforan 50 mg/kg IV every 8 hours for infection. The infant weighs 12 kg.

How many milliliters will you draw from the vial after reconstitution?

719000-2/95

Claforan®

Sterile (sterile cefotaxime sodium)
and
Injection (cefotaxime sodium injection)

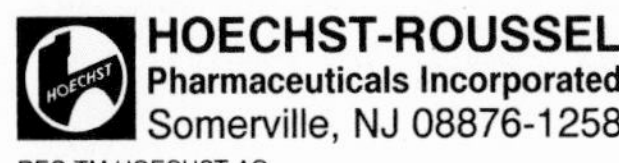

HOECHST-ROUSSEL
Pharmaceuticals Incorporated
Somerville, NJ 08876-1258
REG TM HOECHST AG

Neonates, Infants, and Children
The following dosage schedule is recommended:

Neonates (birth to 1 month):

0-1 week of age	50 mg/kg per dose every 12 hours IV
1-4 weeks of age	50 mg/kg per dose every 8 hours IV

It is not necessary to differentiate between premature and normal-gestational age infants.

Infants and Children (1 month to 12 years): For body weights less than 50 kg, the recommended daily dose is 50 to 180 mg/kg IM or IV body weight divided into four to six equal doses. The higher dosages should be used for more severe or serious infections, including meningitis. For body weights 50 kg or more, the usual adult dosage should be used; the maximum daily dosage should not exceed 12 grams.

Courtesy of Hoechst-Roussel Pharmaceuticals.

Supply: Claforan 1 g/10 mL

The package insert states: Reconstitute vials with at least 10 mL of sterile water for injection.

(Example continues on page 108)

Given quantity = 50 mg/kg
Wanted quantity = mL
Dose on hand = 1 g/10 mL
Weight = 12 kg

Random method:

$$\frac{50\ \cancel{mg}}{\cancel{kg}} \,\Big|\, \frac{1\cancel{0}\ (mL)}{1\ \cancel{g}} \,\Big|\, \frac{1\ \cancel{g}}{100\cancel{0}\ \cancel{mg}} \,\Big|\, \frac{12\ \cancel{kg}}{} \,\Big|\, \frac{5 \times 1 \times 1 \times 12}{1 \times 10} \,\Big|\, \frac{60}{10} = 6\ mL$$

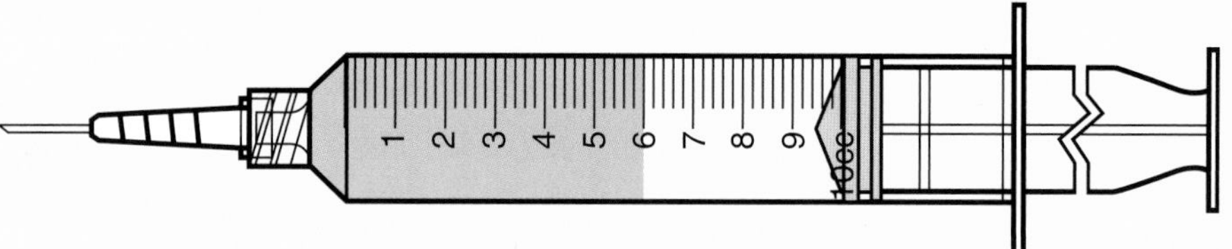

6 mL is the wanted quantity and the answer to the problem.

Exercise 5.2 Medication Problems Involving Reconstitution

(See pages 129–130 for answers)

1. Order: Ancef 500 mg IV every 8 hours for infection.

   How many milliliters will you draw out of the vial after reconstitution? ______

   (Ancef is reconstituted using 50 mL sodium chloride.)

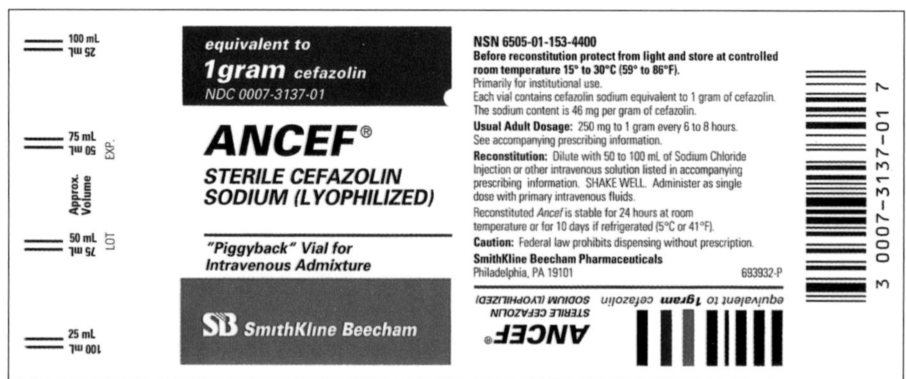

Courtesy of SmithKline Beecham Pharmaceuticals.

2. Order: Primaxin 250 mg IV every 6 hours for infection

   Supply: Primaxin vial labeled 500 mg. Reconstitute with 10 mL of compatible diluent and shake well.

   How many milliliters will you draw from the vial after reconstitution? ______

3. Order: Unasyn (ampicillin) 50 mg/kg IV every 4 hours for infection

   Supply: Unasyn 1.5-g vial

   Nursing drug reference: Reconstitute each Unasyn 1.5-g vial with 4 mL of sterile water to yield 375 mg/mL.

   The child weighs 40 kg.

   How many milliliters will you draw from the vial after reconstitution? __________

4. Order: erythromycin 750 mg IV every 6 hours for infection

   Supply: erythromycin 1-g vial labeled: Reconstitute with 20 mL of sterile water for injection.

   How many milliliters will you draw from the vial after reconstitution? __________

5. Order: Fortaz 30 mg/kg IV every 8 hours for infection

   Supply: Fortaz 500-mg vial labeled: Reconstitute with 5 mL of sterile water for injection

   The child weighs 65 lb.

   How many milliliters will you draw from the vial after reconstitution? __________

MEDICATION PROBLEMS INVOLVING INTRAVENOUS PUMPS

Intravenous medications are administered by drawing a specific amount of medication from a vial or ampule and inserting that medication into an existing intravenous line. All intravenous medications must be given with specific thought to exactly how much *time* it should take to administer the medication. Information regarding time may be obtained from a nursing drug reference, label, or package insert, or may be specifically ordered by the physician.

Although IV medications can be administered IV push, the time involved often requires the use of an intravenous pump (IV pump). All IV pumps deliver milliliters per hour (mL/hr or cc/hr) but may vary in operational capacity or size.

Below is an example of the dimensional analysis problem-solving method with basic terms applied to a medication problem involving an IV pump.

Given Quantity	Unit Path: Conversion Factor for Given Quantity (Numerator)	Conversion Computation	Wanted Quantity
1500 Units	250 mL	15	= 15 mL
hr	25,000 Units	hr	

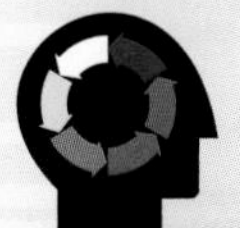

THINKING IT THROUGH

The two-factor–given quantity (the physician's order) contains a **numerator** (the dosage of medication) and a **denominator** (time). The wanted quantity (the answer to the problem) also contains a numerator (mL) and a denominator (time). This is called a two-factor–given quantity to a two-factor–wanted quantity medication problem. The denominator of the given quantity (hr) corresponds with the denominator of the wanted quantity (hr); therefore, only the numerator of the given quantity (units) needs to be canceled from the problem.

After factoring in the dose on hand, the unwanted unit (units) is canceled from the problem and the wanted unit (mL) remains in the numerator to correspond with the wanted quantity. The same number values are canceled from the numerator and denominator leaving 15 mL/hr.

EXAMPLE 5.5

The physician orders heparin 1500 units/hr IV. The pharmacy sends an IV bag labeled: Heparin 25,000 units in 250 mL of D5W.

Calculate the IV pump setting for milliliters per hour.

Given quantity = 1500 units/hr
Wanted quantity = mL/hr
Dose on hand = 25,000 units/250 mL

Sequential method:

Step 1 Begin by identifying the given quantity. Establish the unit path to the wanted quantity.

Unit Path

Given Quantity	Conversion Factor for Given Quantity (Numerator)	Conversion Computation		Wanted Quantity
1500 Units			=	mL
hr				hr

Step 2

Unit Path

Given Quantity	Conversion Factor for Given Quantity (Numerator)	Conversion Computation		Wanted Quantity
1500 ~~Units~~	250 (mL)		=	mL
(hr)	25,000 ~~Units~~			hr

Step 3

Unit Path

Given Quantity	Conversion Factor for Given Quantity (Numerator)	Conversion Computation		Wanted Quantity
1500 ~~Units~~	~~250~~ (mL)	15	=	15 mL
(hr)	~~25,000~~ ~~Units~~			hr

15 mL/hr is the wanted quantity and the answer to the problem.

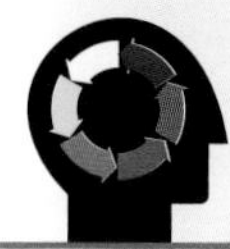

EXAMPLE 5.6

The physician orders 500 mL of 0.45% NS with 20 mEq of KCl to infuse over 8 hours.

Calculate the number of milliliters per hour to set the IV pump.

Given quantity = 500 mL/8 hr
Wanted quantity = mL/hr

Sequential method:

$$\frac{500 \text{ mL}}{8 \text{ hr}} \bigg| \frac{500}{8} = \frac{62.5 \text{ mL}}{\quad} \text{ or } \frac{63 \text{ mL}}{\text{hr}}$$

63 mL/hr is the wanted quantity and the answer to the problem.

THINKING IT THROUGH

In this problem, the needed two factors are already identified in the given quantity and, therefore, require no additional conversions. The 20 mEq of KCl added to the IV bag is included as part of the 500 mL and is additional information for the nurse, but not part of the calculation.

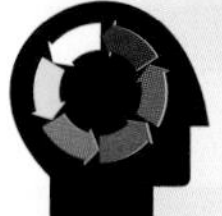

EXAMPLE 5.7

The physician orders aminophylline 44 mg/hr IV. The pharmacy sends an IV bag labeled: Aminophylline 1 g/250 mL NS.

Calculate the milliliters per hour to set the IV pump.

Given quantity = 44 mg/hr
Wanted quantity = mL/hr
Dose on hand = 1 g/250 mL

Random method:

$$\frac{44 \cancel{\text{mg}}}{\text{hr}} \bigg| \frac{25\cancel{0} \text{ mL}}{\cancel{1 \text{ g}}} \bigg| \frac{\cancel{1 \text{ g}}}{100\cancel{0} \cancel{\text{mg}}} \bigg| \frac{44 \times 25}{100} \bigg| \frac{1100}{100} = \frac{11 \text{ mL}}{\text{hr}}$$

11 mL/hr is the wanted quantity and the answer to the problem.

THINKING IT THROUGH

The given quantity has been identified as what the physician orders, but also can be information that the nurse has obtained. The nurse may know that the IV pump is set to deliver 11 mL/hr, but wants to know if the dosage of medication the patient is receiving is within a safe dosage range.

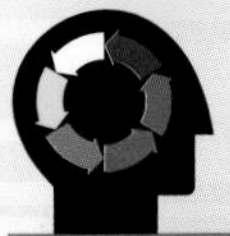

THINKING IT THROUGH

The dose on hand is factored in and allows the unwanted unit (mL) to be canceled.

EXAMPLE 5.8

The nurse checks the IV pump and documents that the pump is set at and delivering 11 mL/hr and that the IV bag hanging is labeled: Aminophylline 1 g/250 mL.

How many milligrams per hour is the patient receiving?

Given quantity = 11 mL/hr
Wanted quantity = mg/hr
Dose on hand = 1 g/250 mL

Sequential method:

Step 1

$$\frac{11\text{ mL}}{\text{hr}} \Bigg| \qquad = \frac{\text{mg}}{\text{hr}}$$

Step 2

$$\frac{11\ \cancel{\text{mL}}}{\text{hr}} \Bigg| \frac{1\text{ g}}{250\ \cancel{\text{mL}}} = \frac{\text{mg}}{\text{hr}}$$

Step 3

$$\frac{11\ \cancel{\text{mL}}}{\text{hr}} \Bigg| \frac{\cancel{1}\ \cancel{\text{g}}}{25\cancel{0}\ \cancel{\text{mL}}} \Bigg| \frac{100\cancel{0}\ \text{mg}}{\cancel{1}\ \cancel{\text{g}}} \Bigg| \frac{11 \times 100}{25} \Bigg| \frac{1100}{25} = \frac{44\text{ mg}}{\text{hr}}$$

44 mg/hr is the wanted quantity and the answer to the problem.

Exercise 5.3 **Medication Problems Involving Intravenous Pumps**
(See page 130 for answers)

1. Order: heparin 1800 units/hr IV

   Supply: heparin 25,000 units/250 mL D5W

   Calculate milliliters per hour to set the IV pump. ____________

2. Order: aminophylline 35 mg/hr IV

   Supply: aminophylline 1 g/250 mL NS

   Calculate milliliters per hour to set the IV pump. ____________

3. Information obtained by the nurse: heparin 25,000 units in 250 mL D5W is infusing at 30 mL/hr.

   How many units per hour is the patient receiving? ______________

4. Information obtained by the nurse: aminophylline 1 g/250 mL NS is infusing at 15 mL/hr.

   How many milligrams per hour is the patient receiving? ______________

5. Order: heparin 900 units/hr IV

   Supply: heparin 25,000 units/500 mL D5W

   Calculate milliliters per hour to set the IV pump. ______________

MEDICATION PROBLEMS INVOLVING DROP FACTORS

Although intravenous pumps are used whenever possible, there are situations (no IV pumps available) and circumstances (outpatient or home care) that arise when IV pumps are not available and IV fluids or medications might be administered using gravity flow. **Gravity flow** involves calculating the drops per minute (gtt/min) required to infuse IV fluids or medications. When IV fluids or medications are administered using gravity flow, it is important to know the drop factor for the IV tubing that is being used. **Drop factor** is the drops per milliliter (gtt/mL) that the IV tubing will produce. Two types of IV tubing are available for gravity flow. *Macrotubing* delivers a large drop and is available in 10 gtt/mL, 15 gtt/mL, and 20 gtt/mL (Table 5.1); and *microtubing* delivers a small drop and is available in 60 gtt/mL.

TABLE 5.1 Examples of Different Macrodrip Factors

MANUFACTURER	DROPS PER MILLILITER (GTT/ML)
Travenol	10
Abbott	15
McGaw	15
Cutter	20

Regardless of the IV tubing used, the problem can be solved by dimensional analysis. Below is an example of a medication problem involving drop factors using the dimensional analysis method.

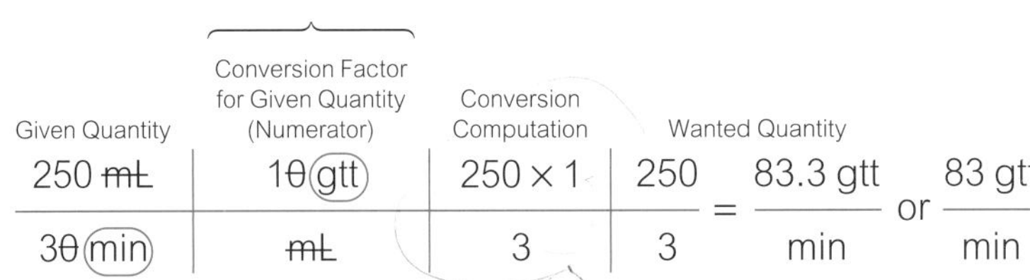

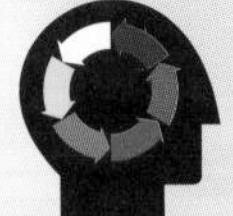

THINKING IT THROUGH

The given quantity and the wanted quantity both include two factors; therefore, this is a two-factor–given quantity to a two-factor–wanted quantity medication problem.

The denominators are the same (min). The numerator in the given quantity (mL) is an unwanted unit and needs to be canceled.

When the drop factor is factored in, the unwanted unit (mL) is canceled, and the wanted unit (gtt) is placed in the numerator to correspond with the wanted quantity.

After you cancel the unwanted units from the problem, multiply the numerators, multiply the denominators, and divide the product of the numerators by the product of the denominators to provide the wanted quantity.

EXAMPLE 5.9

The physician orders 250 mL of normal saline to infuse in 30 minutes. The drop factor listed on the IV tubing box is 10 gtt/mL.

Calculate the number of drops per minute required to infuse the IV bolus.

Given quantity = 250 mL/30 min
Wanted quantity = gtt/min
Drop factor = 10 gtt/mL

Sequential method:

Step 1 Begin by identifying the given quantity and establishing a unit path to the wanted quantity.

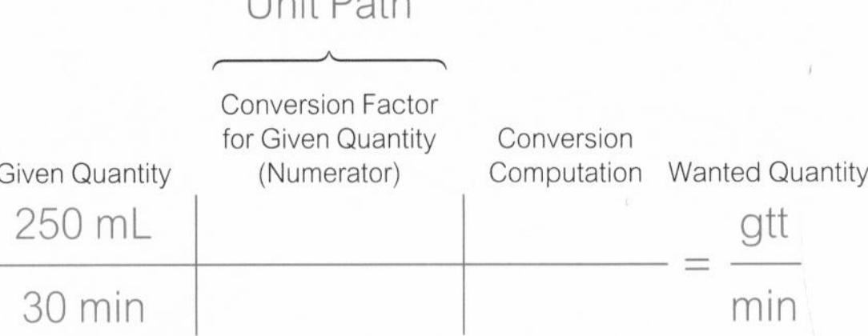

Step 2

Unit Path

Conversion Factor for Given Quantity (Numerator) | Given Quantity | Conversion Computation | Wanted Quantity

250 mL / 30 min | 10 gtt / mL | = gtt / min

▶ Step 3

Given Quantity	Unit Path: Conversion Factor for Given Quantity (Numerator)	Conversion Computation	Wanted Quantity			
250 ~~mL~~	1~~0~~ (gtt)	250 × 1	250	=	83.3 gtt	or 83 gtt
3~~0~~ (min)	~~mL~~	3	3		min	min

83 gtt is the wanted quantity and the answer to the problem.

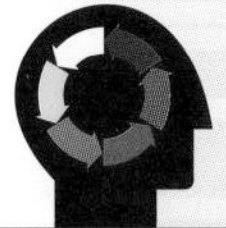

EXAMPLE 5.10

In some situations (home care), it may be important for the nurse to know exactly how long a specific amount of IV fluid will take to infuse. The physician may order a limited amount of IV fluid to infuse at a specific number of drops per minute (gtt/min).

The physician orders 1000 mL of D5W and 0.45% NS to infuse over 8 hours. The drop factor is 20 gtt/mL.

Calculate the number of drops per minute required to infuse the IV volume.

Given quantity = 1000 mL/8 hr
Wanted quantity = gtt/min
Drop factor = 20 gtt/mL

Sequential method:

▶ Step 1

1000 mL	20 gtt	=	gtt
8 hr	mL		min

▶ Step 2

1000 ~~mL~~	20 (gtt)	1 ~~hr~~	=	gtt
8 ~~hr~~	~~mL~~	60 (min)		min

▶ Step 3

1000 ~~mL~~	2~~0~~ (gtt)	1 ~~hr~~	1000 × 2 × 1	2000	=	41.66 gtt
8 ~~hr~~	~~mL~~	6~~0~~ (min)	8 × 6	48		min

41.66 gtt / min or 42 gtt / min

42 gtt/min is the wanted quantity and the answer to the problem.

THINKING IT THROUGH

The unwanted unit (mL) is canceled, and the wanted unit (gtt) is placed in the numerator. Another unwanted unit (hr) needs to be canceled from the unit path.

The conversion factor (1 hr = 60 min) has been factored in to allow the unwanted unit (hr) to be canceled and the wanted unit (min) is placed in the denominator.

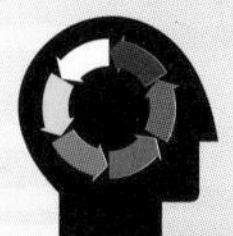

THINKING IT THROUGH

The given quantity and the wanted quantity have been identified and are both in the numerator; therefore, this is a one- factor–given quantity to a one-factor–wanted quantity medication problem.

The drop factor (10 gtt/ mL) has been factored in using the sequential method to cancel the unwanted unit (mL).

The infusing rate of 21 gtt/min has now been factored in to cancel the unwanted unit (gtt).

The conversion factor (1 hr = 60 min) has been factored in to cancel the unwanted unit (min). The wanted unit (hr) remains in the numerator, which corresponds to the wanted quantity.

EXAMPLE 5.11

It is safe nursing practice to monitor an infusing IV every 2 hours to make sure it is infusing without difficulty and on time. It may be necessary to hang the next IV after $7\frac{1}{2}$ hours (before the estimated completion time) to keep the IV from running dry.

The physician orders 1000 mL of D5W. The drop factor is 10 gtt/mL. The infusion is dripping at 21 gtt/min.

How many hours will it take for the IV to infuse?

Given quantity = 1000 mL
Wanted quantity = hr
Drop factor = 10 gtt/mL

Step 1

1000 mL		= hr

Step 2

1000 mL	10 gtt	= hr
	mL	

Step 3

1000 ~~mL~~	10 ~~gtt~~	min	= hr
	~~mL~~	21 ~~gtt~~	

Step 4

1000 ~~mL~~	10 ~~gtt~~	~~min~~	1 (hr)	= hr
	~~mL~~	21 ~~gtt~~	60 ~~min~~	

Step 5

1000 ~~mL~~	1~~0~~ ~~gtt~~	~~min~~	1 (hr)	1000 × 1 × 1	1000	= 7.93 hr or 7.9 hr
	~~mL~~	21 ~~gtt~~	6~~0~~ ~~min~~	21 × 6	126	

8 hours is the wanted quantity and the answer to the problem.

Exercise 5.4 Medication Problems Involving Drop Factors

(See page 130 for answers)

1. Order: 800 mL D5W to infuse in 8 hours

   Drop factor: 15 gtt/mL

   Calculate the number of drops per minute. ____________

2. Order: Infuse 250 mL NS

   Drop factor: 15 gtt/mL

   Infusion rate: 60 gtt/min

   Calculate the hours to infuse. ____________

3. Order: 150 mL over 60 minutes

   Drop factor: 10 gtt/mL

   Calculate the number of drops per minute. ____________

4. Order: 1000 mL D5W/0.9% NS

   Drop factor: 15 gtt/mL

   Infusion rate: 50 gtt/min

   Calculate the number of hours to infuse. ____________

5. Order: 500 mL over 4 hours

   Drop factor: 15 gtt/mL

   Calculate the number of drops per minute. ____________

MEDICATION PROBLEMS INVOLVING INTERMITTENT INFUSION

Intravenous medications can be delivered over a specific amount of time by *intermittent infusion.* These medications require the use of an infusion pump. Some must be reconstituted and further diluted in a specific type and amount of IV fluid and delivered over a limited time. Others do not need to be reconstituted, but must be further diluted in a specific type and amount of IV fluid and delivered over a limited time.

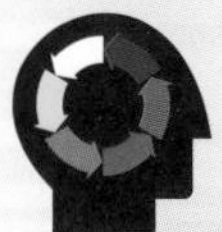

THINKING IT THROUGH

This order contains two problems. The first involves how many milliliters to draw from the vial after reconstitution, and the second involves how many milliliters per hour to set the IV pump.

EXAMPLE 5.12

The physician ordered erythromycin 500 mg IV every 6 hours for infection. The pharmacy sends a vial labeled: Erythromycin 1 g. The nursing drug reference provides information to reconstitute 1 g of erythromycin with 20 mL of sterile water and further dilute in 250 mL of 0.9% NS and to infuse over 1 hour.

How many milliliters will you draw from the vial after reconstitution?

Calculate the milliliters per hour to set the IV pump.

Step 1

How many milliliters will you draw from the vial after reconstitution?

Given quantity = 500 mg
Wanted quantity = mL
Dose on hand = 1 g/20 mL

Random method:

~~500 mg~~	2~~0~~ (mL)	~~1 g~~	5 × 2	10	= 10 mL
	~~1 g~~	1~~000 mg~~	1	1	

The wanted quantity is 10 mL, and is the amount that will need to be drawn from the vial and added to the 250 mL of 0.9% NS. After adding the 10 mL to the IV bag, the IV bag will now contain 260 mL.

Step 2

Calculate the milliliters per hour to set the IV pump.

Given quantity = 260 mL/1 hr
Wanted quantity = mL/hr

Sequential method:

260 (mL)	260	=	260 mL
1 (hr)	1		hr

The IV pump is set at 260 mL/hr to infuse the 500 mg of erythromycin ordered by the physician.

Step 2 (alternative): If an IV pump was unavailable, the infusion could be delivered by gravity using IV tubing with a drop factor of 10 gtt/mL.

Calculate the drops per minute required to infuse the IV volume.

Given quantity = 260 mL/1 hr
Wanted quantity = gtt/min
Drop factor = 10 gtt/mL

Sequential method:

$$\frac{260\ \cancel{mL}}{1\ \cancel{hr}}\left|\frac{1\cancel{0}\ gtt}{\cancel{mL}}\right|\frac{1\ \cancel{hr}}{6\cancel{0}\ min}\left|\frac{260 \times 1 \times 1}{1 \times 6}\right|\frac{260}{6} = \frac{43.3 \text{ or } 43\ gtt}{min}$$

Exercise 5.5 Medication Problems Involving Intermittent Infusion

(See pages 130–131 for answers)

1. Order: ampicillin 250 mg IV every 4 hours for infection

   Supply: ampicillin 1-g vial

   Nursing drug reference: Reconstitute with 10 mL of 0.9% NS and further dilute in 50 mL NS. Infuse over 15 min.

   How many milliliters will you draw from the vial after reconstitution? ____________

   Calculate milliliters per hour to set the IV pump. ____________

   Calculate drops per minute with a drop factor of 10 gtt/mL. ____________

2. Order: clindamycin 0.3 g IV every 6 hours for infection

   Supply: clindamycin 600 mg/4-mL vial

   Nursing drug reference: Dilute with 50 mL 0.9% NS and infuse over 15 min.

   How many milliliters will you draw from the vial? ____________

   Calculate milliliters per hour to set the IV pump. ____________

   Calculate drops per minute with a drop factor of 15 gtt/mL. ____________

(Exercise continues on page 120)

3. Order: Mezlin 3 g IV every 4 hours for infection

   Supply: Mezlin 4-g vial

   Nursing drug reference: Reconstitute each 1-g vial with 10 mL of 0.9% NS and further dilute in 100 mL 0.9% NS to infuse over 1 hr.

   How many milliliters will you draw from the vial after reconstitution? ______________

   Calculate the milliliters per hour to set the IV pump. ______________

   Calculate the drops per minute with a drop factor of 20 gtt/mL. ______________

4. Order: Unasyn 1000 mg IV every 6 hours for infection

   Supply: Unasyn 1.5-g vial

   Nursing drug reference: Reconstitute with 4 mL of 0.9% NS and further dilute with 100 mL NS to infuse over 1 hr.

   How many milliliters will you draw from the vial after reconstitution? ______________

   Calculate the milliliters per hour to set the IV pump. ______________

   Calculate the drops per minute with a drop factor of 20 gtt/mL. ______________

5. Order: Zantac 50 mg IV every 6 hours for ulcers

   Supply: Zantac 25-mg/mL vial

   Nursing drug reference: Dilute with 50 mL 0.9% NS to infuse over 30 min.

   How many milliliters will you draw from the vial? ______________

   Calculate the milliliters per hour to set the IV pump. ______________

   Calculate the drops per minute with a drop factor of 10 gtt/mL. ______________

SUMMARY

This chapter has taught you to calculate two-factor medication problems involving the weight of the patient, reconstitution of medications, and the amount of time over which medications and intravenous fluids can be safely administered. To demonstrate your ability to calculate medication problems accurately, complete the following practice problems.

Practice Problems for Chapter 5 Two-Factor Medication Problems

(See pages 131–132 for answers)

1. Order: verapamil 0.2 mg/kg IV for arrhythmia

   Supply: verapamil (Isoptin) 5 mg/2 mL

   Child's weight: 10 lb

   How many milliliters will you give? ____________

2. Order: Tylenol Elixir 10 mg/kg every 4 hours prn for fever

   Supply: Tylenol Elixir 160 mg/5 mL

   Child's weight: 8 kg

   How many milliliters will you give? ____________

3. Order: Fortaz 1.25 g IV every 8 hours for infection

   Supply: Fortaz 2-g vial

   Nursing drug reference: Dilute each 2 g with 10 mL sterile water for injection.

   How many milliliters will you draw from the vial after reconstitution? ____________

4. Order: Unasyn 750 mg IV every 8 hours for infection

   Supply: Unasyn 1.5-g vial

   Nursing drug reference: Reconstitute with 4 mL of sterile water for injection.

   How many milliliters will you draw from the vial after reconstitution? ____________

5. Order: heparin 700 units/hr for anticoagulation

   Supply: heparin 25,000 units/250 mL NS

   At how many milliliters per hour will you set the IV pump? ____________

(Practice problems continue on page 122)

6. Information obtained by the nurse: Zantac 150 mg in 250 mL NS is infusing at 11 mL/hr.

   How many milligrams per hour is the patient receiving? ______________

7. Order: 1000 mL D5W/0.9% NS to infuse over 8 hours

   Drop factor: 20 gtt/mL

   Calculate the number of drops per minute. ______________

8. Order: Infuse 750 mL NS

   Drop factor: 15 gtt/mL

   Infusion rate: 18 gtt/min

   Calculate the number of hours to infuse. ______________

9. Order: vancomycin 10 mg/kg IV every 8 hours for infection

   Supply: vancomycin 500-mg vial

   Infant's weight: 20 lb

   Nursing drug reference: Dilute each 500-mg vial with 10 mL of sterile water for injection and further dilute in 100 mL of 0.9% NS to infuse over 1 hr.

   How many milliliters will you draw from the vial after reconstitution? ______________

   Calculate milliliters per hour to set the IV pump. ______________

   Calculate drops per minute with a drop factor of 10 gtt/mL. ______________

10. Order: acyclovir 355 mg IV every 8 hours for herpes

    Supply: acyclovir 500-mg vial

    Nursing drug reference: Reconstitute each 500 mg with 10 mL of sterile water for injection and further dilute in 100 mL NS to infuse over 1 hr.

    How many milliliters will you draw from the vial after reconstitution? ______________

    Calculate the milliliters per hour to set the IV pump. ______________

    Calculate the drops per minute with a drop factor of 20 gtt/mL. ______________

POST-TEST FOR CHAPTER 5: TWO-FACTOR MEDICATION PROBLEMS

Name ______________________ **Date** ____________

1. Order: Furosemide 2 mg/kg PO every 8 hours for congestive heart failure

   The child weighs 10 kg.

   How many milliliters will you give? ____________

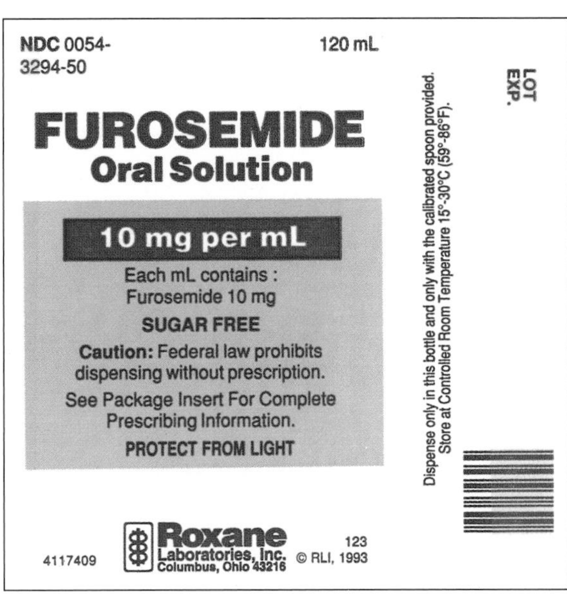

Courtesy of Roxane Laboratories.

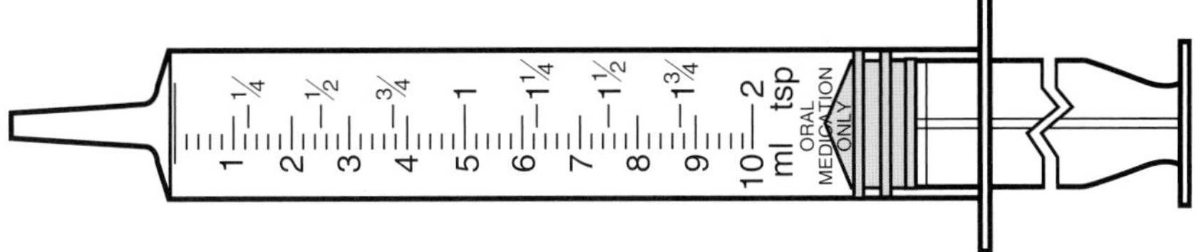

(Post-test continues on page 124)

2. Order: Meperidine 1.5 mg/kg PO every 4 hours for pain

   The child weighs 22 lb.

   How many milliliters will you give? ______________

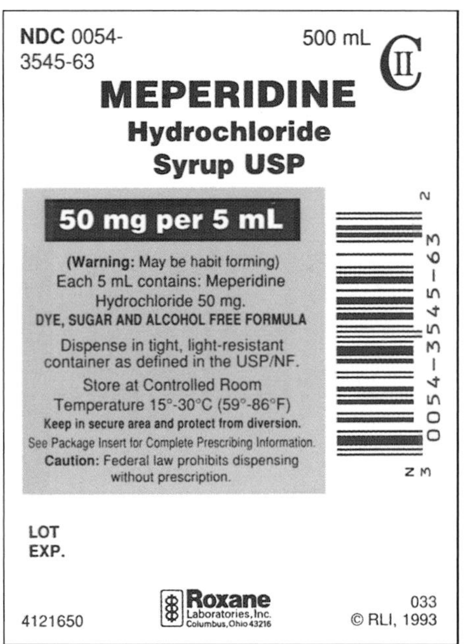
NDC 0054-3545-63 500 mL CII

MEPERIDINE Hydrochloride Syrup USP

50 mg per 5 mL

(Warning: May be habit forming)
Each 5 mL contains: Meperidine Hydrochloride 50 mg.
DYE, SUGAR AND ALCOHOL FREE FORMULA
Dispense in tight, light-resistant container as defined in the USP/NF.
Store at Controlled Room Temperature 15°-30°C (59°-86°F)
Keep in secure area and protect from diversion.
See Package Insert for Complete Prescribing Information.
Caution: Federal law prohibits dispensing without prescription.

3 0054-3545-63 2

LOT
EXP.

4121650 Roxane Laboratories, Inc. Columbus, Ohio 43216 033 © RLI, 1993

Courtesy of Roxane Laboratories.

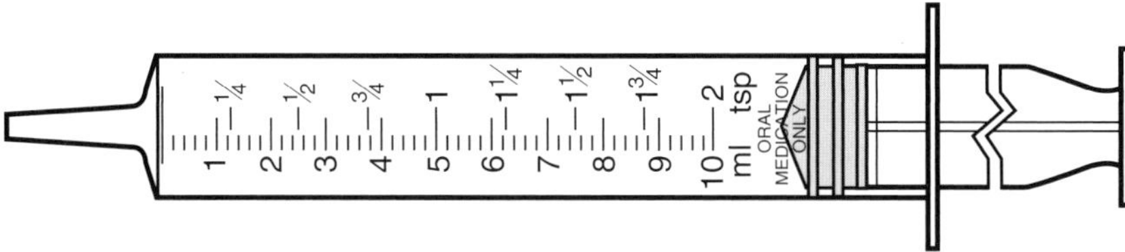

3. Order: Epogen 100 units/kg IV tid for anemia secondary to chronic renal failure

   The patient weighs 160 lb.

   How many milliliters will you give? ______________

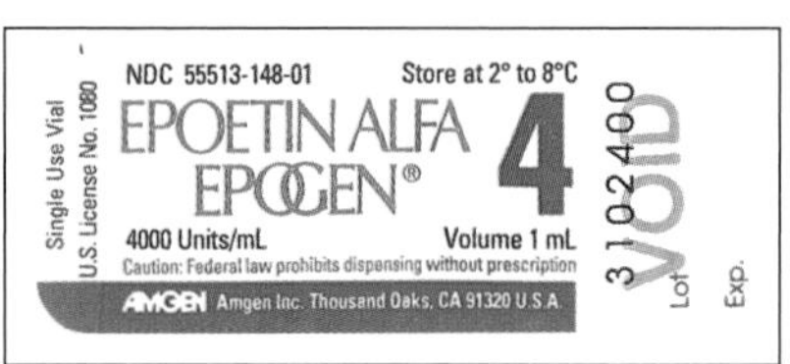

Courtesy of Amgen, Inc.

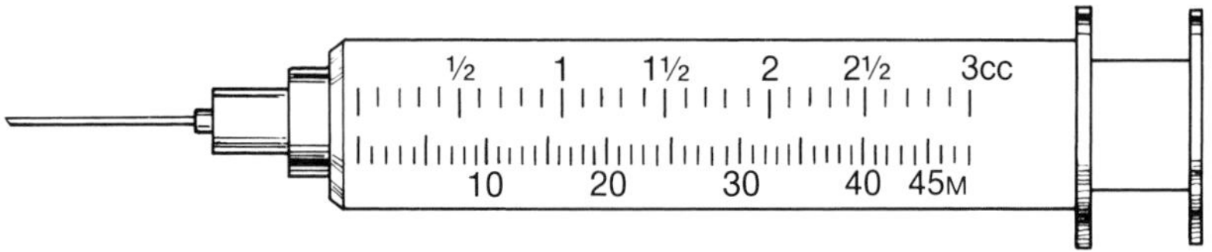

4. Order: Augmentin 10 mg/kg PO every 8 hours for otitis media

   Nursing drug reference states: Dilute with one teaspoon (5 mL) of tap water and shake vigorously to yield 125 mg per 5 mL.

   The child weighs 25 kg.

   How many milliliters will you give after reconstitution? ______________

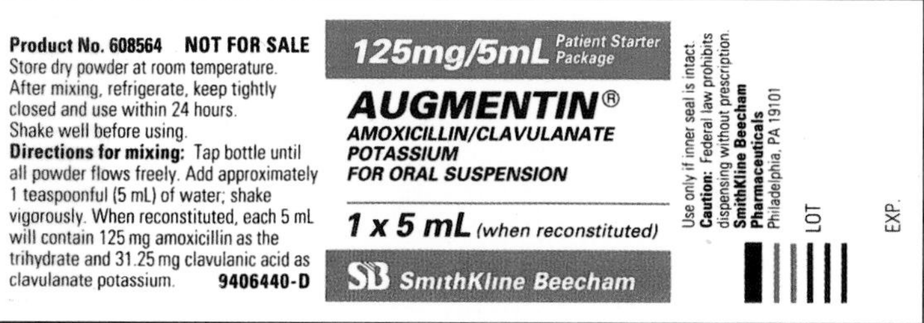

Courtesy of SmithKline Beecham Pharmaceuticals.

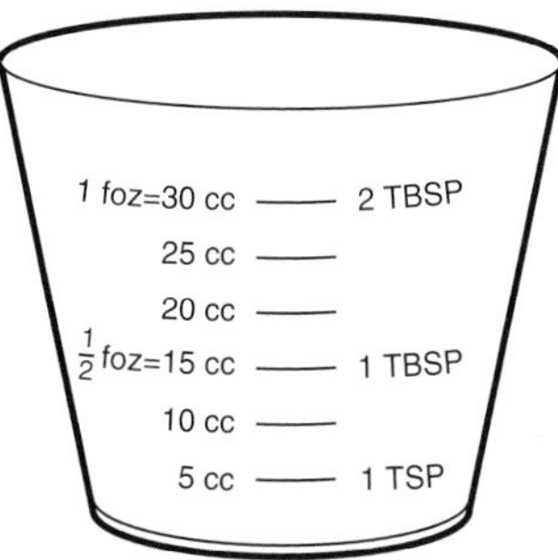

5. The physician orders heparin to infuse at 1300 units/hr continuous IV infusion.

   The pharmacy sends an IV bag labeled heparin 25,000 units in 250 mL.

   Calculate the milliliters per hour to set the IV pump. ______________

6. A patient is receiving heparin 25,000 units in 250 mL infused at 25 mL/hr.

   How many units per hour is the patient receiving? ______________

7. The physician orders morphine sulfate 2 mg/hr continuous IV for intractable pain related to end-stage lung cancer.

   The pharmacy sends an IV bag labeled morphine sulfate 100 mg in 250 mL.

   Calculate milliliters per hour to set the IV pump. ______________

(Post-test continues on page 126)

8. Order: 1000 mL D5W/1/2 NS with 20 mEq of KCl to infuse in 12 hours

   Drop factor: 20 gtt/mL

   Calculate the number of drops per minute. ______________

9. Order: Azactam 500 mg IV every 12 hours for septicemia

   Supply: Azactam 1-g vials

   Nursing drug reference states: Dilute each 1-g vial with 10 mL of sterile water for injection and further dilute in 100 mL of NS to infuse over 60 minutes.

   How many milliliters will you draw from the vial after reconstitution? ______________

   Calculate milliliters per hour to set the IV pump. ______________

   Calculate drops per minute with a drop factor of 20 gtt/mL. ______________

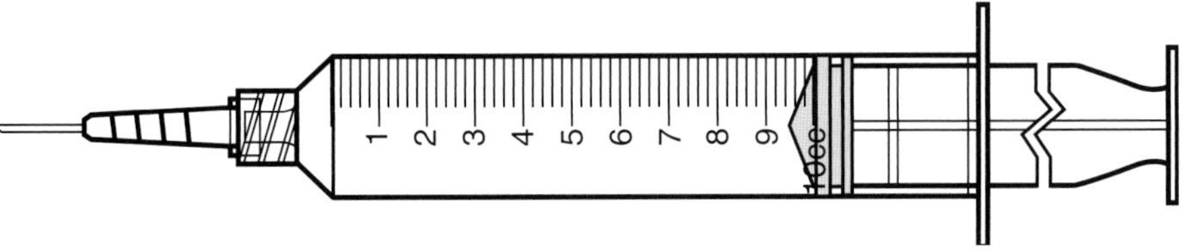

10. Order: Ancef 6.25 mg/kg IV every 6 hours for pneumonia

The child weighs 38.2 kg.

Nursing drug reference states: Dilute each 1-g vial with 10 mL of sterile water for injection and further dilute 50 mL of NS to infuse over 30 minutes.

How many milliliters will you draw from the vial after reconstitution? ______________

Calculate milliliters per hour to set the IV pump. ______________

Calculate drops per minute with a drop factor of 10 gtt/mL. ______________

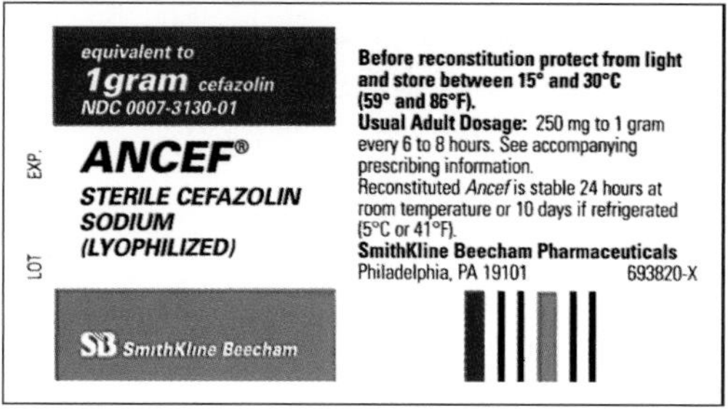

Courtesy of SmithKline Beecham Pharmaceuticals.

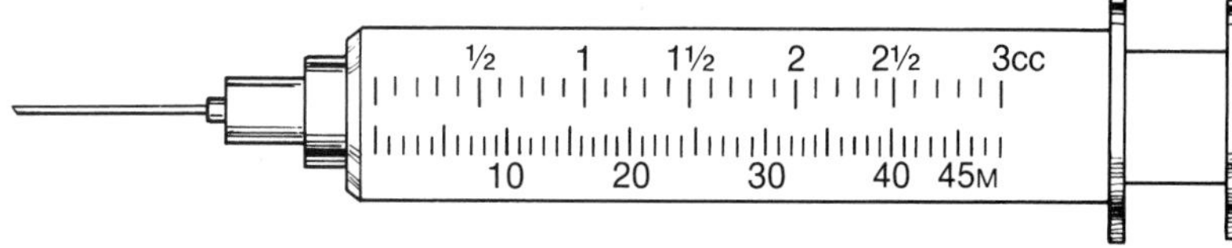

ANSWER KEY FOR CHAPTER 5: TWO-FACTOR MEDICATION PROBLEMS

Exercise 5.1 Medication Problems Involving Weight

1. Sequential method:

1 ~~mg~~	(mL)	1 ~~kg~~	45 ~~lb~~	1 × 1 × 45	45	= 2.04 or 2 mL
~~kg~~	10 ~~mg~~	2.2 ~~lb~~		10 × 2.2	22	

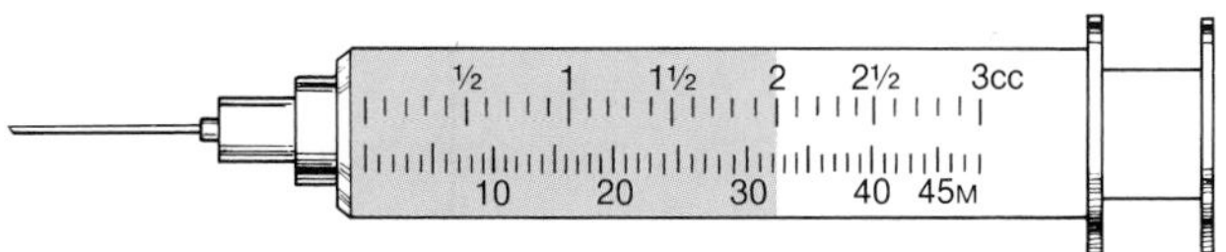

2. Sequential method:

0.01 ~~mg~~	(mL)	1 ~~kg~~	20 ~~lb~~	0.01 × 1 × 20	0.2	= 0.9 mL
~~kg~~	0.1 ~~mg~~	2.2 ~~lb~~		0.1 × 2.2	0.22	

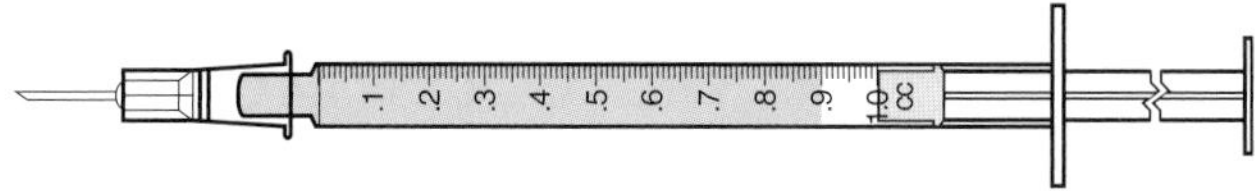

3. Sequential method:

0.5 ~~mg~~	(mL)	1 ~~kg~~	45 ~~lb~~	0.5 × 1 × 45	22.5	= 0.4 mL
~~kg~~	25 ~~mg~~	2.2 ~~lb~~		25 × 2.2	55	

4. Random method:

50 ~~mcg~~	(mL)	1 ~~mg~~	1 ~~kg~~	75 ~~lb~~	5 × 1 × 1 × 75	375	= mL
~~kg~~	8 ~~mg~~	1000 ~~mcg~~	2.2 ~~lb~~		8 × 100 × 2.2	1760	

$$\frac{375}{1760} = 0.2 \text{ mL}$$

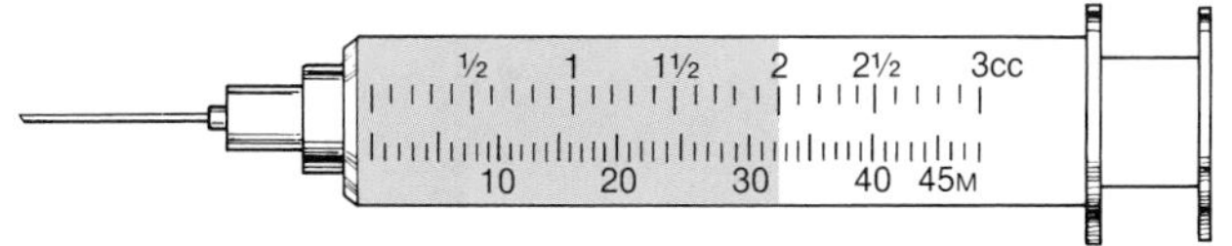

5. Random method:

10 ~~mg~~	1 ~~kg~~	70 ~~lb~~	5 (mL)	10 × 1 × 7 × 5	350	= 5.3 or 5 mL
~~kg~~	2.2 ~~lb~~		300 ~~mg~~	2.2 × 30	66	

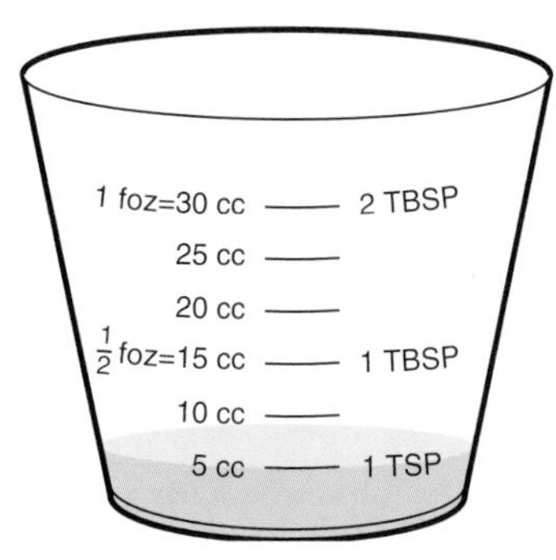

Exercise 5.2 Medication Problems Involving Reconstitution

1. Random method:

500 ~~mg~~	50 (mL)	1 ~~g~~	5 × 5	25	= 25 mL
	1 ~~g~~	1000 ~~mg~~	1	1	

2. Sequential method:

250 ~~mg~~	10 (mL)	25 × 1	25	= 5 mL
	500 ~~mg~~	5	5	

3. Random method:

50 ~~mg~~	4 (mL)	1 ~~g~~	40 ~~kg~~	5 × 4 × 1 × 4	80	= 5.33 or 5 mL
~~kg~~	1.5 ~~g~~	1000 ~~mg~~		1.5 × 10	15	

Random method using yield:

50 ~~mg~~	1 (mL)	40 ~~kg~~	50 × 1 × 40	2000	= 5.33 or 5 mL
~~kg~~	375 ~~mg~~		375	375	

4. Random method:

750 ~~mg~~	20 (mL)	1 ~~g~~	75 × 2 × 1	150	= 15 mL
	1 ~~g~~	1000 ~~mg~~	1 × 10	10	

5. Sequential method:

3~~0~~ ~~mg~~	5 (mL)	1 ~~kg~~	65 ~~lb~~	3 × 5 × 1 × 65	975	=	8.86 or
~~kg~~	50~~0~~ ~~mg~~	2.2 ~~lb~~		50 × 2.2	110		8.9 mL

Exercise 5.3 Medication Problems Involving Intravenous Pumps

1. Sequential method:

18~~00~~ ~~units~~	~~250~~ (mL)	18	=	18 mL
(hr)	~~25,000~~ ~~units~~			hr

2. Random method:

35 ~~mg~~	25~~0~~ (mL)	~~1 g~~	35 × 25	875	=	8.75 or 9 mL
(hr)	~~1 g~~	100~~0~~ ~~mg~~	100	100		hr

3. Sequential method:

30 ~~mL~~	25,00~~0~~ (units)	30 × 2500	75,000	=	3000 units
(hr)	25~~0~~ ~~mL~~	25	25		hr

4. Sequential method:

15 ~~mL~~	~~1 g~~	100~~0~~ (mg)	15 × 100	1500	=	60 mg
(hr)	25~~0~~ ~~mL~~	~~1 g~~	25	25		hr

5. Sequential method:

90~~0~~ ~~units~~	5~~00~~ (mL)	90 × 5	450	=	18 mL
(hr)	25,~~000~~ ~~units~~	25	25		hr

Exercise 5.4 Medication Problems Involving Drop Factors

1. Sequential method:

80~~0~~ ~~mL~~	15 (gtt)	1 ~~hr~~	80 × 15 × 1	1200	=	25 gtt
8 ~~hr~~	~~mL~~	6~~0~~ (min)	8 × 6	48		min

2. Sequential method:

250 ~~mL~~	15 ~~gtt~~	~~min~~	1 (hr)	250 × 15 × 1	3750	=	1.04 or
	~~mL~~	60 ~~gtt~~	60 ~~min~~	60 × 60	3600		1 hr

3. Sequential method

150 ~~mL~~	1~~0~~ (gtt)	150 × 1	150	=	25 gtt
6~~0~~ (min)	~~mL~~	6	6		min

4. Sequential method:

10~~00~~ ~~mL~~	15 ~~gtt~~	~~min~~	1 (hr)	10 × 15 × 1	150	= 5 hr
	~~mL~~	5~~0~~ ~~gtt~~	6~~0~~ ~~min~~	5 × 6	30	

5. Sequential method:

50~~0~~ ~~mL~~	15 (gtt)	1 ~~hr~~	50 × 15 × 1	750	=	31.25 or 31 gtt
4 ~~hr~~	~~mL~~	6~~0~~ (min)	4 × 6	24		min

Exercise 5.5 Medication Problems Involving Intermittent Infusion

1. Random method:

25~~0~~ ~~mg~~	1~~0~~ (mL)	~~1 g~~	25 × 1	25	= 2.5 mL
	~~1 g~~	10~~00~~ ~~mg~~	10	10	

Calculate milliliters per hour to set the IV pump.
Sequential method:

52.5 (mL)	60 ~~min~~	52.5 × 60	3150	=	210 mL
15 ~~min~~	1 (hr)	15 × 1	15		hr

Calculate drops per minute with a drop factor of 10 gtt/mL.
Sequential method:

52.5 ~~mL~~	10 (gtt)	52.5 × 10	525	=	35 gtt
15 (min)	~~mL~~	15	15		min

2. Random method:

0.3 ~~g~~	4 (mL)	10~~00~~ ~~mg~~	0.3 × 4 × 10	12	= 2 mL
	6~~00~~ ~~mg~~	1 ~~g~~	6 × 1	6	

Calculate milliliter per hour to set the IV pump.
Sequential method:

52 (mL)	60 ~~min~~	52 × 60	3120	=	208 mL
15 ~~min~~	1 (hr)	15 × 1	15		hr

Calculate drops per minute with a drop factor of 15 gtt/mL.
Sequential method:

52 ~~mL~~	~~15~~ (gtt)	52	= 52 gtt
~~15~~ (min)	~~mL~~		min

3. Sequential method:

3 ~~g~~	40 (mL)	3 × 40	120	= 30 mL
	4 ~~g~~	4	4	

Calculate milliliters per hour to set the IV pump.
Sequential method:

130 (mL)	130	= 130 mL
1 (hr)	1	hr

Calculate drops per minute with a drop factor of 20 gtt/mL.
Sequential method:

130 ~~mL~~	~~20~~ (gtt)	~~1 hr~~	130 × 2	260	= 43.33 or 43 gtt
~~1 hr~~	~~mL~~	~~60~~ (min)	6	6	min

4. Random method:

~~1000 mg~~	4 (mL)	1 ~~g~~	4 × 1	4	= 2.66 or
	1.5 ~~g~~	~~1000 mg~~	1.5	1.5	2.7 mL

Calculate milliliters per hour to set the IV pump.
Sequential method:

102.7 (mL)	102.7	= 102.7 or 103 mL
1 (hr)	1	hr

Calculate drops per minute with a drop factor of 20 gtt/mL.
Sequential method:

102.7 ~~mL~~	~~20~~ (gtt)	~~1 hr~~	102.7 × 2	205.4	= 34.2 or 34 gtt
~~1 hr~~	~~mL~~	~~60~~ (min)	6	6	min

5. Sequential method:

50 ~~mg~~	(mL)	50	= 2 mL
	25 ~~mg~~	25	

Calculate milliliters per hour to set the IV pump.
Random method:

52 (mL)	~~60~~ ~~min~~	52 × 6	312	= 104 mL
~~30~~ ~~min~~	1 (hr)	3 × 1	3	hr

Calculate drops per minute with a drop factor of 10 gtt/mL.
Sequential method:

52 ~~mL~~	~~10~~ (gtt)	52 × 1	52	= 17.3 or 17 gtt
~~30~~ (min)	~~mL~~	3	3	min

Practice Problems

1. Sequential method:

0.2 ~~mg~~	2 (mL)	1 ~~kg~~	10 ~~lb~~	0.2 × 2 × 1 × 10	4	= 0.36 or
~~kg~~	5 ~~mg~~	2.2 ~~lb~~		5 × 2.2	11	0.4 mL

2. Sequential method:

~~10 mg~~	5 (mL)	8 ~~kg~~	1 × 5 × 8	40	= 2.5 mL
~~kg~~	~~160 mg~~		16	16	

3. Sequential method:

1.25 ~~g~~	10 (mL)	1.25 × 10	12.5	= 6.25 or 6.3 mL
	2 ~~g~~	2	2	

4. Random method:

75~~0 mg~~	4 (mL)	1 ~~g~~	75 × 4 × 1	300	= 2 mL
	1.5 ~~g~~	100~~0 mg~~	1.5 × 100	150	

5. Sequential method:

$$\frac{\cancel{700\text{ units}}}{\text{hr}}\;\Big|\;\frac{25\cancel{0}\text{ mL}}{\cancel{25{,}000\text{ units}}}\;\Big|\;7=\frac{7\text{ mL}}{\text{hr}}$$

6. Sequential method:

$$\frac{11\,\cancel{\text{mL}}}{\text{hr}}\;\Big|\;\frac{15\cancel{0}\text{ mg}}{25\cancel{0}\,\cancel{\text{mL}}}\;\Big|\;\frac{11\times 15}{25}\;\Big|\;\frac{165}{25}=\frac{6.6\text{ mg}}{\text{hr}}$$

7. Sequential method:

$$\frac{1000\,\cancel{\text{mL}}}{8\,\cancel{\text{hr}}}\;\Big|\;\frac{2\cancel{0}\text{ gtt}}{\cancel{\text{mL}}}\;\Big|\;\frac{1\,\cancel{\text{hr}}}{6\cancel{0}\text{ min}}\;\Big|\;\frac{1000\times 2\times 1}{8\times 6}\;\Big|\;\frac{2000}{48}=\frac{41.66\text{ or }42\text{ gtt}}{\text{min}}$$

8. Sequential method:

$$\frac{75\cancel{0}\,\cancel{\text{mL}}}{}\;\Big|\;\frac{15\,\cancel{\text{gtt}}}{\cancel{\text{mL}}}\;\Big|\;\frac{\cancel{\text{min}}}{18\,\cancel{\text{gtt}}}\;\Big|\;\frac{1\text{ hr}}{6\cancel{0}\,\cancel{\text{min}}}\;\Big|\;\frac{75\times 15\times 1}{18\times 6}\;\Big|\;\frac{1125}{108}=10.41\text{ or }10\text{ hr}$$

9. Sequential method:

$$\frac{1\cancel{0}\,\cancel{\text{mg}}}{\cancel{\text{kg}}}\;\Big|\;\frac{1\cancel{0}\text{ mL}}{50\cancel{0}\,\cancel{\text{mg}}}\;\Big|\;\frac{1\,\cancel{\text{kg}}}{2.2\,\cancel{\text{lb}}}\;\Big|\;\frac{20\,\cancel{\text{lb}}}{}\;\Big|\;\frac{1\times 1\times 20}{5\times 2.2}\;\Big|\;\frac{20}{11}=1.8\text{ mL}$$

Sequential method:

$$\frac{101.8\text{ mL}}{1\text{ hr}}\;\Big|\;\frac{101.8}{1}=\frac{101.8\text{ or }102\text{ mL}}{\text{hr}}$$

Sequential method:

$$\frac{101.8\,\cancel{\text{mL}}}{\cancel{1}\,\cancel{\text{hr}}}\;\Big|\;\frac{1\cancel{0}\text{ gtt}}{\cancel{\text{mL}}}\;\Big|\;\frac{\cancel{1}\,\cancel{\text{hr}}}{6\cancel{0}\text{ min}}\;\Big|\;\frac{101.8\times 1}{6}\;\Big|\;\frac{101.8}{6}=\frac{16.96\text{ or }17\text{ gtt}}{\text{min}}$$

10. Sequential method:

$$\frac{355\,\cancel{\text{mg}}}{}\;\Big|\;\frac{1\cancel{0}\text{ mL}}{50\cancel{0}\,\cancel{\text{mg}}}\;\Big|\;\frac{355\times 1}{50}\;\Big|\;\frac{355}{50}=7.1\text{ or }7\text{ mL}$$

Calculate mL per hour to set the IV pump.

$$\frac{107\text{ mL}}{1\text{ hr}}\;\Big|\;\frac{107}{1}=\frac{107\text{ mL}}{\text{hr}}$$

Calculate drops per minute with a drop factor of 20 gtt/mL.

Sequential method:

$$\frac{107\,\cancel{\text{mL}}}{\cancel{1}\,\cancel{\text{hr}}}\;\Big|\;\frac{2\cancel{0}\text{ gtt}}{\cancel{\text{mL}}}\;\Big|\;\frac{\cancel{1}\,\cancel{\text{hr}}}{6\cancel{0}\text{ min}}\;\Big|\;\frac{107\times 2}{6}\;\Big|\;\frac{214}{6}=\frac{35.66\text{ or }36\text{ gtt}}{\text{min}}$$

When medications are ordered for infants and children, the **dosage** of medication (g, mg, mcg, gr) based on the **weight** of the child must be considered as well as how much medication the child can receive per **dose** or **day**. Although the physician orders the medications, the nurse must be aware of the safe dosage range for administration of medications.

When medications are ordered by physicians for critically ill patients, the patients must be closely monitored by the nurse for effectiveness of the medications. Often, the medications or intravenous fluids must be *titrated* for effectiveness, with an increase or decrease in the dosage based on the patient's response. Factors involved in the safe administration of medications or intravenous fluids for the critically ill patient include the **dosage** of medication based on the **weight** of the patient and the **time** required for administration. The medication may need reconstitution or preparation by the nurse for immediate administration in a critical situation. The weight of the patient also may need to be obtained daily to ensure accurate correlation with the dosage of medication ordered.

To be able to calculate three-factor–given quantity to one-factor–, two-factor–, or three-factor–wanted quantity medication problems, it is necessary to understand all of the components of the medication order and to be able to calculate medication problems in a critical situation. This chapter will teach you to calculate medication problems involving the dosage of medication based on the weight of the patient and the time required for safe administration using dimensional analysis.

6

THREE-FACTOR MEDICATION PROBLEMS

Outline

Objectives

After completing this chapter, you will be able to:

1. Calculate three-factor–given quantity to one-factor–, two-factor–, or three-factor–wanted quantity medication problems involving a specific amount of medication or intravenous fluid based on the weight of the patient and the time required for safe administration.
2. Calculate problems requiring reconstitution or preparation of medications using information from a nursing drug reference, label, or package insert.

Three-factor–given quantity medication problems can be solved implementing the sequential method or the random method of dimensional analysis. The *given quantity* or the physician's order now contains three parts, including a **numerator** (the *dosage* of medication ordered) and two **denominators** (the *weight* of the patient and the *time* required for safe administration).

Below is an example of this problem-solving method showing placement of basic dimensional analysis terms applied to a three-factor medication problem.

Unit Path

Given Quantity	Conversion Factor for Given Quantity (Numerator)	Conversion Factor for Given Quantity (Denominator)	Conversion Computation		Wanted Quantity
30 mg	5 mL	22 kg	30 × 5 × 22	3300	= 11 mL
kg/day	300 mg		300	300	day

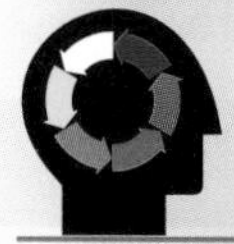

THINKING IT THROUGH

The three-factor–given quantity has been set up with a numerator (30 mg) and two denominators (kg/day) leading across the unit path to a two-factor– wanted quantity, with a numerator (mL) and a denominator (day). The conversion factors can now be factored into the unit path to allow cancellation of unwanted units.

The *dose on hand* (300 mg/ 5 mL) has been factored in and placed so that the wanted unit (mL) correlates with the *wanted quantity* (mL) and the unwanted unit (mg) is canceled.

The child's weight (22 kg) has been factored in and set up to allow the unwanted unit (kg) to be canceled.

All the unwanted units have been canceled, and the wanted units are placed to correlate with the two-factor–wanted quantity (mL/day). Multiply numerators, multiply denominators, and divide the product of the numerators by the product of the denominators to provide the numerical

EXAMPLE 6.1

The physician orders Tagamet for gastrointestinal ulcers 30 mg/kg/day PO in four divided doses for a child weighing 22 kg. The dose on hand is Tagamet 300 mg/5 mL.

How many milliliters per day will the child receive?

Given quantity = 30 mg/kg/day
Wanted quantity = mL/day
Dose on hand = 300 mg/5 mL
Weight = 22 kg

Step 1 Identify the three-factor–given quantity (the physician's order), which contains three parts: a *numerator* (30 mg) and two *denominators* (kg/day). Establish the unit path from the *given quantity* (30 mg/kg/day) to the *two-factor–wanted quantity* (mL/day) using the sequential method of dimensional analysis and the necessary conversion factors.

Sequential method:

30 mg		= mL
kg/day		day

Step 2

Unit Path

Given Quantity	Conversion Factor for Given Quantity (Numerator)	Conversion Factor for Given Quantity (Denominator)	Conversion Computation		Wanted Quantity
30 ~~mg~~	5 (mL)				= mL
kg/(day)	300 ~~mg~~				day

answer. The wanted quantity is 11 mL/day.

The child is to receive 11 mL/day in four divided doses; therefore, the *conversion factor* involves how many doses are in a day (4 divided doses = day).

Step 3

Unit Path

Given Quantity	Conversion Factor for Given Quantity (Numerator)	Conversion Factor for Given Quantity (Denominator)	Conversion Computation			Wanted Quantity
30 ~~mg~~	5 (mL)	22 ~~kg~~			=	mL
~~kg~~/(day)	300 ~~mg~~					day

Step 4

Unit Path

Given Quantity	Conversion Factor for Given Quantity (Numerator)	Conversion Factor for Given Quantity (Denominator)	Conversion Computation			Wanted Quantity
3~~0~~ ~~mg~~	5 (mL)	22 ~~kg~~	3 × 5 × 22	330	=	11 mL
~~kg~~/(day)	30~~0~~ ~~mg~~		30	30		day

Step 5 Using dimensional analysis, calculate how many milliliters per dose the child should receive.

Given quantity = 11 mL/day
Wanted quantity = mL/dose

11 mL		=	mL
day			dose

Step 6

11 (mL)	~~day~~	11	= 2.75 or	2.8 mL
~~day~~	4 (doses)	4		dose

The wanted quantity is 2.8 mL/dose, and the child will receive this orally (PO) four times a day (qid).

The problem could have been set up to find the wanted quantity of milliliters per dose.

Step 6 (alternative).

Given quantity = 30 mg/kg/day
Wanted quantity = mL/dose
Dose on hand = 300 mg/5 mL
Weight = 22 kg

Sequential method:

3~~0~~ ~~mg~~	5 (mL)	22 ~~kg~~	day	3 × 5 × 22	330	= 2.75 or	2.8 mL
~~kg~~/~~day~~	30~~0~~ ~~mg~~		4 (doses)	30 × 4	120		dose

The wanted quantity is 2.8 mL/dose, and the child will receive this orally (PO) four times a day (qid).

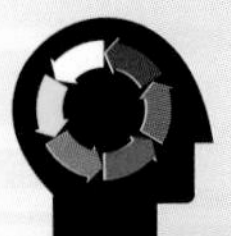

THINKING IT THROUGH

The *two-factor–given quantity* (2.8 mL/dose) has been factored in with a *numerator* (2.8 mL) and a *denominator* (dose). The *three-factor–wanted quantity* (mg/kg/day) also has been factored in with a *numerator* (mg) and two *denominators* (kg/day).

The *conversion factors* have been added, and all unwanted units have been canceled from the problem. The wanted unit (mg) is placed in the numerator to correlate with the *wanted quantity* (mg) also in the numerator. The wanted units (kg and day) are in the denominator to correlate with the wanted quantity (kg and day) in the denominator.

EXAMPLE 6.2

As a prudent nurse, you are concerned that the child may be receiving an unsafe dosage of Tagamet; therefore, you want to identify how many milligrams per kilogram per day (mg/kg/day) the child weighing 22 kg is receiving. The dosage of medication being given four times a day is 2.8 mL/dose. The dosage on hand is 300 mg/5 mL.

How many milligrams per kilogram per day is the child receiving?

Given quantity = 2.8 mL/dose
Wanted quantity = mg/kg/dose
Dose on hand = 300 mg/5 mL
Child's weight = 22 kg

Sequential method:

Step 1

$$\frac{2.8\ \text{mL}}{\text{dose}} \Bigg| \qquad = \frac{\text{mg}}{\text{kg/day}}$$

Step 2

$$\frac{2.8\ \text{mL}}{\text{dose}} \Bigg| \frac{300\ \text{mg}}{5\ \text{mL}} \Bigg| \frac{4\ \text{doses}}{\text{day}} \Bigg| \frac{}{22\ \text{kg}} = \frac{\text{mg}}{\text{kg/day}}$$

Step 3

$$\frac{2.8\ \cancel{\text{mL}}}{\cancel{\text{dose}}} \Bigg| \frac{300\ \text{mg}}{5\ \cancel{\text{mL}}} \Bigg| \frac{4\ \cancel{\text{doses}}}{\text{day}} \Bigg| \frac{}{22\ \text{kg}} \Bigg| \frac{2.8 \times 300 \times 4}{5 \times 22} \Bigg| \frac{3360}{110} = \frac{30.54\ \text{or}\ 30.5\ \text{mg}}{\text{kg/day}}$$

The three-factor–wanted quantity is 30.5 mg/kg/day. The nursing drug reference identifies that 20 to 40 mg/kg/day in four divided doses is a safe dosage of Tagamet for children. Therefore, the nurse is assured that the child is receiving a correct dosage. Dimensional analysis assists you to critically think through any type of medication problem.

EXAMPLE 6.3

The physician orders dobutamine 5 mcg/kg/min IV for cardiac failure. The pharmacy sends an IV bag labeled: dobutamine 250 mg/50 mL D5W/0.45% NS. The patient weighs 165 lb.

Calculate the milliliters per hour at which to set the IV pump.

Given quantity = 5 mcg/kg/min
Wanted quantity = mL/hr
Dose on hand = 250 mg/50 mL
Weight = 165 lb

Step 1 Identify the *three-factor–given quantity* (the physician's order) containing three parts, including the *numerator* (5 mg) and *two denominators* (kg/min). Establish the unit path from the three-factor–given quantity to the two-factor–wanted quantity (mL/hr).

Random method:

5 mcg		=	mL
kg/min			hr

Step 2

5 mcg	60 ~~min~~	=	mL
kg/~~min~~	1 hr		hr

Step 3

5 mcg	60 ~~min~~	50 (mL)	=	mL
kg/~~min~~	1 (hr)	250 mg		hr

Step 4

5 ~~mcg~~	60 ~~min~~	50 (mL)	1 ~~mg~~	=	mL
kg/~~min~~	1 (hr)	250 ~~mg~~	1000 ~~mcg~~		hr

Step 5

5 ~~mcg~~	60 ~~min~~	50 (mL)	1 ~~mg~~	1 ~~kg~~	165 ~~lb~~	=	mL
~~kg/min~~	1 (hr)	250 ~~mg~~	1000 ~~mcg~~	2.2 ~~lb~~			hr

(Example continues on page 140)

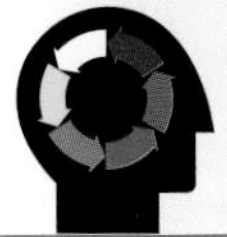

THINKING IT THROUGH

The three-factor–given quantity has been set up with a *numerator* (5 mg) and *two denominators* (kg/min) leading across the unit path to a two-factor–wanted quantity with a *numerator* (mL) and a *denominator* (hr). By using the random method of dimensional analysis, the *conversion factors* are factored to cancel out unwanted units.

The unwanted unit (min) has been canceled by factoring the *conversion factor* (1 hr = 60 min), and the wanted unit corresponds with the *wanted quantity denominator* (hr).

The *dose on hand* (250 mg/50 mL) has been factored in and placed so that the *wanted unit* (mL) corresponds with the wanted quantity numerator (mL).

The *conversion factor* (1 mg = 1000 mcg) has been factored in to cancel the unwanted units (mg and mcg).

The final *conversion factors* (1 kg = 2.2 lb) and the *weight* of the patient have been factored in to cancel the remaining unwanted units (kg and lb). All the unwanted units have been canceled and the wanted units (mL and hr) remain in position to correlate with the *two-factor–wanted quantity* (mL/hr). Multiply the numerators, multiply the denominators, and divide the product of the numerators by the product of the denominators to provide the numerical value for the two-factor–wanted quantity.

Step 6

$$\frac{5\,\cancel{mcg}}{\cancel{kg/min}}\left|\frac{6\cancel{0}\,\cancel{min}}{\cancel{1}\,(hr)}\right|\frac{5\cancel{0}\,(mL)}{25\cancel{0}\,\cancel{mg}}\left|\frac{\cancel{1\,mg}}{100\cancel{0}\,\cancel{mcg}}\right|\frac{1\,\cancel{kg}}{2.2\,\cancel{lb}}\left|\frac{165\,\cancel{lb}}{}\right| = \frac{mL}{hr}$$

$$\frac{5 \times 6 \times 5 \times 1 \times 165}{25 \times 100 \times 2.2}\left|\frac{24{,}750}{5500}\right| = \frac{4.5\text{ mL}}{hr}$$

The 4.5 mL/hr is the wanted quantity and is the answer to the problem. Intravenous pumps used in critical care can be set to deliver amounts including decimal points so it is not necessary to round up the answer.

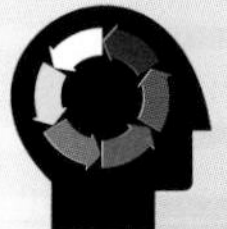

THINKING IT THROUGH

The *two-factor–given quantity* is identified as the information that the nurse obtained from the IV pump, and the *three-factor–wanted quantity* is the information that the physician has requested.

The *dose on hand* (the IV fluid that is presently infusing) has been factored in to cancel the unwanted unit (mL).

The *conversion factor* (1 mg = 1000 mcg) has been factored in to cancel the unwanted unit (mg). The wanted unit (mcg) remains and corresponds with the wanted quantity in the *numerator*.

The *conversion factor* (1 hr = 60 min) has been factored in to cancel the unwanted unit (hr). The wanted unit (min) remains placed in the *denominator*.

The *conversion factor* (1 kg = 2.2 lb) has been factored in to correspond with the *wanted quantity denominator* (kg). The *weight* of the patient also is factored in to cancel the unwanted unit (lb). After all unwanted units have been canceled and the wanted units identified, multiply

EXAMPLE 6.4

The nurse has been monitoring the hemodynamic readings of a patient weighing 165 lb receiving dobutamine, 250 mg in 50 mL of D5W/0.45% NS, and has received additional orders from the physician to *titrate* for effectiveness.

The IV pump is now set at 9 mL/hr, and the physician wants to know how many micrograms per kilogram per minute the patient is now receiving.

Given quantity = 9 mL/hr
Wanted quantity = mcg/kg/min
Dose on hand = 250 mg/50 mL
Weight = 165 lb

Step 1

$$\frac{9\text{ mL}}{hr}\Bigg| \qquad = \frac{mcg}{kg/min}$$

Step 2

Sequential method:

$$\frac{9\,\cancel{mL}}{hr}\left|\frac{250\text{ mg}}{50\,\cancel{mL}}\right| = \frac{mcg}{kg/min}$$

Step 3

$$\frac{9\,\cancel{mL}}{hr}\left|\frac{250\text{ mg}}{50\,\cancel{mL}}\right|\frac{1000\,(mcg)}{1\,\cancel{mg}} = \frac{mcg}{kg/min}$$

the numerators, multiply the denominators, and divide the product of the numerators by the product of the denominators to provide the numerical value for the *wanted quantity*.

Step 4

9 ~~mL~~	250 ~~mg~~	1000 (mcg)	1 ~~hr~~	=	mcg
~~hr~~	50 ~~mL~~	1 ~~mg~~	60 (min)		kg/min

Step 5

9 ~~mL~~	250 ~~mg~~	1000 (mcg)	1 ~~hr~~	2.2 ~~lb~~		=	mcg
~~hr~~	50 ~~mL~~	1 ~~mg~~	60 (min)	1 (kg)	165 ~~lb~~		kg/min

Step 6

9 ~~mL~~	25~~0~~ ~~mg~~	100~~0~~ (mcg)	~~1~~ ~~hr~~	2.2 ~~lb~~		=	mcg
~~hr~~	5~~0~~ ~~mL~~	~~1~~ ~~mg~~	6~~0~~ (min)	1 (kg)	165 ~~lb~~		kg/min

9 × 25 × 100 × 2.2	49,500	=	10 mcg
5 × 6 × 1 × 165	4950		kg/min

The nurse can inform the physician that the patient is now receiving 10 mcg/kg/min infusing at 9 mL/hr.

Dimensional analysis is a problem-solving method that uses critical thinking. When implementing the *sequential method* or the *random method* of dimensional analysis, the medication problem can be set up in a number of different ways, with a focus on the correct placement of *conversion factors* to allow unwanted units to be canceled from the unit path.

Dimensional analysis is a problem-solving method that nurses can use to calculate a variety of medication problems in the hospital, outpatient, or home care environment. The medication problems may involve one-factor–, two-factor–, or three-factor–given quantity medication orders, resulting in one-factor–, two-factor–, or three-factor–wanted quantity answers.

With advanced nursing and home care nursing resulting in increased autonomy, it is more important than ever that nurses be able to accurately calculate medication problems. Dimensional analysis provides the opportunity to use one problem-solving method for any type of medication problem, thereby increasing consistency and decreasing confusion when calculating medication problems.

Exercise 6.1 Medication Problems Involving Dosage, Weight, and Time

(See pages 157–158 for answers)

1. Order: furosemide 2 mg/kg/day PO in two divided doses for congestive heart failure

   Supply: furosemide 40 mg/5 mL

   Child's weight: 20 kg

   How many milliliters per dose will you give? ____________

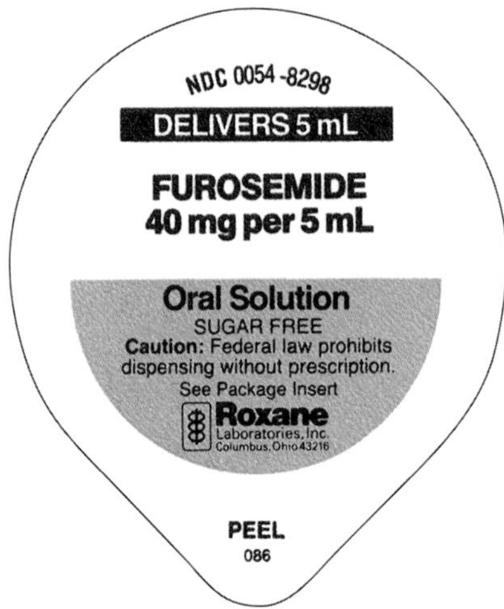

Courtesy of Roxane Laboratories.

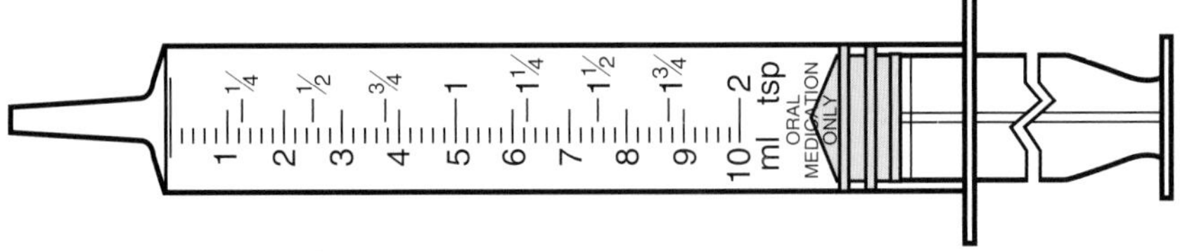

2. Order: Ancef 40 mg/kg/day in divided doses every 8 hours for infection

   Supply: Ancef 1 g

   Child's weight: 30 lb

   Nursing drug reference: Reconstitute with 10 mL of sterile water for injection.

   How many milliliters per dose will you draw from the vial after reconstitution? ______________

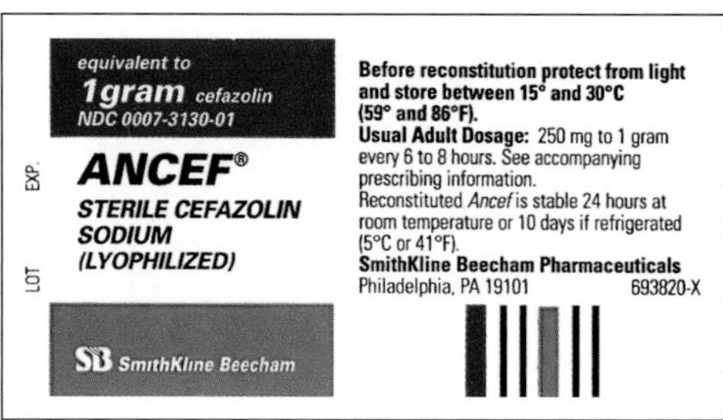

Courtesy of SmithKline Beecham Pharmaceuticals.

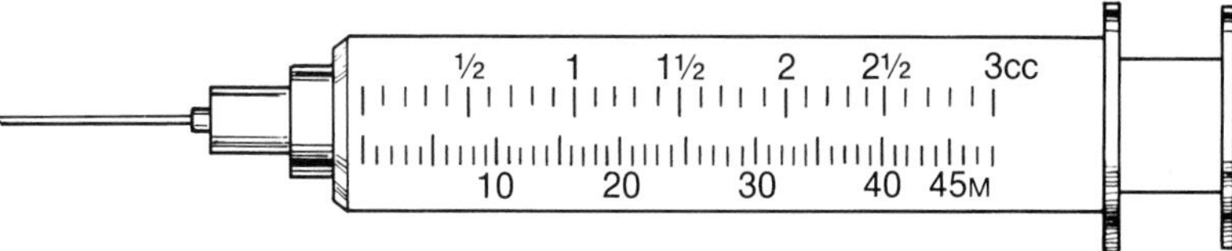

3. Order: Dilantin 6 mg/kg/day in divided doses every 12 hours for seizures

   Supply: Dilantin 125 mg/5 mL

   Child's weight: 45 lb

   How many milliliters per dose will you give? ______________

(Exercise continues on page 144)

4. Order: prednisolone 1.5 mg/kg/day in four divided doses for inflammation

Supply: prednisolone 6.7 mg/5 mL

Child's weight: 20 kg

How many milliliters per dose will you give? ____________

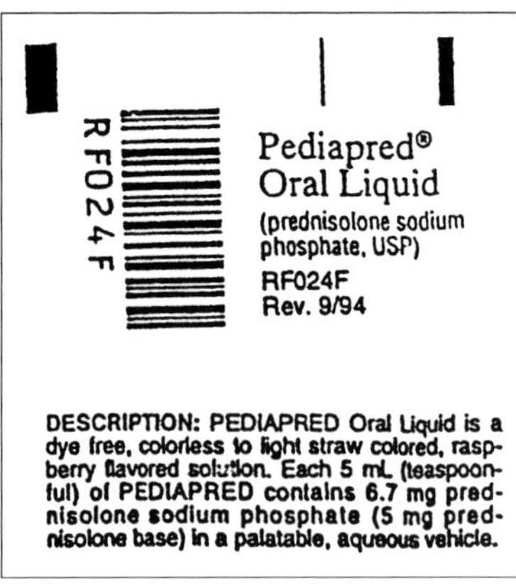

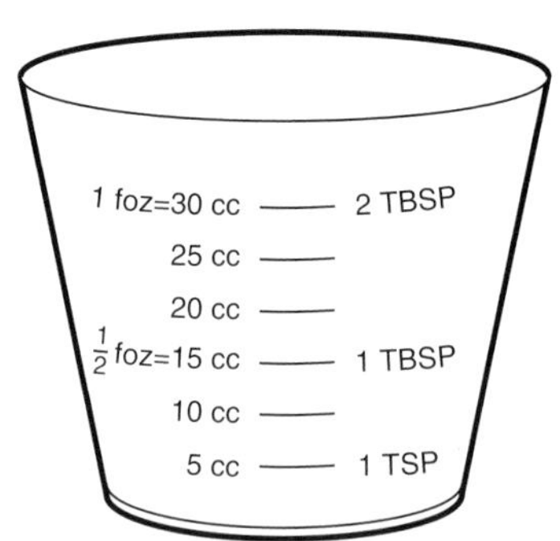

Courtesy of Fisons Pharmaceuticals.

5. Order: Cleocin 10 mg/kg/day IV in divided doses every 8 hours for infection

Supply: Cleocin 300 mg/2 mL

Child's weight: 50 lb

How many milliliters per dose will you give? ____________

Upjohn

Cleocin Phosphate®

brand of clindamycin phosphate sterile solution and clindamycin phosphate IV solution

(clindamycin phosphate injection, USP and clindamycin phosphate injection in 5% dextrose)

Sterile Solution is for Intramuscular and Intravenous Use

CLEOCIN PHOSPHATE in the ADD-Vantage™ Vial is For Intravenous Use Only

DESCRIPTION

CLEOCIN PHOSPHATE Sterile Solution in vials contains clindamycin phosphate, a water soluble ester of clindamycin and phosphoric acid. Each mL contains the equivalent of 150 mg clindamycin, 0.5 mg disodium edetate and 9.45 mg benzyl alcohol added as preservative in each mL. Clindamycin is a semisynthetic antibiotic produced by a 7(S)-chloro-substitution of the 7(R)-hydroxyl group of the parent compound lincomycin.

Courtesy of Upjohn Company.

6. Order: dopamine 5 mcg/kg/min IV to increase blood pressure

Supply: dopamine 400-mg vial

Supply: 250 cc D5W

Patient's weight: 200 lb

How many milliliters will you draw from the vial to equal 400 mg? ____________

Calculate milliliters per hour to set the IV pump. ____________

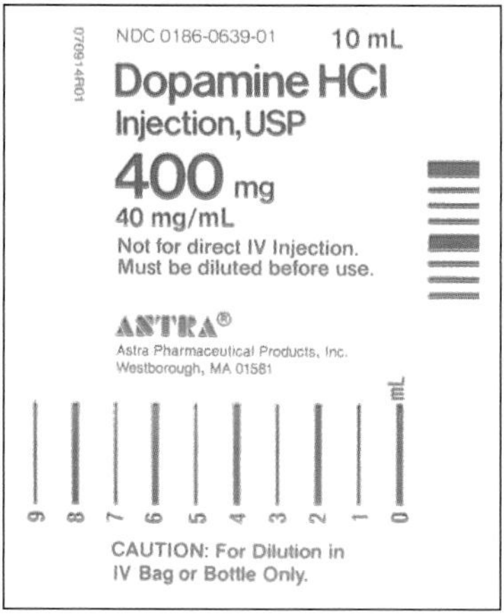

Courtesy of Astra Pharmaceutical Products.

(Exercise continues on page 146)

Dopamine Hydrochloride Injection, USP

DOSAGE AND ADMINISTRATION

WARNING: **This is a potent drug. It must be diluted before administration to patient.**

Suggested Dilution

Transfer contents of one or more additive syringes of dopamine hydrochloride by aseptic technique to either a 250 mL, or 500 mL container of one of the following sterile intravenous solutions:

1. Sodium Chloride Injection, USP
2. Dextrose 5% Injection, USP
3. Dextrose (5%) and Sodium Chloride (0.9%) Injection, USP
4. Dextrose (5%) and Sodium Chloride (0.45%) Injection, USP
5. Dextrose (5%) in Lactated Ringer's Injection
6. Sodium Lactate (1/6 Molar) Injection, USP
7. Lactated Ringer's Injection, USP

Dopamine HCl has been found to be stable for a minimum of 24 hours after dilution in the sterile intravenous solutions listed above. However, as with all intravenous admixtures, dilution should be made just prior to administration.

Do NOT add dopamine HCl to 5% Sodium Bicarbonate or other alkaline intravenous solution, since the drug is inactivated in alkaline solution.

Rate of Administration

Dopamine HCl, after dilution, is administered intravenously through a suitable intravenous catheter or needle. An IV drip chamber or other suitable metering device is essential for controlling the rate of flow in drops/minute. Each patient must be individually titrated to the desired hemodynamic and/or renal response with dopamine HCl. In titrating to the desired increase in systolic blood pressure, the optimum dosage rate for renal response may be exceeded, thus necessitating a reduction in rate after the hemodynamic condition is stabilized.

Administration at rates greater than 50 mcg/kg/minute have safely been used in advanced circulatory decompensation states. If unnecessary fluid expansion is of concern, adjustment of drug concentration may be preferred over increasing the flow rate of a less concentrated dilution.

Suggested Regimen

1. When appropriate, increase blood volume with whole blood or plasma until central venous pressure is 10 to 15 cm H_2O or pulmonary wedge pressure is 14 to 18 mm Hg.
2. Begin administration of diluted solution at doses of 2–5 mcg/kg/minute dopamine HCl in patients who are likely to respond to modest increments of heart force and renal perfusion.

   In more seriously ill patients, begin administration of diluted solution at doses of 5 mcg/kg/minute dopamine HCl and increase gradually using 5–10 mcg/kg/minute increments up to 20–50 mcg/kg/minute as needed. If doses of dopamine HCl in excess of 50 mcg/kg/minute are required, it is suggested that urine output be checked frequently. Should urine flow begin to decrease in the absence of hypotension, reduction of dopamine HCl dosage should be considered. Multiclinic trials have shown that more than 50% of the patients were satisfactorily maintained on doses of dopamine HCl of less than 20 mcg/kg/minute. In patients who do not respond to these doses with adequate arterial pressures or urine flow, additional increments of dopamine HCl may be employed in an effort to produce an appropriate arterial pressure and central perfusion.
3. Treatment of all patients requires constant evaluation of therapy in terms of the blood volume, augmentation of myocardial contractility, and distribution of peripheral perfusion. Dosage of dopamine HCl should be adjusted according to the patient's response, with particular attention to diminution of established urine flow rate, increasing tachycardia or development of new dysrhythmias as indices for decreasing or temporarily suspending the dosage.
4. As with all potent administered drugs, care should be taken to control the rate of administration to avoid inadvertent administration of a bolus of drug.

Parenteral drug products should be inspected visually for particulate matter and discoloration prior to administration, whenever solution and container permit.

HOW SUPPLIED

Dopamine HCl 200 mg is supplied in the following form:
Additive Syringe 5 mL (40 mg/mL) NDC 0186-0638-01

Dopamine HCl 400 mg is supplied in the following forms:
Additive Syringe 5 mL (80 mg/mL) NDC 0186-0641-01
10 mL (40 mg/mL) NDC 0186-0639-01

Dopamine HCl 800 mg is supplied in the following form:
Additive Syringe 5 mL (160 mg/mL) NDC 0186-0642-01

Packages are color coded according to the total dosage content; 200 mg coded blue/white, 400 mg coded green/white and 800 mg coded yellow/white.
Store at controlled room temperature 15°–30°C (59°–86°F). Protect from light.
Avoid contact with alkalies (including sodium bicarbonate), oxidizing agents, or iron salts.
NOTE: Do not use the Injection if it is darker than slightly yellow or discolored in any way.

ASTRA® | Astra Pharmaceutical Products, Inc. Westborough, MA 01581 021861R07 3/92 (7)

Courtesy of Astra Pharmaceutical Products.

7. Information obtained by the nurse: Nipride 50 mg/250 mL D5W is infusing at 22 mL/hr.

   Patient's weight: 160 lb

   How many micrograms per kilogram per minute is the patient receiving? ______________

8. Order: Inocor 5 mcg/kg/min IV for congestive heart failure

   Supply: Inocor 100 mg/100 mL of 0.9% NS

   Patient's weight: 180 lb

   Calculate milliliters per hour to set the IV pump. ______________

9. Information obtained by the nurse: Nipride 50 mg/250 mL D5W is infusing at 46 mL/hr.

   Patient's weight: 160 lb

   How many micrograms per kilogram per minute is the patient receiving? ____________

10. Order: bretylium 5 mg/kg in 50 mL D5W IV over 30 minutes for arrhythmia

    Supply: bretylium 500-mg vial

    Patient's weight: 240 lb

    How many milliliters will you draw from the vial to equal 500 mg? ____________

    Calculate milliliters per hour to set the IV pump. ____________

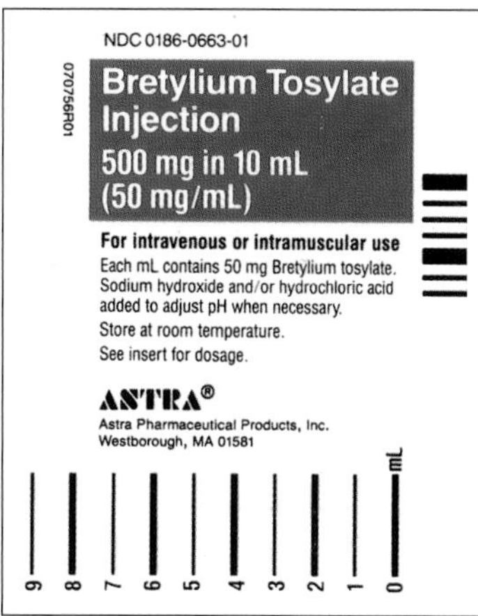

Courtesy of Astra Pharmaceutical Products.

Bretylium Tosylate Injection

For Intramuscular or Intravenous Use.

Suggested Bretylium Tosylate Admixture Dilutions and Administration Rates for Continuous Infusion Maintenance Therapy Arranged in Descending Order of Concentration

PREPARATION				ADMINISTRATION		
Amount of Bretylium Tosylate	Volume of IV Fluid*	Final Volume	Final conc. (mg/mL)	Dose mg/min	Microdrops per min	mL/hour
FOR FLUID RESTRICTED PATIENTS:						
500 mg (10 mL)	50 mL	60 mL	8.3	1.0	7	7
				1.5	11	11
				2.0	14	14
2 g (40 mL)	500 mL	540 mL	3.7	1.0	16	16
1 g (20 mL)	250 mL	270 mL	3.7	1.5	24	24
				2.0	32	32
1 g (20 mL)	500 mL	520 mL	1.9	1.0	32	32
500 mg (10 mL)	250 mL	260 mL	1.9	1.5	47	47
				2.0	63	63

*IV fluid may be either Dextrose Injection, USP or Sodium Chloride Injection, USP. This table does not consider the overfill volume present in the IV fluids.

Courtesy of Astra Pharmaceutical Products.

SUMMARY

This chapter has taught you to calculate three-factor medication problems involving the **dosage** of medication, the **weight** of the patient, and the amount of **time** over which medications or intravenous fluids can be safely administered. Using the sequential method or the random method of dimensional analysis, demonstrate your ability to calculate medication problems accurately by completing the following practice problems.

Practice Problems for Chapter 6 — Three-Factor Medication Problems

(See pages 158–159 for answers)

1. Order: amrinone 8 mcg/kg/min IV for congestive heart failure

   Supply: amrinone 100 mg/100 mL of 0.9% NS

   Patient's weight: 198 lb

   Calculate milliliters per hour to set the IV pump. __________

2. Order: Tagamet 40 mg/kg/day PO in four divided doses for gastrointestinal ulcers

   Supply: Tagamet 300 mg/5 mL

   Child's weight: 80 lb

   How many milliliters per dose will you give? __________

3. Information obtained by the nurse: dopamine 200 mg in 500 mL D5W is infusing at 45 mL/hr for a patient weighing 60 kg.

   How many micrograms per kilogram per minute is the patient receiving? __________

4. Order: dopamine 2 mcg/kg/min IV for decreased cardiac output

   Supply: dopamine 400 mg/500 mL

   Patient's weight: 176 lb

   Calculate milliliters per hour to set the IV pump. __________

5. Order: Neupogen 5 mcg/kg/day SQ for 2 weeks for neutropenia

   Supply: Neupogen 300 mcg/mL

   Patient's weight: 130 lb

   How many micrograms per day will you give? __________

6. Order: aminophylline 0.5 mg/kg/hr IV loading dose for bronchodilation

   Supply: aminophylline 250 mg/250 mL D5W

   Patient's weight: 132 lb

   Calculate milliliters per hour to set the IV pump. ______________

7. Order: furosemide 2 mg/kg/day PO for congestive heart failure

   Supply: furosemide 10 mg/mL

   Child's weight: 40 kg

   How many milliliters per day will you give? ______________

8. Information obtained by the nurse: Nipride 200 mg in 1000 mL D5W is infusing at 15 mL/hr for a patient weighing 100 kg.

   How many micrograms per kilogram per minute is the patient receiving? ______________

9. Information obtained by the nurse: A child weighing 65 lb is receiving 10 mL of Tagamet PO qid from a stock bottle labeled: Tagamet 300 mg/5 mL.

   How many milligrams per kilogram per day is the child receiving? ______________

10. Information obtained by the nurse: aminophylline 250 mg/250 mL 0.9% NS is infusing at 25 mL/hr for a patient weighing 50 kg.

    How many milligrams per kilogram per hour is the patient receiving? ______________

POST-TEST FOR CHAPTER 6: THREE-FACTOR MEDICATION PROBLEMS

Name ______________________ **Date** ____________

1. Order: morphine sulfate 0.3 mg/kg/dose PO every 4 hours for pain

   Supply: morphine sulfate 10 mg/5 mL

   Child's weight: 20 lb

   How many milliliters per dose will you give? ____________

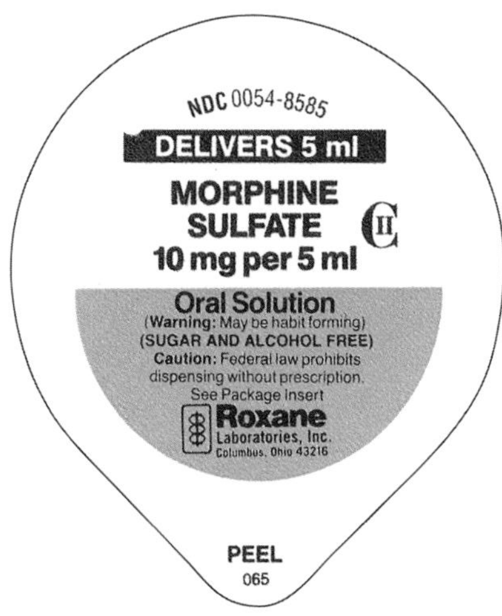

Courtesy of Roxane Laboratories, Inc.

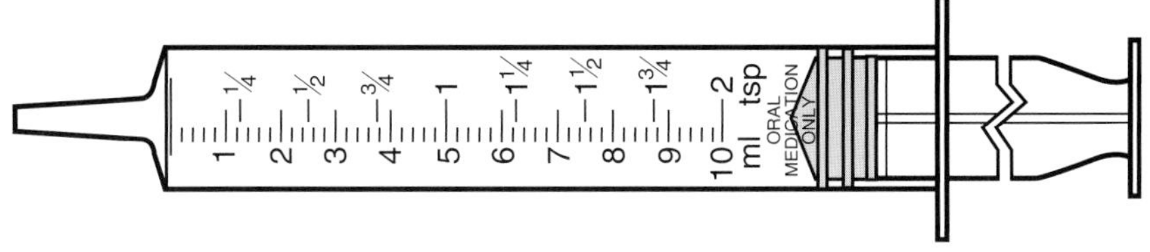

(Post-test continues on page 152)

2. Order: filgrastim 5 mcg/kg/day for myelosuppression secondary to chemotherapy administration

   Supply: filgrastim 480 mcg/1.6 mL

   Patient's weight: 100 lb

   How many milliliters per day will you give? __________

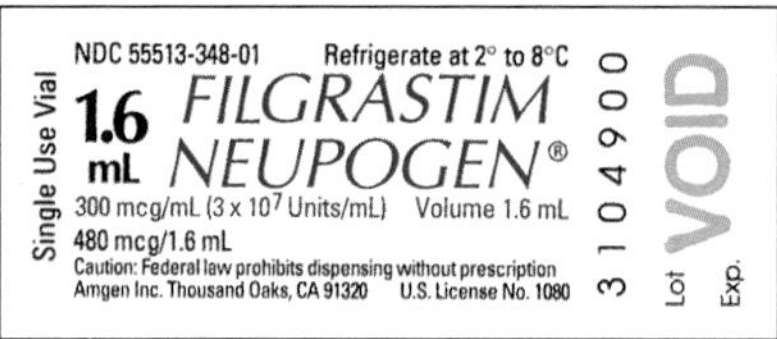

Courtesy of Amgen, Inc.

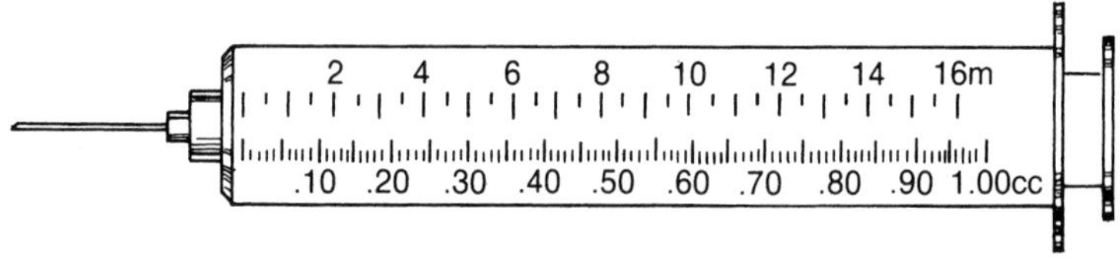

3. Order: Epogen 100 units/kg/day SQ three times weekly for anemia secondary to AZT administration

   Supply: Epogen 10,000 units/mL

   Patient's weight: 180 lb

   How many milliliters per day will you give? __________

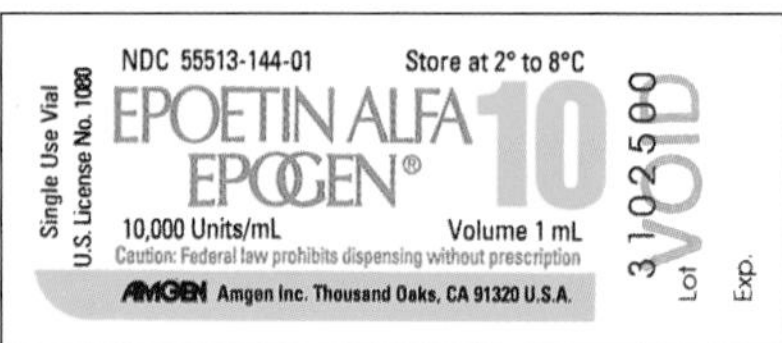

Courtesy of Amgen, Inc.

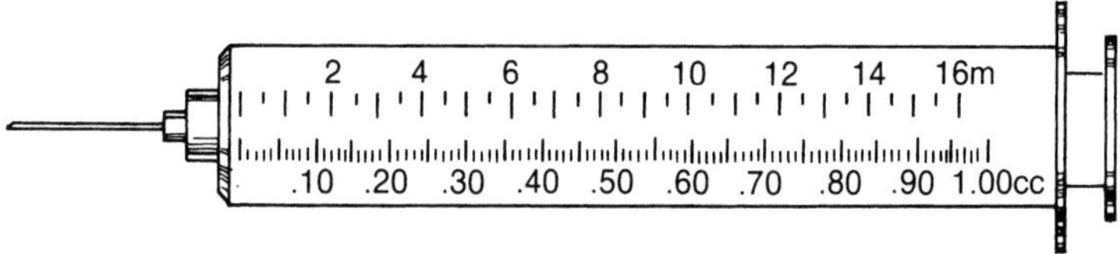

4. Order: digoxin 25 mcg/kg/day PO every 8 hours for congestive heart failure

   Supply: digoxin 0.25 mg/5 mL

   Child's weight: 25 lb

   How many milliliters will you give per day? ______________

   How many milliliters will you give per dose? ______________

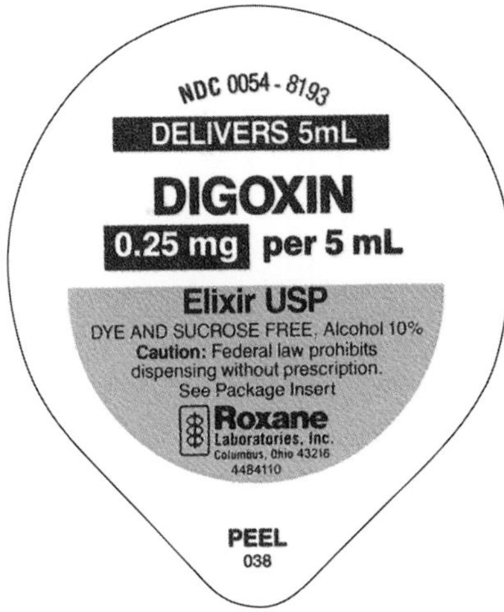

Courtesy of Roxane Laboratories, Inc.

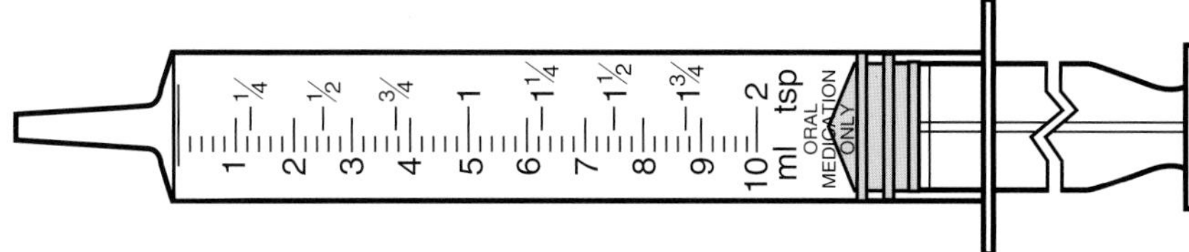

(Post-test continues on page 154)

5. Order: clindamycin 10 mg/kg/day IV in three divided doses for respiratory tract infection

   Supply: clindamycin 150 mg/mL

   Child's weight: 10 kg

   How many milliliters per dose will you draw from the vial? ____________

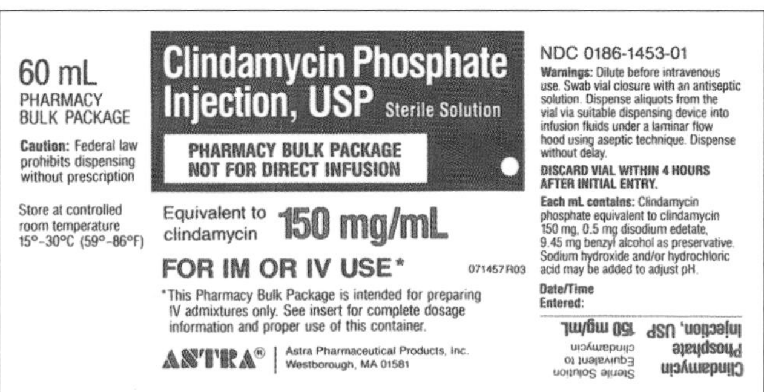

Courtesy of Astra Pharmaceutical Products.

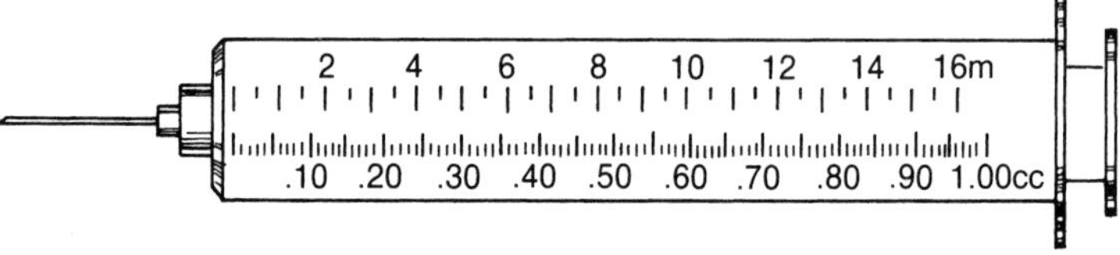

6. Order: Claforan 100 mg/kg/day IV in two divided doses for infection

   Supply: Claforan 1 g/10 mL

   Neonate's weight: 2045 g

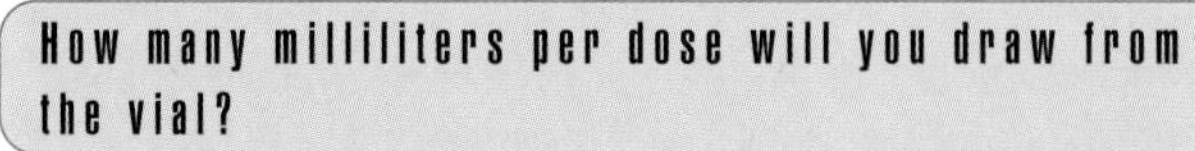

   How many milliliters per dose will you draw from the vial? ____________

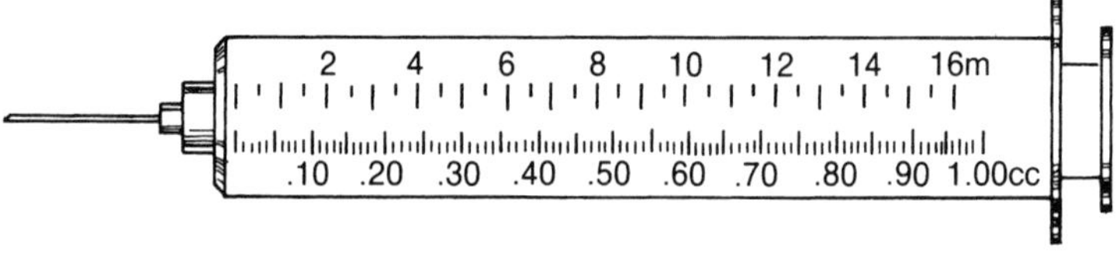

7. Order: gentamicin 2.5 mg/kg/dose IV every 12 hours for gram-negative bacillary infection

   Supply: gentamicin 40 mg/mL

   Neonate's weight: 1182 g

   How many milligrams per dose will the neonate receive? ____________

8. Order: ampicillin 100 mg/kg/day IV in divided doses every 12 hours for respiratory tract infection

   Supply: ampicillin 125 mg/5 mL

   Neonate's weight: 1182 g

   How many milligrams per dose will the neonate receive? ______________

   How many milliliters per dose will you draw from the vial? ______________

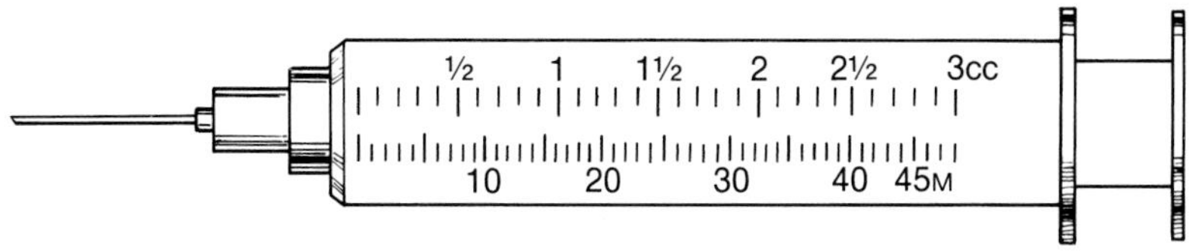

9. Order: Solu-Medrol 5.4 mg/kg/hr IV for acute spinal cord injury

   Supply: Solu-Medrol 125 mg/2 mL

   Patient's weight: 160 lb

   How many milligrams per hour will the patient receive? ______________

10. Order: aminophylline 0.8 mg/kg/hr IV for respiratory distress

    Supply: aminophylline 250 mg/100 mL

    Child's weight: 65 lb

    Calculate milliliters per hour to set the IV pump. __________

ANSWER KEY FOR CHAPTER 6: THREE-FACTOR MEDICATION PROBLEMS

Exercise 6.1 Medication Problems Involving Dosage, Weight, and Time

1. Sequential method:

2 ~~mg~~	5 (mL)	20 ~~kg~~	~~day~~	2 × 5 × 2	20	=	2.5 mL
~~kg/day~~	40 ~~mg~~		2 (doses)	4 × 2	8		dose

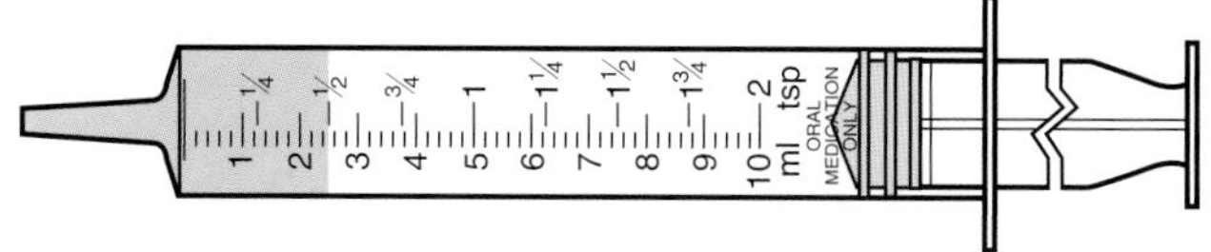

2. Random method:

40 ~~mg~~	10 (mL)	~~day~~	~~1 kg~~	30 ~~lb~~	~~1 g~~	=	mL
~~kg/day~~	~~1 g~~	3 (doses)	2.2 ~~lb~~		~~1000 mg~~		dose

4 × 1 × 3	12	=	1.81 or 1.8 mL
3 × 2.2	6.6		dose

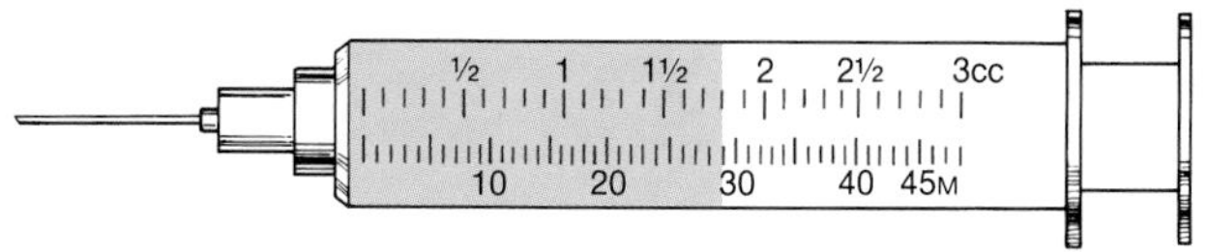

3. Sequential method:

6 ~~mg~~	5 (mL)	1 ~~kg~~	45 ~~lb~~	~~day~~	=	mL
~~kg/day~~	125 ~~mg~~	2.2 ~~lb~~		2 (doses)		dose

6 × 5 × 1 × 45	1350	=	2.45 or 2.5 mL
125 × 2.2 × 2	550		dose

4. Sequential method:

1.5 ~~mg~~	5 (mL)	20 ~~kg~~	~~day~~	1.5 × 5 × 20	=	mL
~~kg/day~~	6.7 ~~mg~~		4 (doses)	6.7 × 4		dose

$$\frac{150}{26.8} = 5.59 \text{ or } 5.6 \ \frac{\text{mL}}{\text{dose}}$$

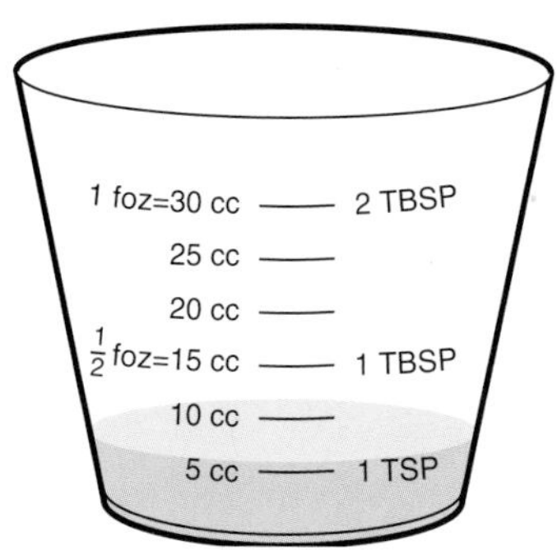

5. Sequential method:

10 ~~mg~~	2 (mL)	1 ~~kg~~	1 ~~day~~	50 ~~lb~~	1 × 2 × 1 × 1 × 5	10	=	0.5 mL
~~kg/day~~	300 ~~mg~~	2.2 ~~lb~~	3 (doses)		3 × 2.2 × 3	19.8		dose

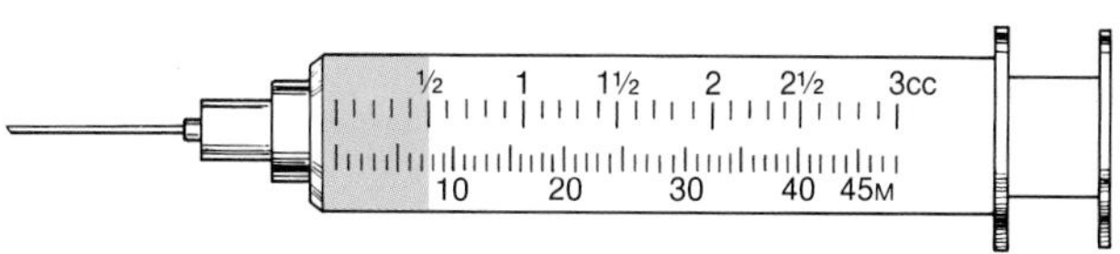

6. Sequential method:

400 ~~mg~~	(mL)	40	= 10 mL
	40 ~~mg~~	4	

Random method:

5 ~~mcg~~	60 ~~min~~	~~1 kg~~	200 ~~lb~~	260 (mL)	1 ~~mg~~	=	mL
~~kg/min~~	~~1~~ (hr)	2.2 ~~lb~~		400 ~~mg~~	1000 ~~mcg~~		hr

5 × 6 × 2 × 26 × 1	1560	=	17.7 or 18 mL
2.2 × 4 × 10	88		hr

7. Sequential method:

22 mL	50 mg	1 hr	1000 (mcg)	2.2 lb		= mcg
hr	250 mL	60 (min)	1 mg	1 (kg)	160 lb	kg/min

22 × 5 × 10 × 2.2	2420	= 1.008 or 1 mcg
25 × 6 × 1 × 16	2400	kg/min

8. Random method:

5 mcg	100 (mL)	1 mg	1 kg	180 lb	60 min	= mL
kg/min	100 mg	1000 mcg	2.2 lb		1 (hr)	hr

5 × 1 × 18 × 6	540	= 24.5 or 25 mL
10 × 2.2	22	hr

9. Sequential method:

46 mL	50 mg	1 hr	1000 (mcg)	2.2 lb		= mcg
hr	250 mL	60 (min)	1 mg	1 (kg)	160 lb	kg/min

46 × 5 × 10 × 2.2	5060	= 2.1 or 2 mcg
25 × 6 × 1 × 16	2400	kg/min

10. Sequential method:

500 mg	(mL)	50	= 10 mL
	50 mg	5	

Sequential method:

5 mg	60 (mL)	1 kg	240 lb	60 min	= mL
kg/30 min	500 mg	2.2 lb		1 (hr)	hr

5 × 6 × 24 × 6	4320	= 130.9 or 131 mL
3 × 5 × 2.2	33	hr

Practice Problems

1. Random method:

8 mcg	100 (mL)	1 mg	1 kg	198 lb	60 min	= mL
kg/min	100 mg	1000 mcg	2.2 lb		1 (hr)	hr

8 × 1 × 198 × 6	9504	= 43.2 mL
100 × 2.2	220	hr

2. Sequential method:

40 mg	5 (mL)	1 kg	80 lb	day	= mL
kg/day	300 mg	2.2 lb		4 (doses)	dose

4 × 5 × 1 × 8	160	= 6.06 or 6 mL
3 × 2.2 × 4	26.4	dose

3. Sequential method:

45 mL	200 mg	1000 (mcg)	1 hr		= mcg
hr	500 mL	1 mg	60 (min)	60 (kg)	kg/min

45 × 2 × 10	900	= 5 mcg
5 × 6 × 6	180	kg/min

4. Random method:

2 mcg	500 (mL)	1 mg	60 min	1 kg	176 lb	= mL
kg/min	400 mg	1000 mcg	1 (hr)	2.2 lb		hr

2 × 5 × 6 × 1 × 176	10,560	= 12 mL
4 × 100 × 2.2	880	hr

5. Random method:

5 (mcg)	1 kg	130 lb	5 × 1 × 130	650	= 295.45 or 296 mcg
kg/(day)	2.2 lb		2.2	2.2	day

6. Sequential method:

0.5 ~~mg~~	~~250~~ (mL)	1 ~~kg~~	132 ~~lb~~	0.5 × 1 × 132	66	=	30 mL
~~kg~~/(hr)	~~250 mg~~	2.2 ~~lb~~		2.2	2.2		hr

7. Sequential method:

2 ~~mg~~	(mL)	4~~0~~ ~~kg~~	2 × 4	8	=	8 mL
~~kg~~/(day)	1~~0~~ ~~mg~~		1	1		day

8. Sequential method:

15 ~~mL~~	~~200~~ ~~mg~~	~~1 hr~~	~~1000~~ (mcg)		15 × 2	30	=	0.5 mcg
~~hr~~	~~1000 mL~~	60 (min)	~~1 mg~~	1~~00~~ (kg)	60	60		kg/min

9. Sequential method:

10 ~~mL~~	300 (mg)	4 ~~doses~~	2.2 ~~lb~~		=	mg
~~dose~~	5 ~~mL~~	(day)	1 (kg)	65 ~~lb~~		kg/day

10 × 300 × 4 × 2.2	26,400	=	81.23 or 81 mg
5 × 1 × 65	325		kg/day

10. Sequential method:

25 ~~mL~~	~~250~~ (mg)		25	=	0.5 mg
(hr)	~~250 mL~~	50 (kg)	50		kg/hr

SECTION

2

PRACTICE PROBLEMS

Practice Problems — One-Factor Practice Problems

(See pages 197–200 for answers)

1. Order: Tigan 200 mg qid IM for nausea and vomiting

How many milliliters will you give? ____________

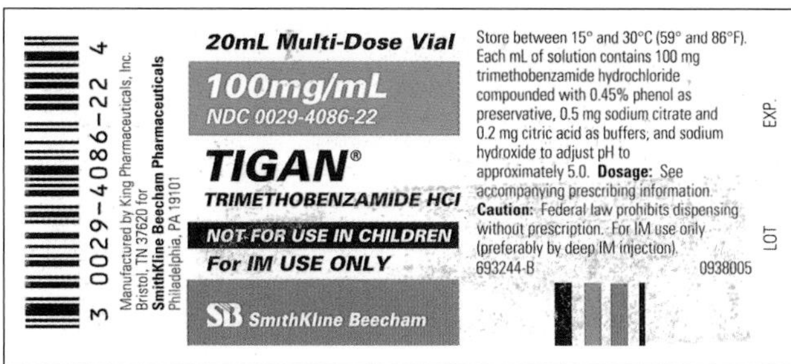

Courtesy of SmithKline Beecham Pharmaceuticals.

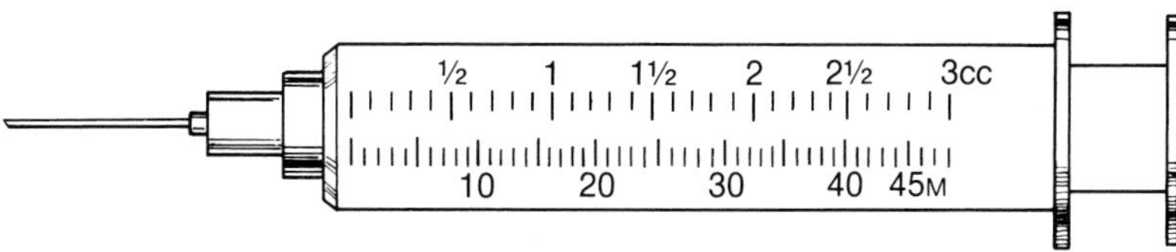

2. Order: morphine 30 mg PO every 4 hours for pain

How many tablets will you give? ____________

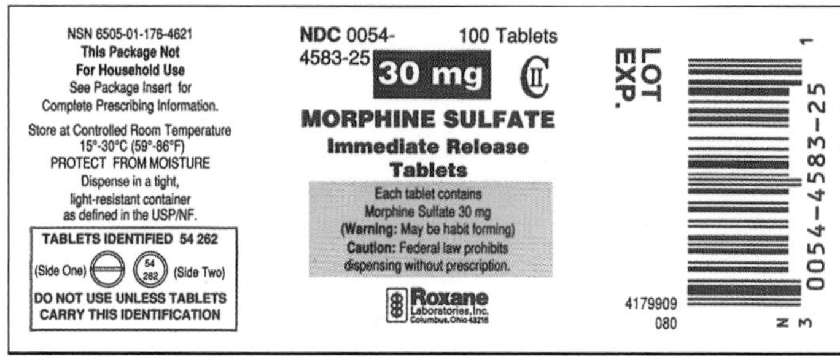

Courtesy of Roxane Laboratories.

(Practice problems continue on page 164)

3. Order: prednisone 7.5 mg PO bid for inflammation

How many tablets will you give? ____________

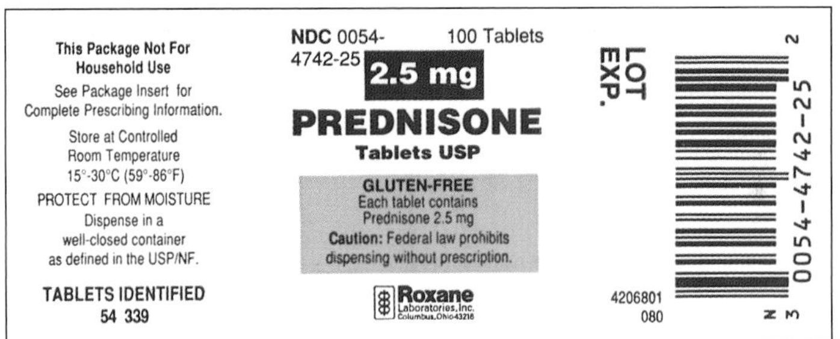

Courtesy of Roxane Laboratories.

4. Order: acetaminophen 160 mg PO every 4 hours for fever

How many teaspoons will you give? ____________

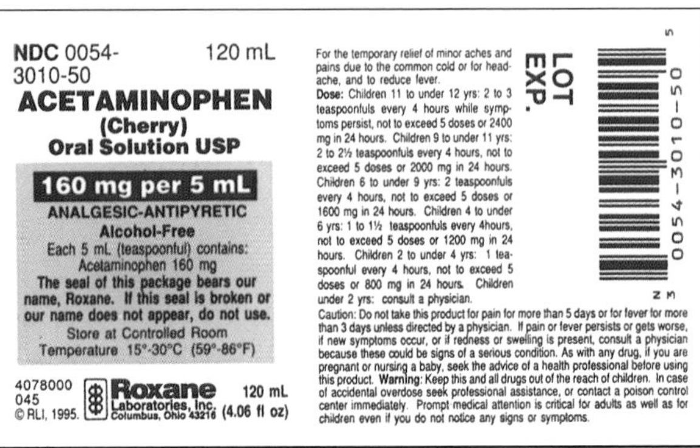

Courtesy of Roxane Laboratories.

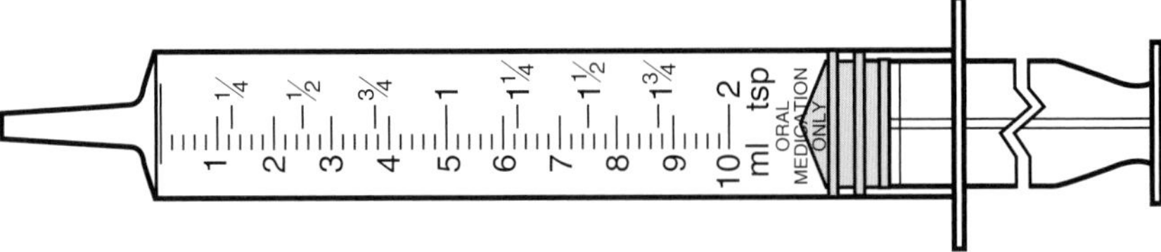

5. Order: Xanax 0.5 mg PO tid for anxiety

How many tablets will you give? ___________

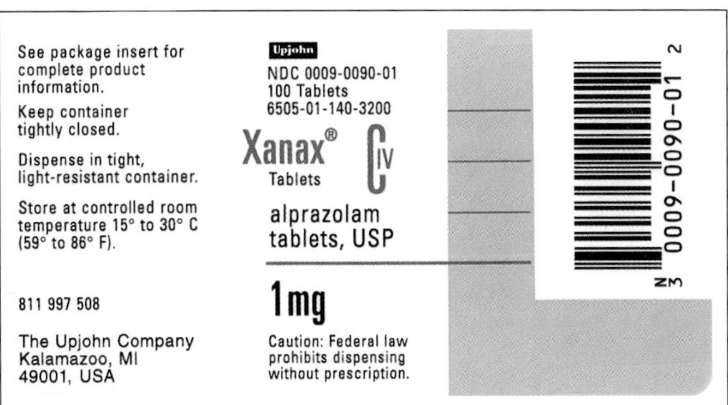

Courtesy of the Upjohn Company.

6. Order: Adalat 60 mg PO daily for hypertension

How many tablets will you give? ___________

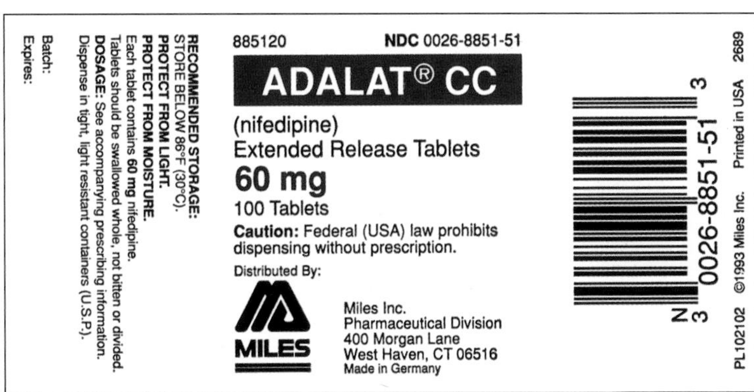

Courtesy of Miles Inc.

7. Order: Halcion 0.25 mg PO at hs for insomnia

How many tablets will you give? ___________

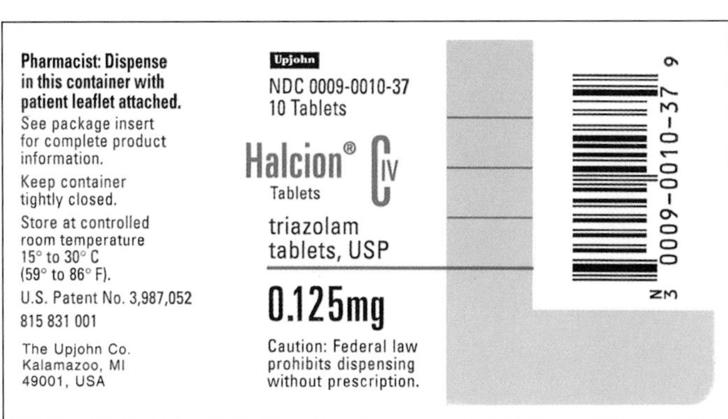

Courtesy of the Upjohn Company.

(Practice problems continue on page 166)

8. Order: furosemide 80 mg PO daily for congestive heart failure

How many tablets will you give? ______________

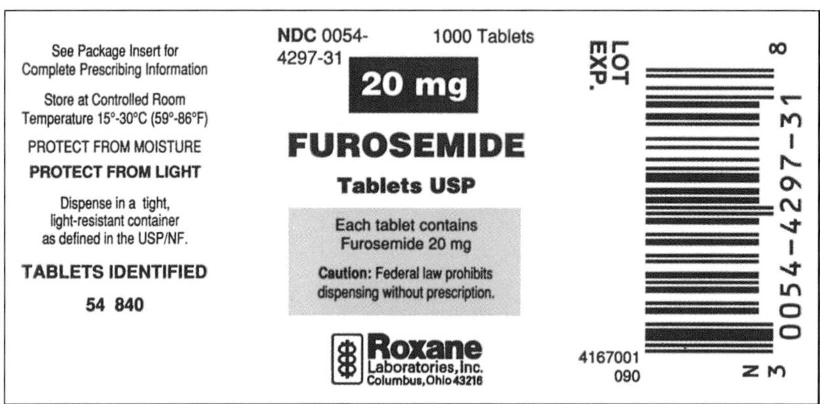

Courtesy of Roxane Laboratories.

9. Order: morphine sulfate 10 mg IM prn for pain

How many milliliters will you give? ______________

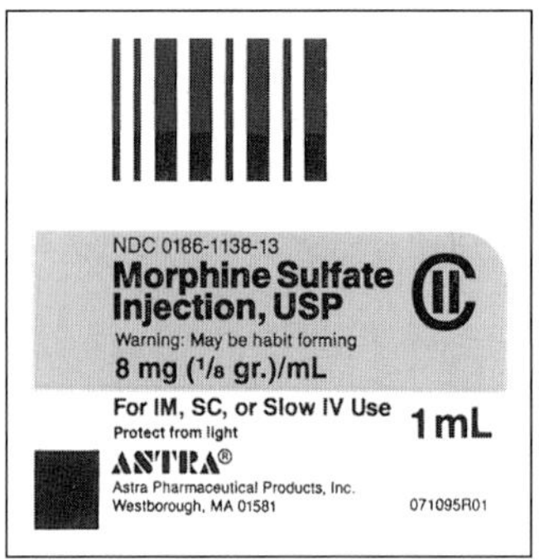

Courtesy of Astra Pharmaceutical Products.

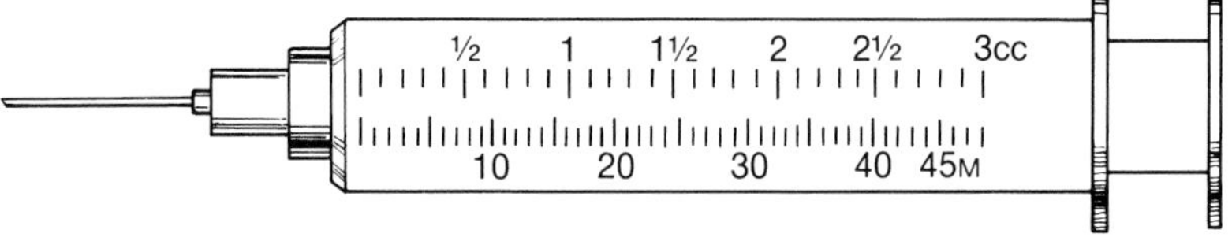

10. Order: naloxone HCl 100 mcg IVP prn for respiratory depression

How many milliliters will you give? ____________

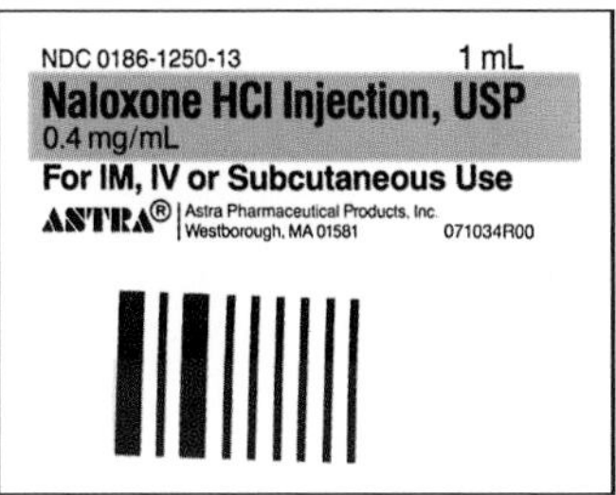

Courtesy of Astra Pharmaceutical Products.

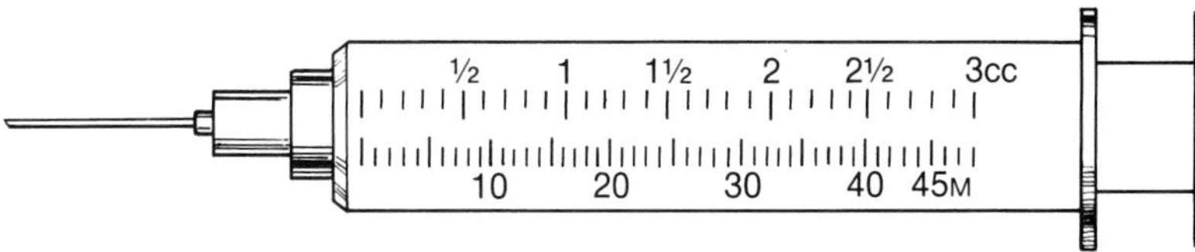

11. Order: Solu-Medrol 80 mg IVP every 4 hours for inflammation

How many milliliters will you give? ____________

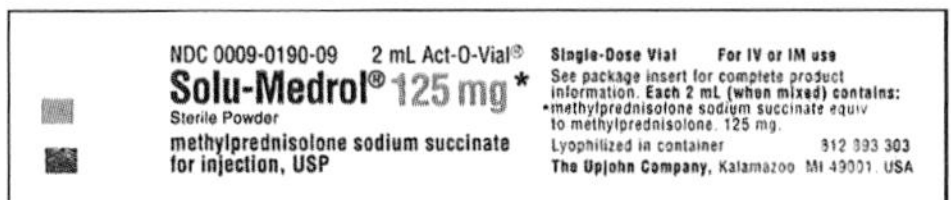

Courtesy of the Upjohn Company.

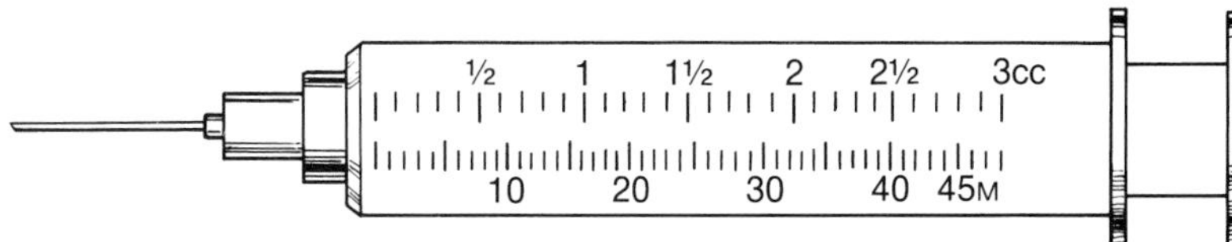

(Practice problems continue on page 168)

12. Order: lactulose 20 g PO daily for constipation

How many milliliters will you give? ____________

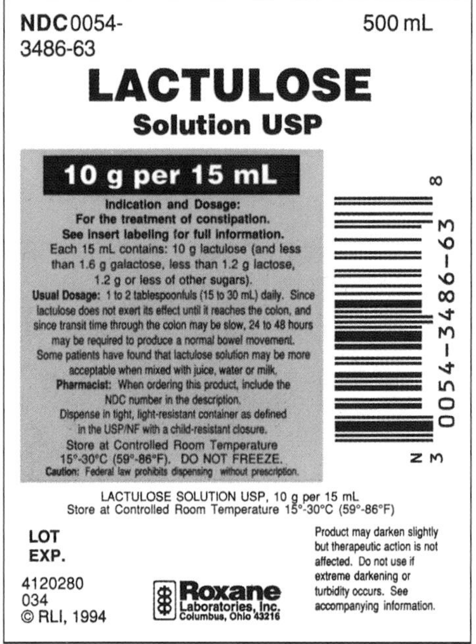

Courtesy of Roxane Laboratories.

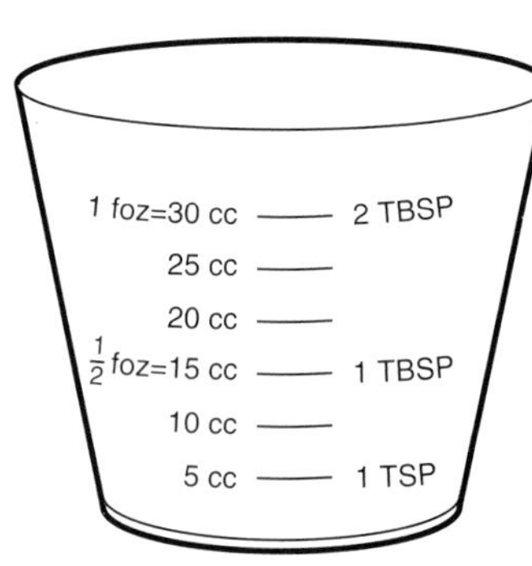

13. Order: Compazine 5 mg IM tid for nausea and vomiting

How many milliliters will you give? ____________

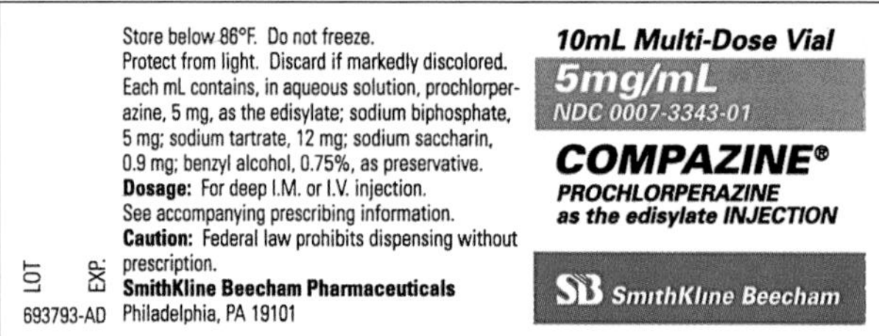

Courtesy of SmithKline Beecham Pharmaceuticals.

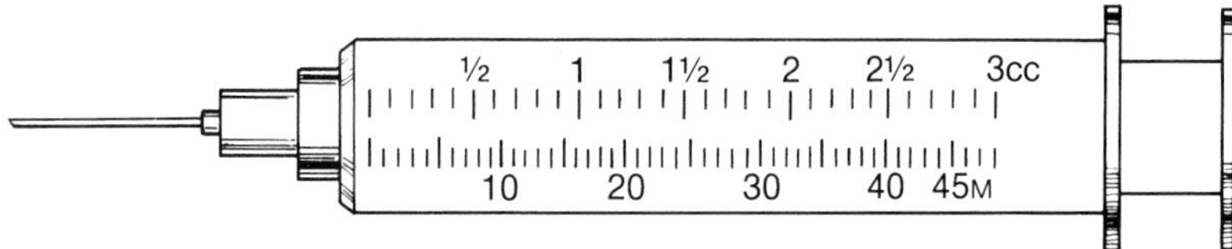

14. Order: Augmentin 250 mg PO every 8 hours for infection

How many milliliters will you give? ___________

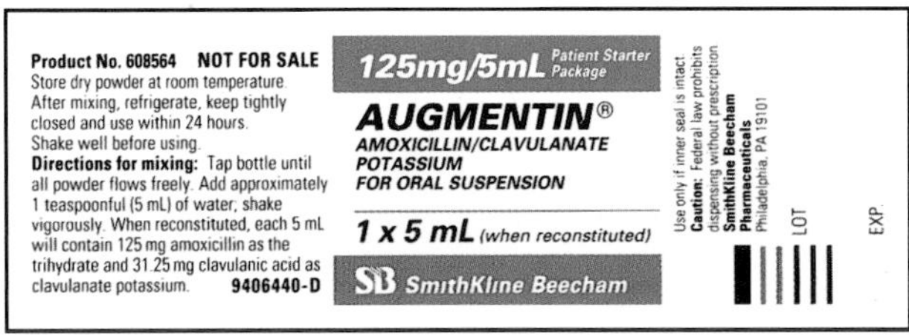

Courtesy of SmithKline Beecham Pharmaceuticals.

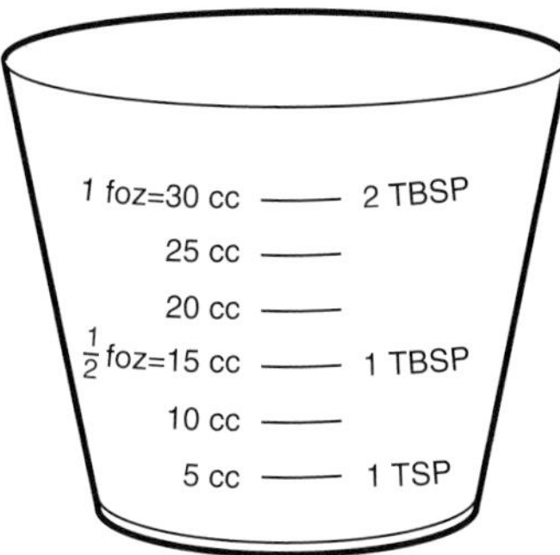

15. Order: Tigan 200 mg PO tid for nausea and vomiting

How many capsules will you give? ___________

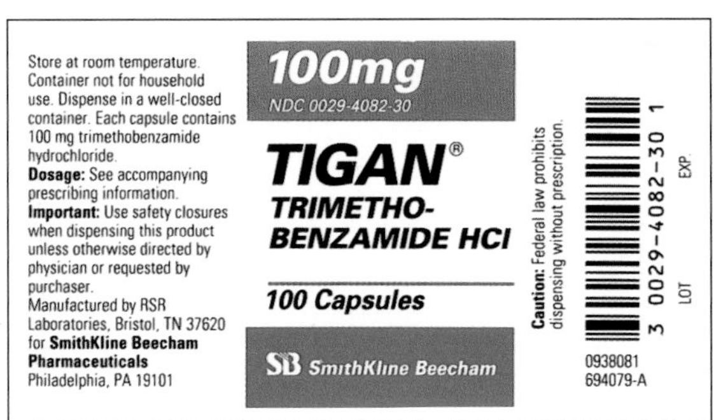

Courtesy of SmithKline Beecham Pharmaceuticals.

16. Order: prednisone 10 mg PO bid for adrenal insufficiency

How many tablets will you give? ___________

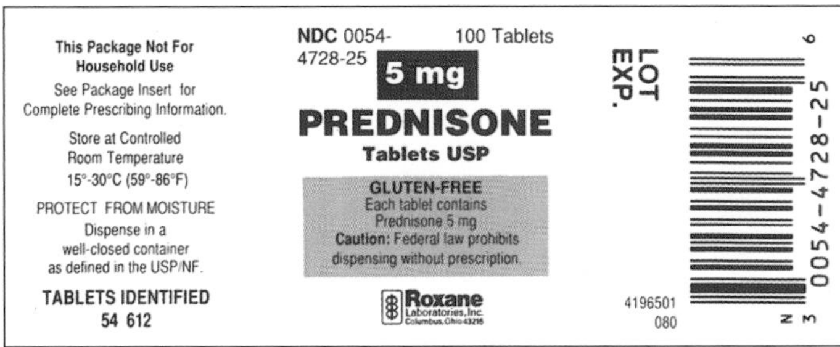

Courtesy of Roxane Laboratories.

(Practice problems continue on page 170)

17. Order: hydromorphone 3 mg IM every 4 hours for pain

How many milliliters will you give? ____________

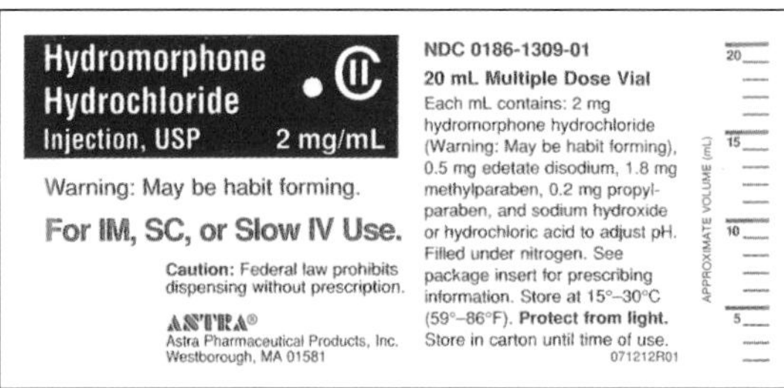

Courtesy of Astra Pharmaceutical Products.

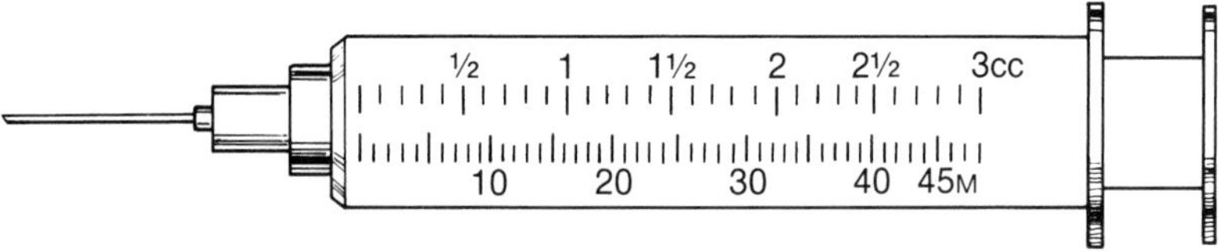

18. Order: acetaminophen 400 mg PO every 4 hours prn for fever

How many milliliters will you give? ____________

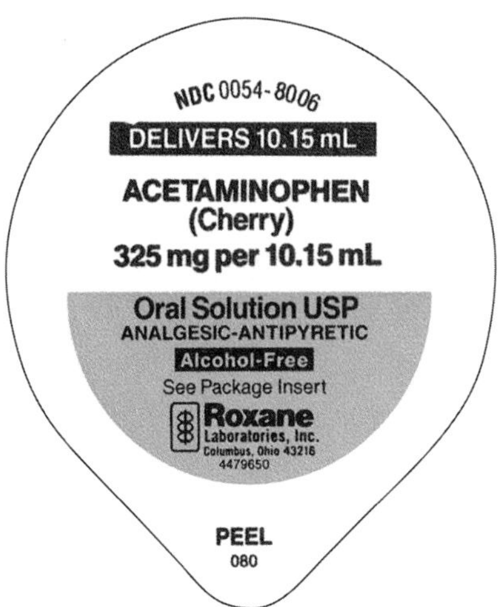

Courtesy of Roxane Laboratories.

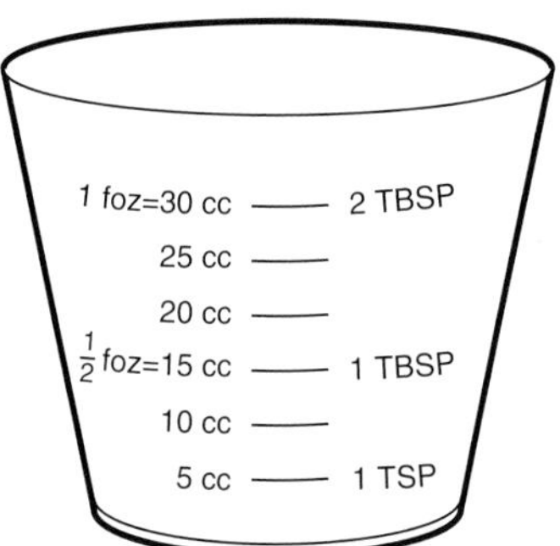

19. Order: magnesium sulfate 1000 mg IM times four doses for hypomagnesemia

How many milliliters will you give? ______________

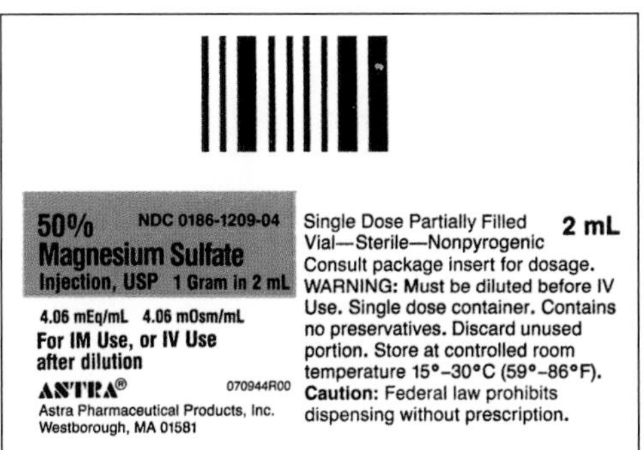
50% NDC 0186-1209-04
Magnesium Sulfate
Injection, USP 1 Gram in 2 mL
4.06 mEq/mL 4.06 mOsm/mL
For IM Use, or IV Use after dilution
ASTRA®
070944R00
Astra Pharmaceutical Products, Inc.
Westborough, MA 01581
Single Dose Partially Filled Vial—Sterile—Nonpyrogenic 2 mL
Consult package insert for dosage.
WARNING: Must be diluted before IV Use. Single dose container. Contains no preservatives. Discard unused portion. Store at controlled room temperature 15°–30°C (59°–86°F).
Caution: Federal law prohibits dispensing without prescription.

Courtesy of Astra Pharmaceutical Products.

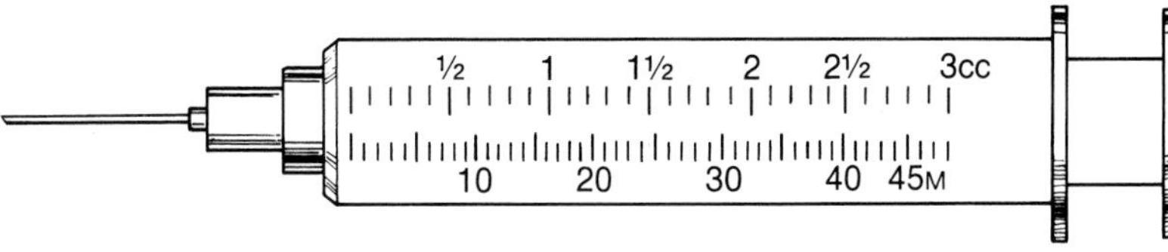

20. Order: Compazine 10 mg PO qid prn for nausea and vomiting

How many teaspoons will you give? ______________

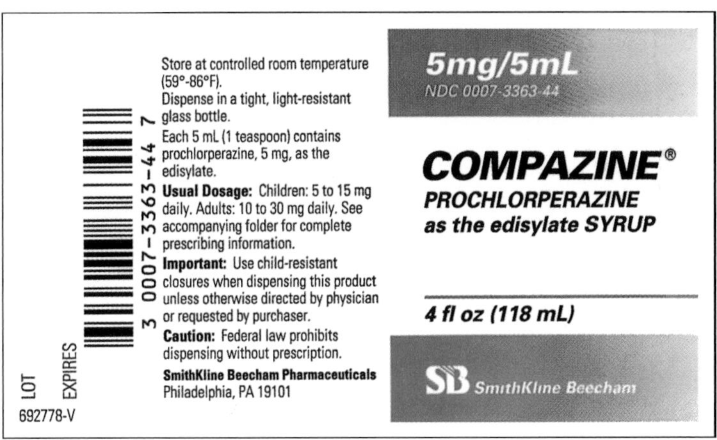
Store at controlled room temperature (59°-86°F).
Dispense in a tight, light-resistant glass bottle.
Each 5 mL (1 teaspoon) contains prochlorperazine, 5 mg, as the edisylate.
Usual Dosage: Children: 5 to 15 mg daily. Adults: 10 to 30 mg daily. See accompanying folder for complete prescribing information.
Important: Use child-resistant closures when dispensing this product unless otherwise directed by physician or requested by purchaser.
Caution: Federal law prohibits dispensing without prescription.
SmithKline Beecham Pharmaceuticals
Philadelphia, PA 19101
3 0007-3363-44 7
LOT
EXPIRES
692778-V
5mg/5mL
NDC 0007-3363-44
COMPAZINE®
PROCHLORPERAZINE
as the edisylate SYRUP
4 fl oz (118 mL)
SB SmithKline Beecham

Courtesy of SmithKline Beecham Pharmaceuticals.

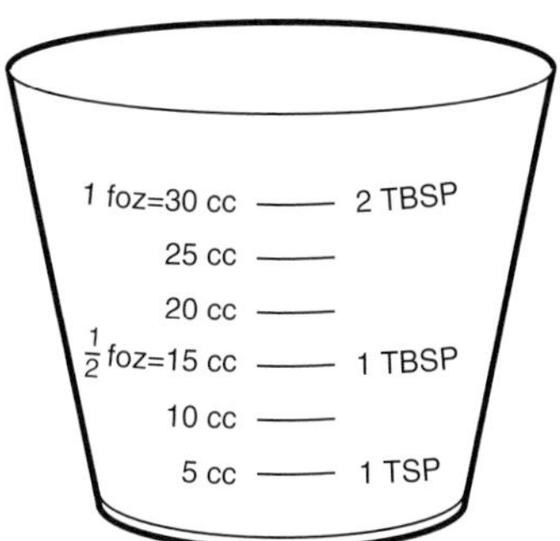

(Practice problems continue on page 172)

21. Order: Hemabate 0.25 mg IM to control postpartum bleeding

How many milliliters will you give? ____________

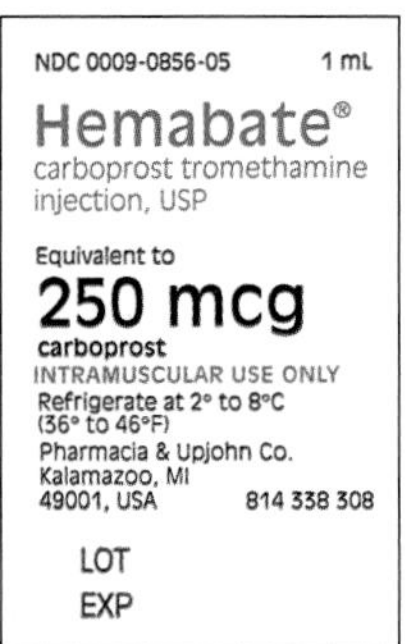

Courtesy of Pharmacia & Upjohn Company.

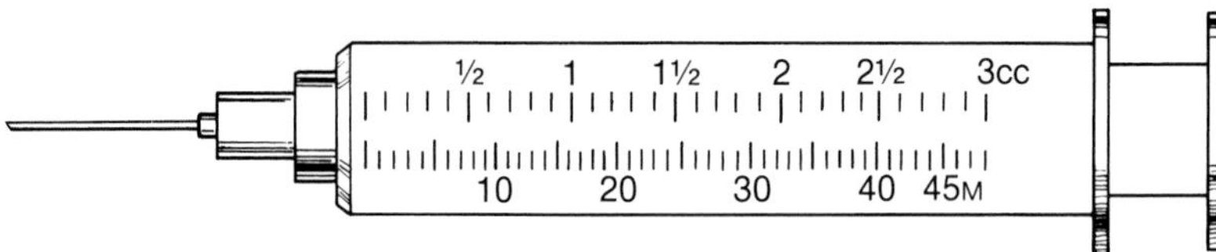

22. Order: Lincocin 500 mg every 8 hours IV for infection

How many milliliters will you draw from the vial? ____________

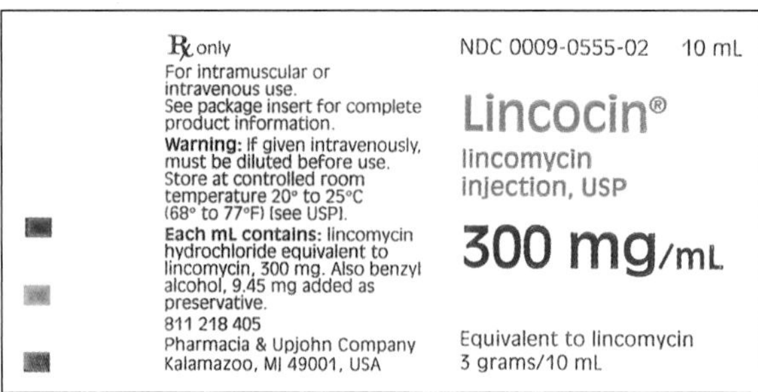

Courtesy of Pharmacia & Upjohn Company.

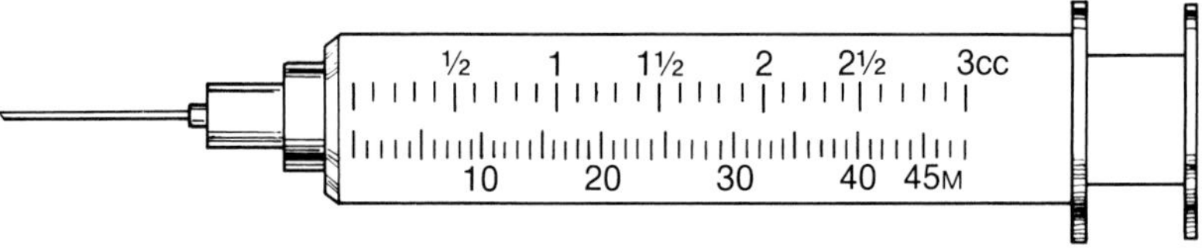

23. Order: Fragmin 2500 IU SQ daily for 10 days for thromboembolism prophylaxis

How many milliliters will you give? ____________

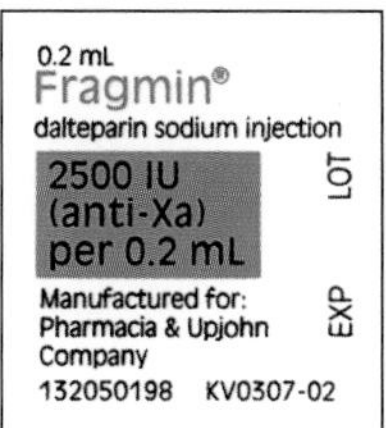

Courtesy of Pharmacia & Upjohn Company.

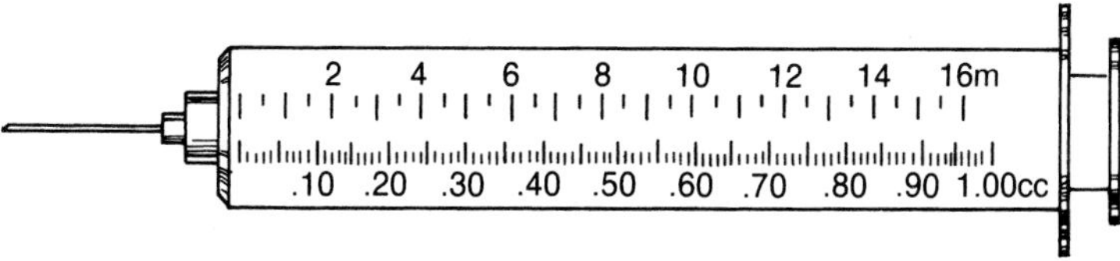

24. Order: Vantin 200 mg every 12 hours PO for infection

How many milliliters will you give? ____________

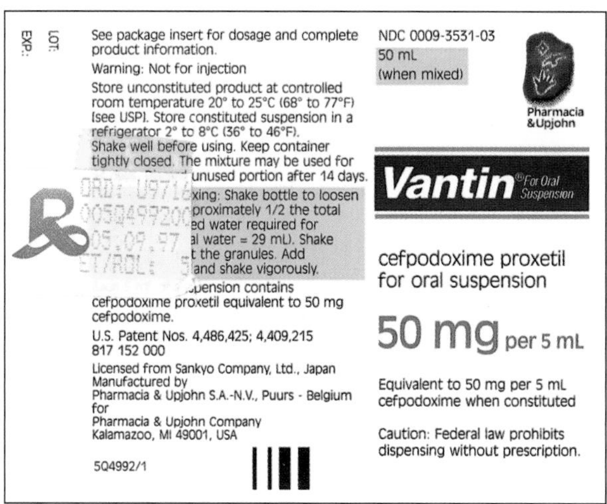

Courtesy of Pharmacia & Upjohn Company.

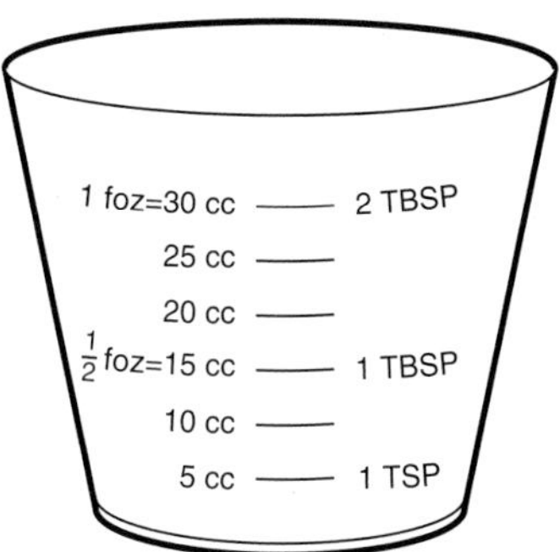

(Practice problems continue on page 174)

25. Order: Cleocin 300 mg PO daily for *P. carinii* pneumonia

How many capsules will you give? ________

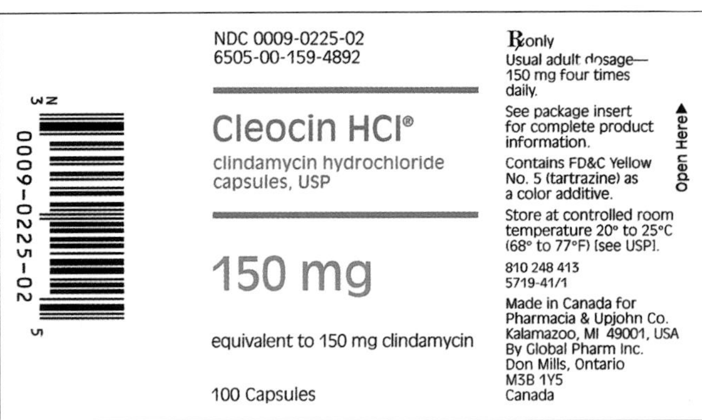

Courtesy of Pharmacia & Upjohn Company.

26. Order: Azulfidine 500 mg PO every 12 hours for management of inflammatory bowel disease

How many tablets will you give? ________

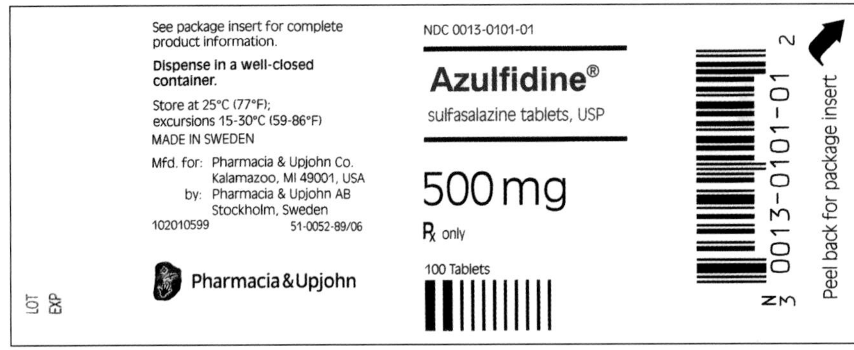

Courtesy of Pharmacia & Upjohn Company.

27. Order: Mirapex 0.25 mg PO tid for signs/symptoms of idiopathic Parkinson's disease

How many tablets will you give? ________

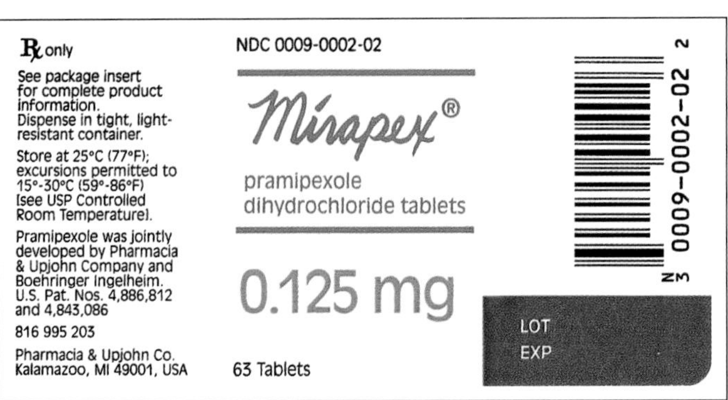

Courtesy of Pharmacia & Upjohn Company.

28. Order: Glyset 25 mg PO tid at the start of each meal for management of type 2 diabetes mellitus

How many tablets will you give? ________

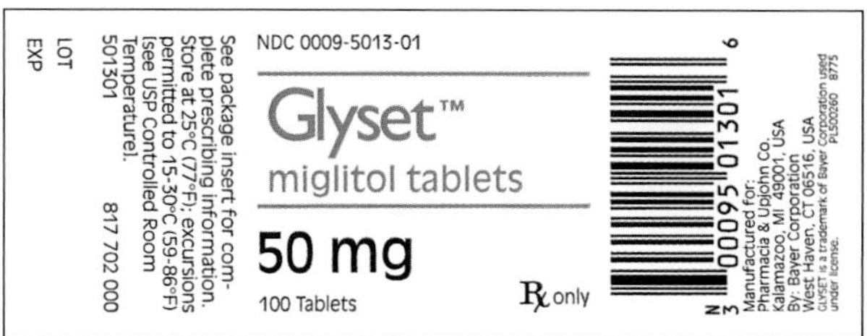

Courtesy of Pharmacia & Upjohn Company.

29. Order: Micronase 5 mg PO daily for control of blood sugars associated with noninsulin-dependent diabetes mellitus

How many tablets will you give? ________

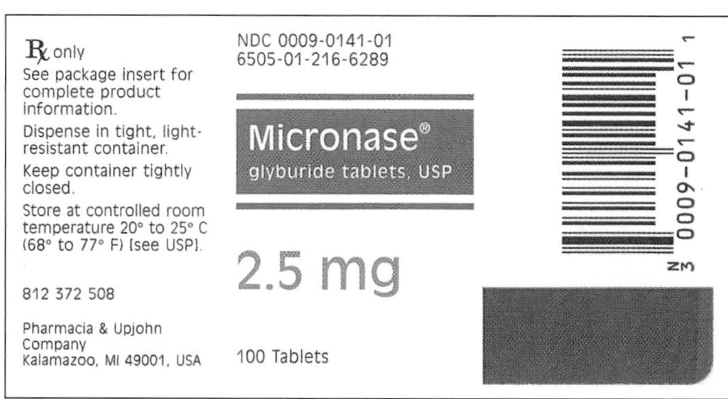

Courtesy of Pharmacia & Upjohn Company.

30. Order: Xanax 0.5 mg PO tid for panic attacks

How many tablets will you give? ________

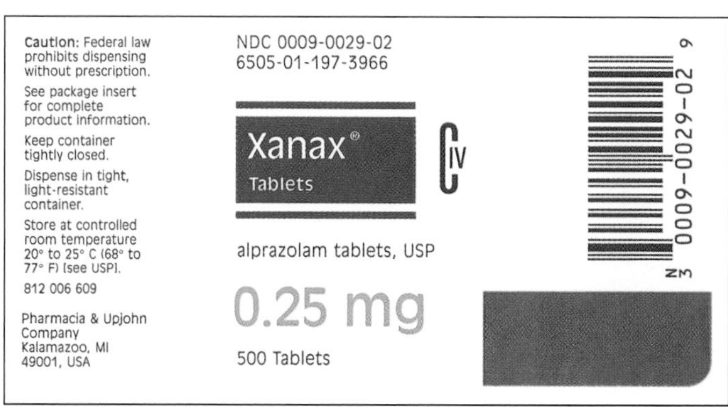

Courtesy of Pharmacia & Upjohn Company.

(Practice problems continue on page 176)

31. Order: Depo-Provera 150 mg IM within the first 5 days of menses for contraception

How many milliliters will you give? ____________

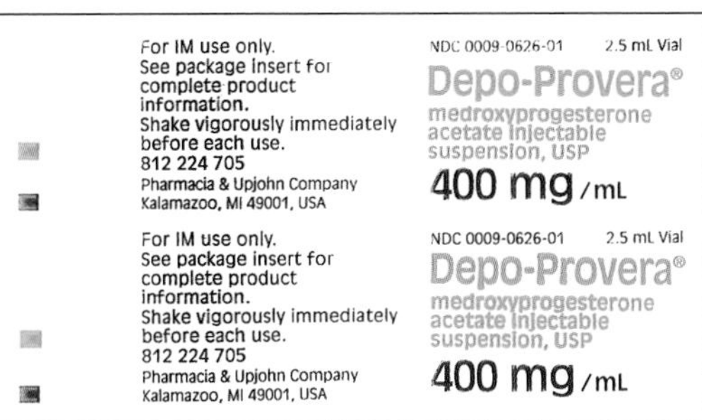

Courtesy of Pharmacia & Upjohn Company.

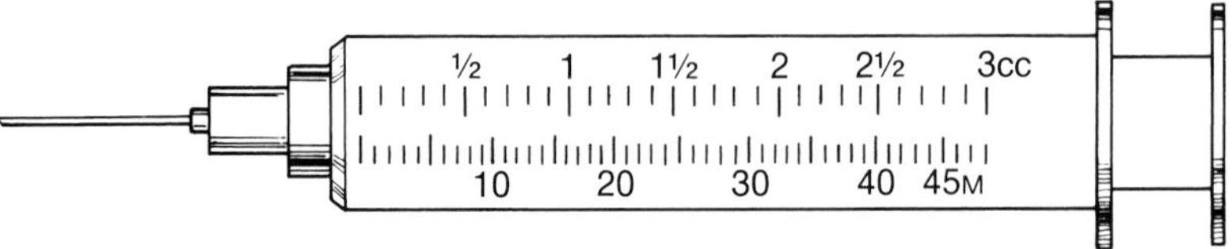

32. Order: Eskalith 600 mg PO tid initial dose followed by 300 mg PO qid for treatment of bipolar affective disorder. Check lithium levels every 3 months.

How many tablets will you give? ____________

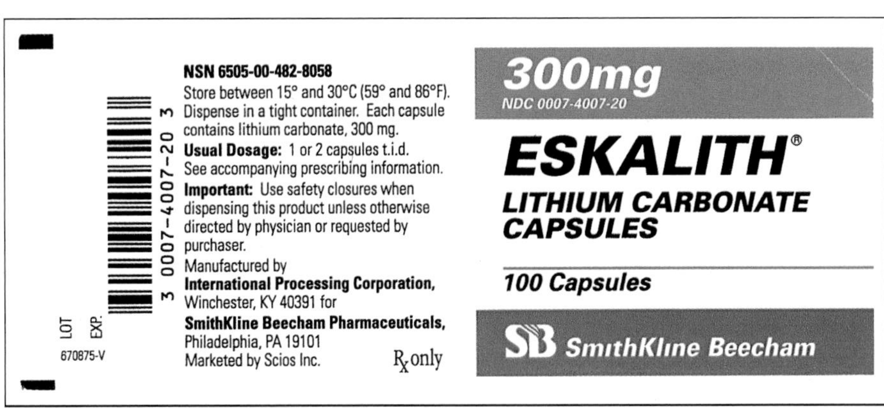

Courtesy of SmithKline Beecham Pharmaceuticals.

Practice Problems

Two-Factor Practice Problems

(See pages 200–203 for answers)

1. Order: digoxin elixir 25 mcg/kg for congestive heart failure

   Child's weight: 25 lb

   How many milliliters will you give? __________

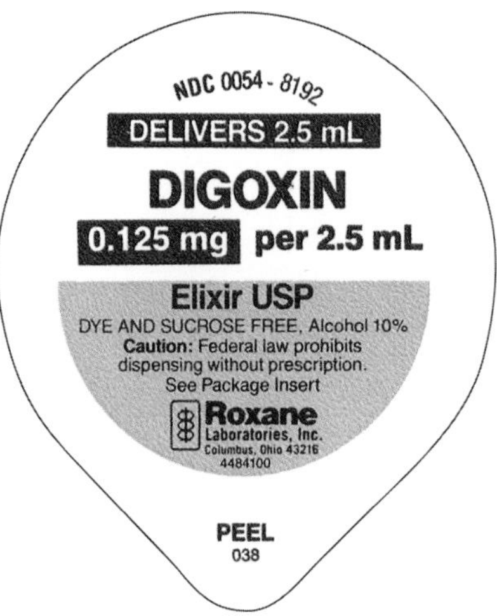

Courtesy of Roxane Laboratories.

2. Order: atropine sulfate 0.02 mg/kg IV every 4 hours for bradycardia

   Child's weight: 35 lb

   How many milliliters will you give? __________

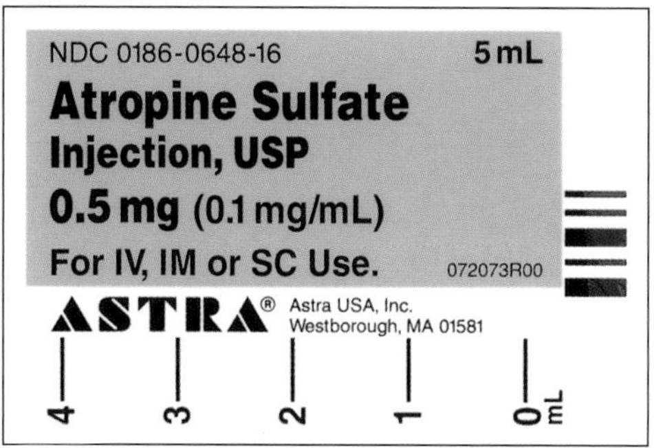

Courtesy of Astra Pharmaceutical Products.

(Practice problems continue on page 178)

3. Order: lidocaine 2 mg/min IV for arrhythmia

   Supply: lidocaine 2 g/500 mL D5W

   Calculate milliliters per hour to set the IV pump. ______________

4. Order: Mezlin 1.5 g IV every 4 hours for infection

   Nursing drug reference: Reconstitute each 1 g with 10 mL of normal saline.

   How many milliliters will you draw from the vial after reconstitution? ______________

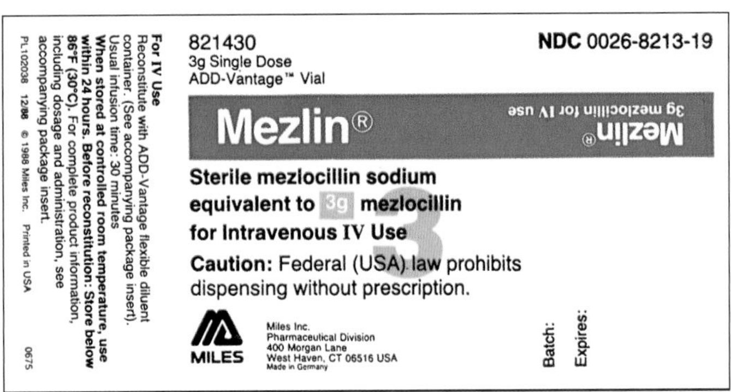

Courtesy of Miles.

5. Order: gentamicin 1 mg/kg IV every 8 hours for infection

   Supply: gentamicin 40 mg/mL

   Child's weight: 94 lb

   How many milliliters will you draw from the vial? ______________

6. Order: morphine 15 mg/hr IV for intractable pain

   Supply: morphine 300 mg/500 mL NS

   Calculate milliliters per hour to set the IV pump. ______________

7. Information obtained by the nurse: Dilaudid 50 mg in 250 mL NS is infusing at 25 mL/hr.

   How many milligrams per hour is the patient receiving? ______________

8. Order: add 10 mEq KCl to 1000 mL D5W

   Supply: KCl 20 mEq/20 mL

   How many milliliters will you draw from the vial to add to the IV bag? ____________

9. Information obtained by the nurse: nitroglycerin 50 mg in 500 mL D5W is infusing at 3 mL/hr.

   How many micrograms per minute is the patient receiving? ____________

10. Information obtained by the nurse: 1000 mL D5W with 10 mEq KCl is infusing at 100 mL/hr.

    How many milliequivalents of KCl is the patient receiving per hour? ____________

11. Order: infuse 1000 mL D5W at 250 mL/hr

    Drop factor: 20 gtt/mL

    Calculate the number of drops per minute. ____________

12. Order: infuse 750 mL NS over 5 hours

    Drop factor: 10 gtt/mL

    Calculate the number of drops per minute. ____________

13. Order: infuse 500 mL D5W over 8 hours

    Drop factor: 60 gtt/mL

    Calculate the number of drops per minute. ____________

14. Order: infuse 750 mL D5W

    Drop factor: 15 gtt/mL

    Infusion rate: 18 gtt/min

    Calculate the number of hours to infuse. ____________

(Practice problems continue on page 180)

15. Order: infuse 250 mL NS

    Drop factor: 15 gtt/mL

    Infusion rate: 50 gtt/min

    Calculate the number of hours to infuse. ______________

16. Order: infuse 1000 mL D5W/0.45% NS

    Drop factor: 15 gtt/mL

    Infusion rate: 25 gtt/min

    Calculate the number of hours to infuse. ______________

17. Order: Fortaz 1.25 g IV every 12 hours for urinary tract infection

    Supply: Fortaz 2-g vial

    Nursing drug reference: Dilute each 1 g with 10 mL of sterile water and further dilute in 100 mL 0.9% NS to infuse over 1 hour.

    How many milliliters will you draw from the vial after reconstitution? ______________

    Calculate the milliliters per hour to set the IV pump. ______________

    Calculate the drops per minute with a drop factor of 10 gtt/mL. ______________

18. Order: vancomycin 275 mg IV every 8 hours for infection

    Supply: vancomycin 500-mg vial

    Nursing drug reference: Reconstitute each 500-mg vial with 10 mL NS and further dilute with 250 mL NS to infuse over 1 hour.

    How many milliliters will you draw from the vial after reconstitution? ______________

    Calculate milliliters per hour to set the IV pump. ______________

    Calculate the drops per minute with a drop factor of 10 gtt/mL. ______________

19. Order: Mezlin 450 mg IV every 4 hours for infection

    Supply: Mezlin 4-g vial

    Nursing drug reference: Reconstitute each 1 g with 10 mL of sterile water and further dilute in 100 mL NS to infuse over 30 minutes.

    How many milliliters will you draw from the vial after reconstitution? ______________

    Calculate milliliters per hour to set the IV pump. ______________

    Calculate the drops per minute with a drop factor of 10 gtt/mL. ______________

20. Order: gentamicin 23 mg IV every 8 hours for infection

    Supply: gentamicin 40 mg/mL

    Nursing drug reference: Dilute with 100 mL NS and infuse over 1 hour.

    How many milliliters will you draw from the vial? ______________

    Calculate the milliliters per hour to set the IV pump. ______________

    Calculate the drops per minute with a drop factor of 15 gtt/mL. ______________

(Practice problems continue on page 182)

21. Order: Cortef 0.56 mg/kg PO daily for adrenal insufficiency

How many milliliters will you give a child weighing 18 kg? ______________

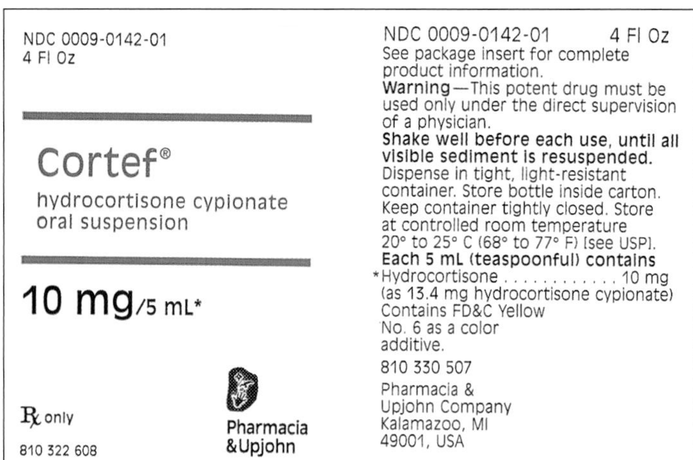

Courtesy of Pharmacia & Upjohn Company.

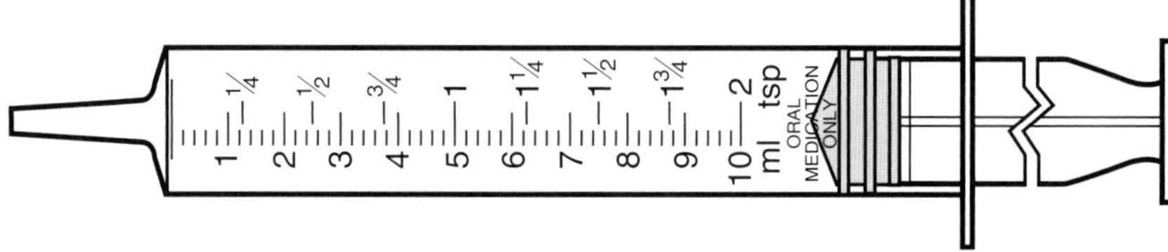

22. Order: Colestid 30 g/day PO in four divided doses for hypercholesterolemia or management of cholesterol

How many packets/dose will you give? ______________

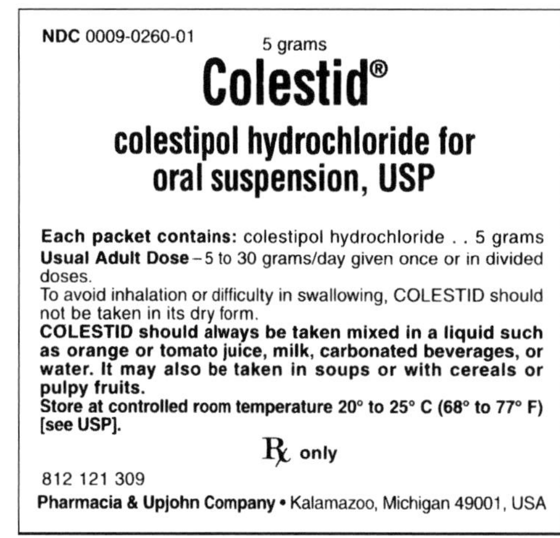

Courtesy of Pharmacia & Upjohn Company.

23. Order: vincristine 10 mcg/kg IV weekly for treatment of Hodgkin's lymphoma

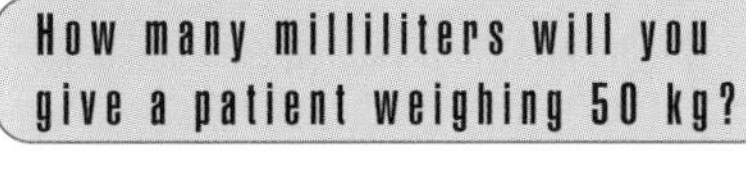

____

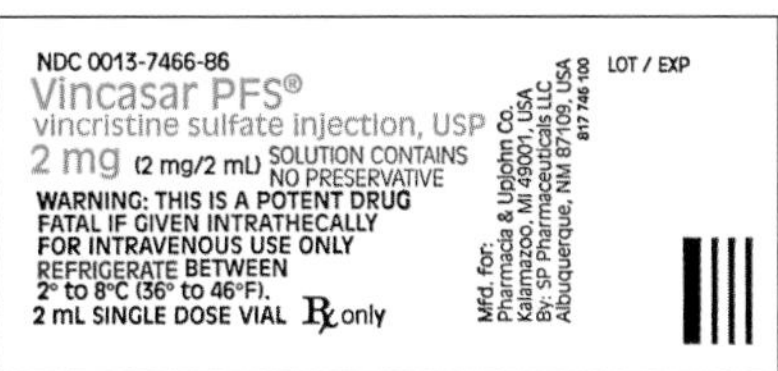

Courtesy of Pharmacia & Upjohn Company.

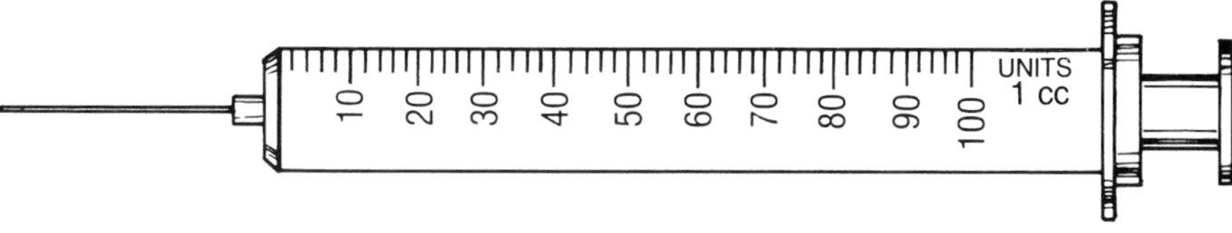

24. Order: Tagamet 1600 mg/day PO in two divided doses for gastroesophageal reflux disease

How many tablets per dose will you give? _______________

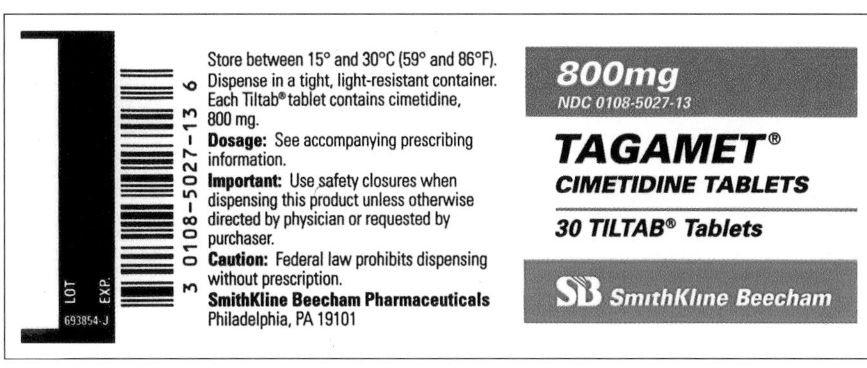

Courtesy of SmithKline Beecham Pharmaceuticals.

(Practice problems continue on page 184)

25. Order: Thorazine 1 g/day PO in three divided doses for psychoses

How many milliliters per dose will you give? ________

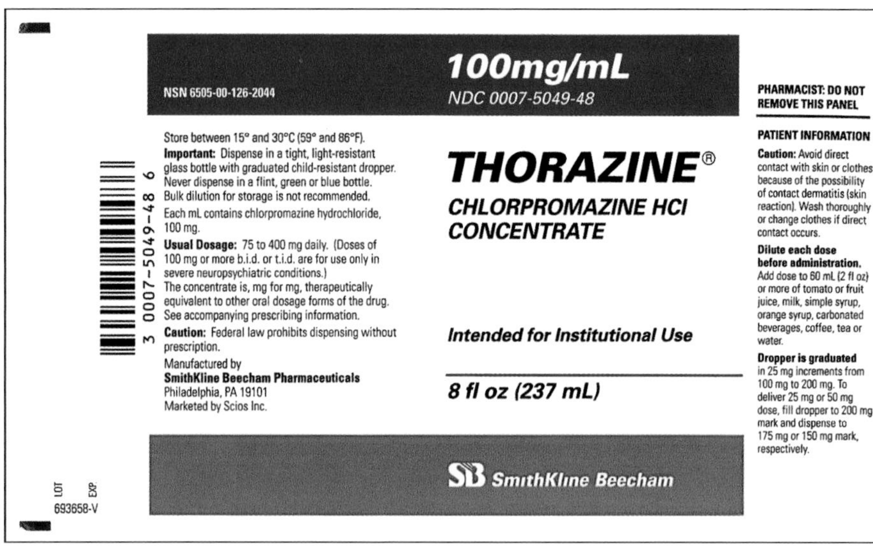

Courtesy of SmithKline Beecham Pharmaceuticals.

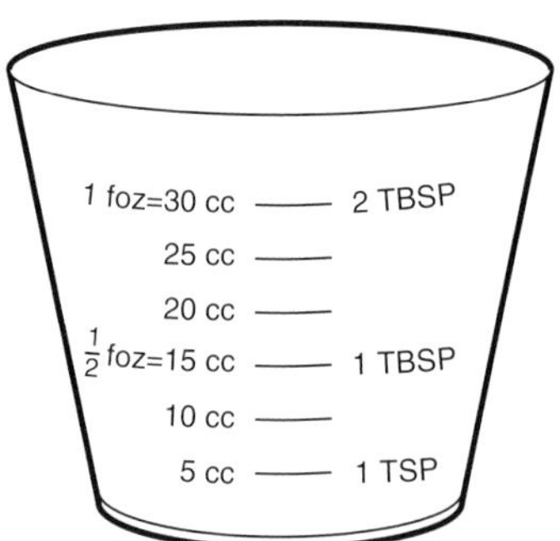

26. Order: Epivir 4 mg/kg PO bid for treatment of HIV infection

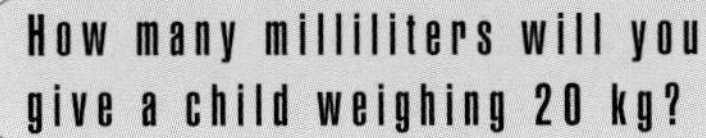
How many milliliters will you give a child weighing 20 kg? _______________

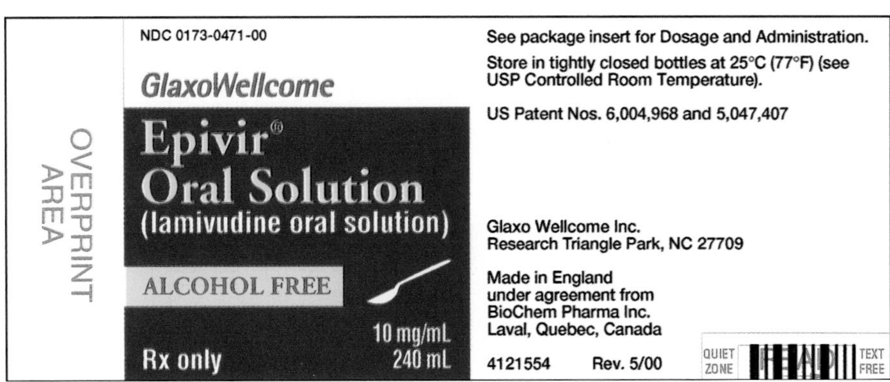

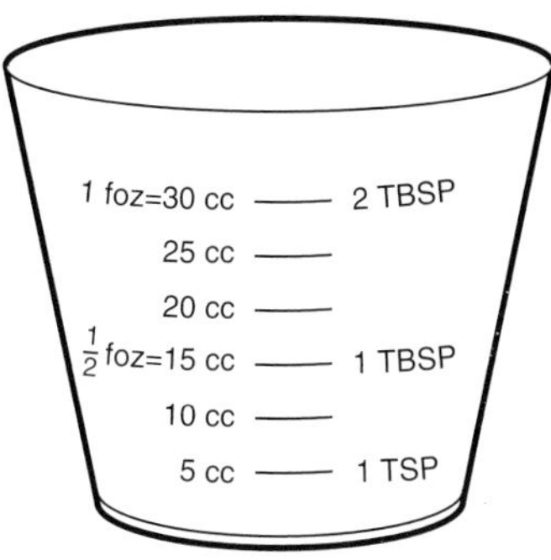

27. Order: Zofran 0.15 mg/kg IV 15 to 30 minutes prior to administration of chemotherapy for prevention of nausea and vomiting

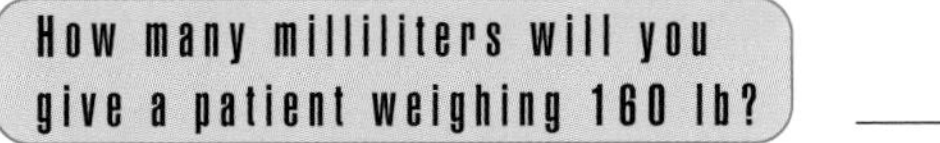
How many milliliters will you give a patient weighing 160 lb? _______________

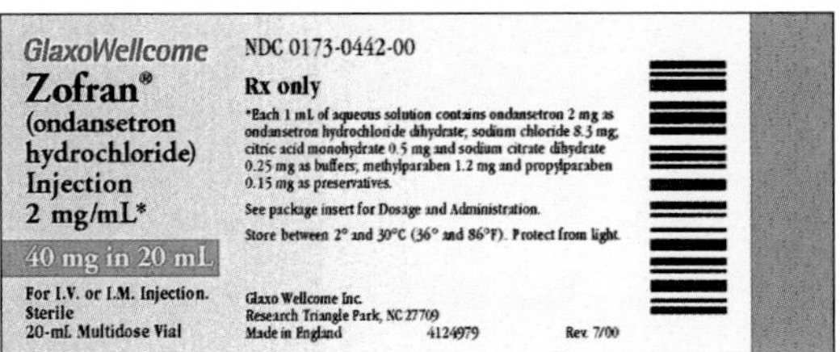

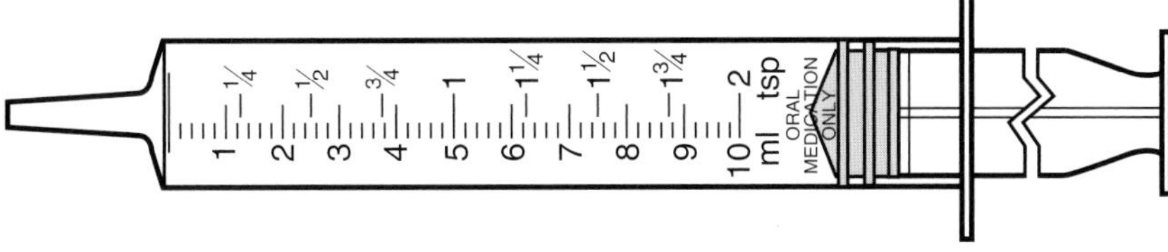

(Practice problems continue on page 186)

28. Order: Epivir 2 mg/kg PO twice daily for treatment of HIV infection

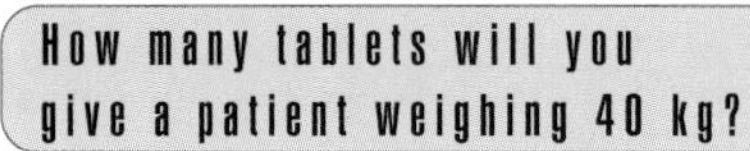

____

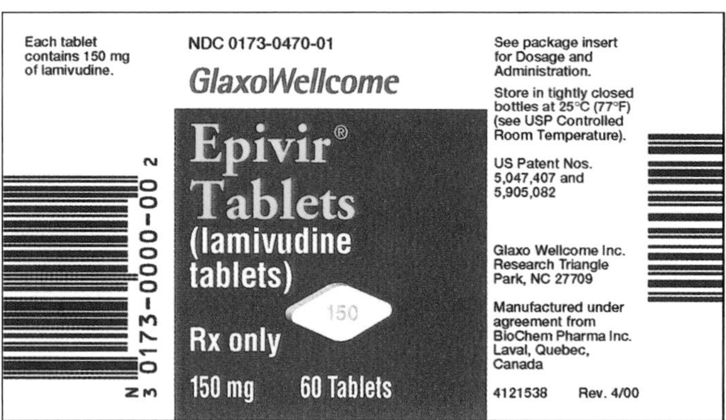

29. Order: Zovirax 20 mg/kg PO qid for 5 days for treatment of chickenpox

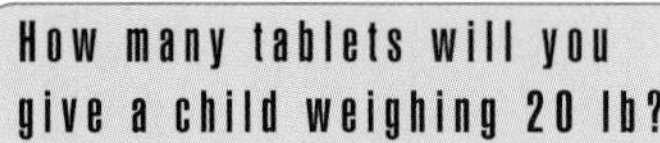

____

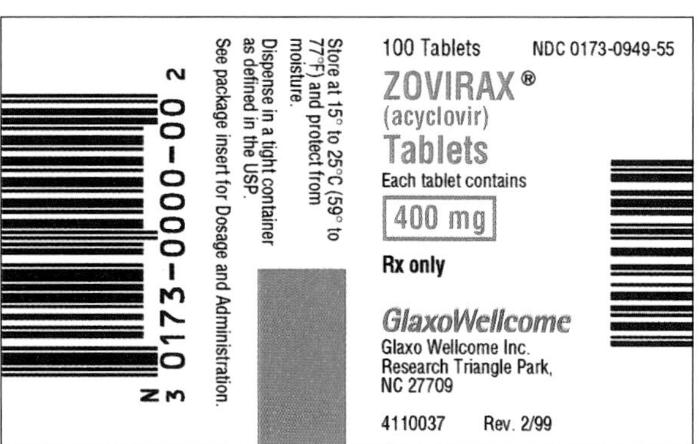

30. Order: Wellbutrin SR 450 mg/day PO in three divided doses for treatment of depression

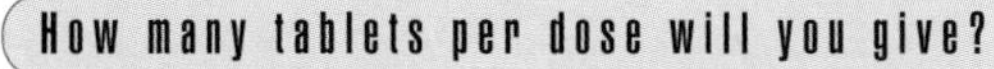

____

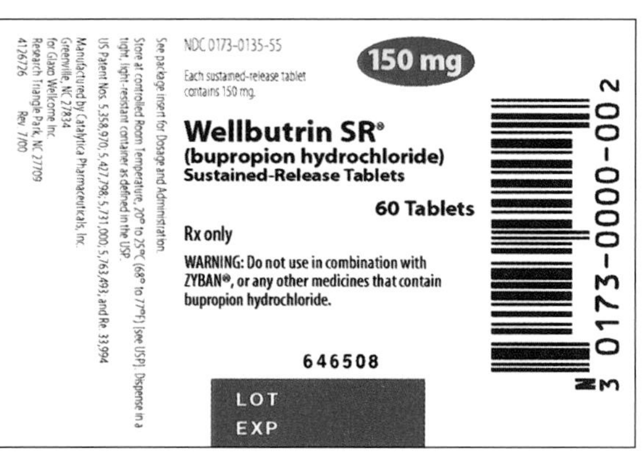

31. Order: Zantac 2.4 g/day PO in four divided doses for treatment of duodenal ulcer

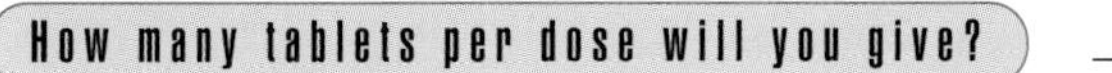

____

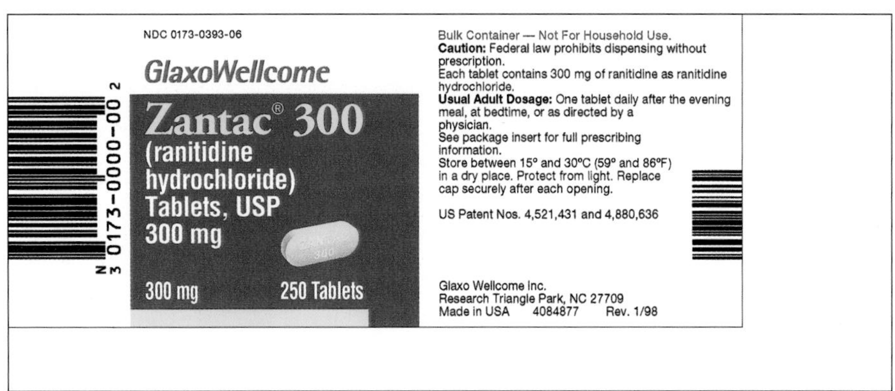

32. Order: Zinacef 500 mg/day IV in two divided doses for urinary tract infection

How many milliliters per dose will you give? _______________

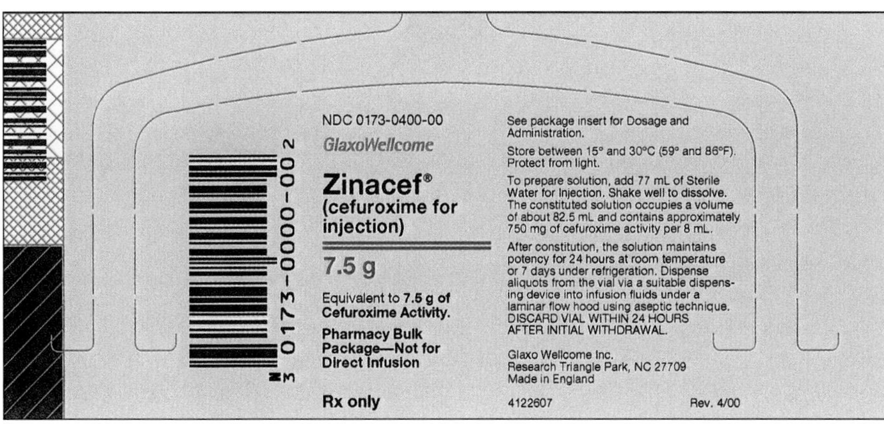

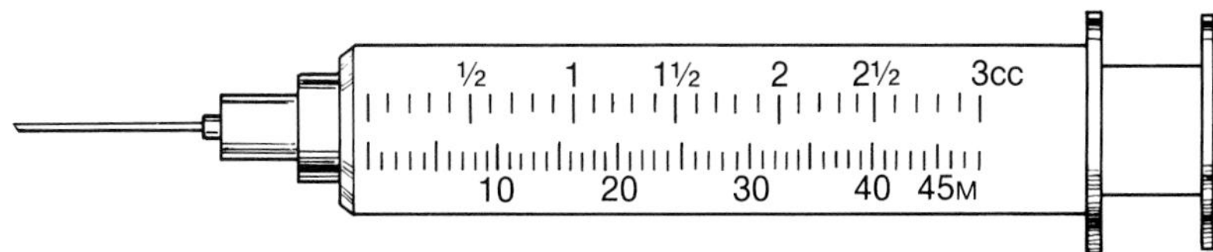

(Practice problems continue on page 188)

33. Order: Ceptaz 1000 mg/day IV in two divided doses for treatment of respiratory tract infection

Nursing drug reference: Dilute each 1-g vial with 10 mL of normal saline.

How many milliliters per dose will you give? ______________

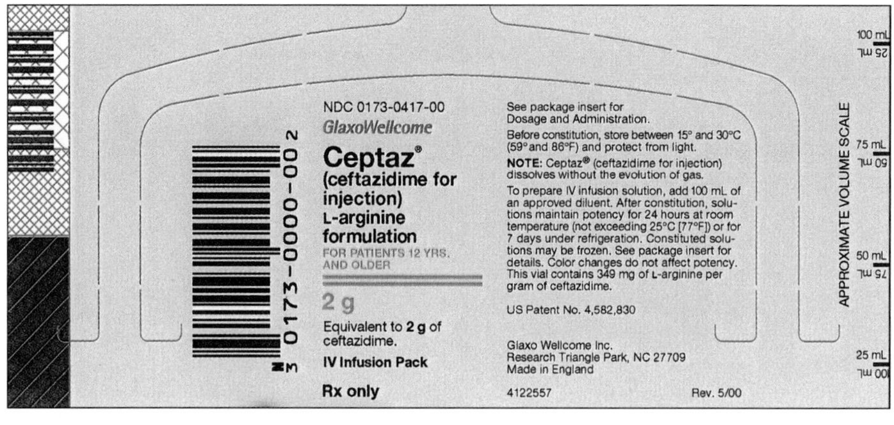

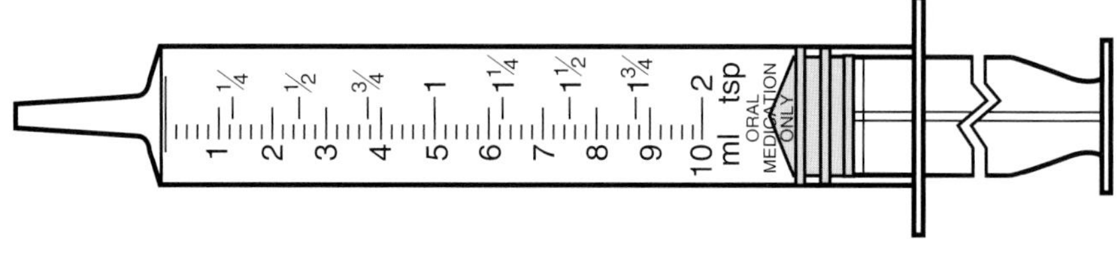

Practice Problems

Three-Factor Practice Problems

(See pages 203–205 for answers)

1. Order: Tagamet 40 mg/kg/day PO in four divided doses for treatment of active ulcer

Child's weight: 60 kg

How many milliliters per day will you give? ______________

How many milliliters per dose will you give? ______________

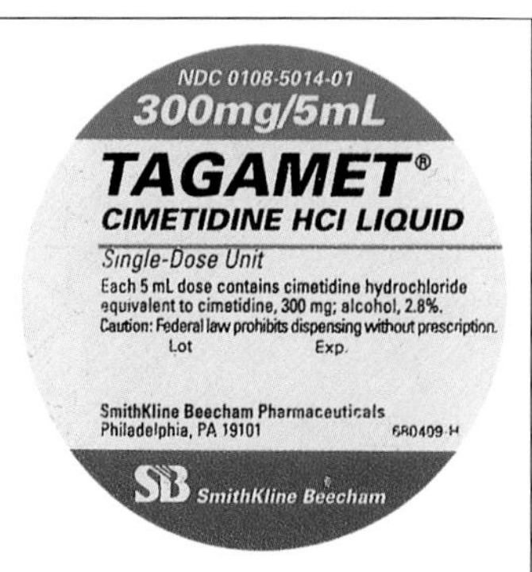

Courtesy of SmithKline Beecham Pharmaceuticals.

2. Order: furosemide 4 mg/kg/day IV for management of hypercalcemia of malignancy

   Child's weight: 60 lb

   How many milliliters per day will you give? __________

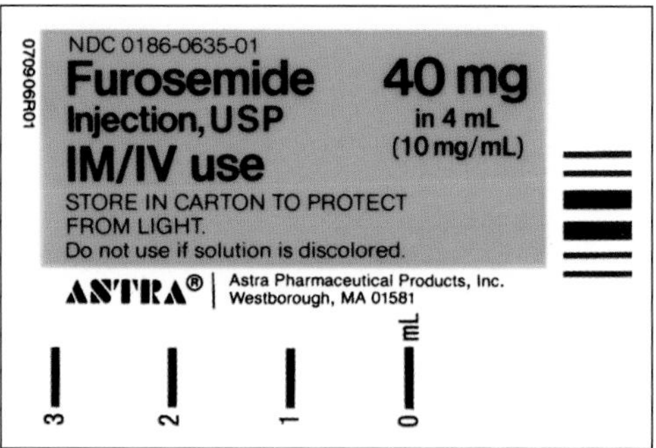

Courtesy of Astra Pharmaceutical Products.

3. Order: Cleocin 30 mg/kg/day IV in divided doses every 8 hours for infection

   Child's weight: 50 kg

   How many milliliters per day will you give? __________

   How many milliliters per dose will you give? __________

Single Dose Container
See package insert for complete product information. Store at controlled room temperature 15° to 30° C (59° to 86° F).
Do not refrigerate.
812 728 205
The Upjohn Company
Kalamazoo, MI 49001, USA
Upjohn NDC 0009-0870-21
2 mL Vial
Cleocin Phosphate®
Sterile Solution
clindamycin phosphate injection, USP
300mg Equivalent to 300mg clindamycin

Courtesy of the Upjohn Company.

4. Information obtained by the nurse: A child is receiving 0.575 mL/dose of gentamicin IV every 8 hours from a supply of gentamicin 40 mg/mL.

   Child's weight: 45 lb

   How many milligrams per kilogram per day is the patient receiving? __________

5. Information obtained by the nurse: A child is receiving 0.125 mL/dose of diphenhydramine (Benadryl) IV every 8 hours from a supply of Benadryl 50 mg/mL.

   Child's weight: 20 lb

   How many milligrams per kilogram per day is the child receiving? __________

(Practice problems continue on page 190)

6. Order: dopamine 5 mcg/kg/min IV for decreased cardiac output

   Supply: dopamine 400-mg vial

   Nursing drug reference: Dilute each 400-mg vial in 250 mL NS

   Patient's weight: 110 lb

   How many milliliters will you draw from the vial? ______

   Calculate the milliliters per hour to set the IV pump. ______

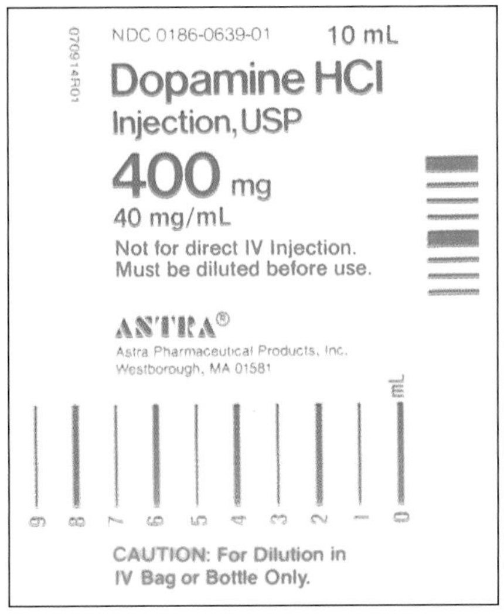

Courtesy of Astra Pharmaceutical Products.

7. Order: Nipride 0.8 mcg/kg/min IV for hypertensive crisis

   Supply: Nipride 50 mg/500 mL NS

   Patient's weight: 143 lb

   Calculate the milliliters per hour to set the IV pump. ______

8. Information obtained by the nurse: Nipride 50 mg in 250 mL NS is infusing at 68 mL/hr.

   Patient's weight: 250 lb

   How many micrograms per kilogram per minute is the patient receiving? ______

9. Order: Hydrea 30 mg/kg/day PO for ovarian carcinoma

   Patient's weight: 157 lb

   How many grams per day is the patient receiving? ______

10. Order: Venoglobulin-S 0.01 mL/kg/min for treatment of immunodeficiency syndrome.

    Patient's weight: 180 lb

    Calculate milliliters per hour to set the IV pump. ______________

11. Information obtained by the nurse: dopamine 400 mg in 250 mL D5W is infusing at 28 mL/hr.

    Patient's weight: 15 kg

    How many micrograms per kilogram per minute is the patient receiving? ______________

12. Order: Inocor 3 mcg/kg/min IV for congestive heart failure

    Supply: Inocor 100 mg/100 mL of 0.9% NS

    Patient's weight: 160 lb

    Calculate milliliters per hour to set the IV pump. ______________

13. Order: Nipride 2 mcg/kg/min.

    Supply: Nipride 50 mg/250 mL NS

    Patient's weight: 250 lb

    Calculate milliliters per hour to set the IV pump. ______________

14. Order: Nipride 1 mcg/kg/min IV for hypertensive crisis

    Supply: Nipride 50 mg/250 mL NS

    Patient's weight: 160 lb

    Calculate milliliters per hour to set the IV pump. ______________

15. Order: dopamine 2.5 mcg/kg/min IV for hypotension

    Supply: dopamine 400 mg/500 mL D5W

    Patient's weight: 65 kg

    Calculate milliliters per hour to set the IV pump. ______________

(Practice problems continue on page 192)

16. Information obtained by the nurse: Isuprel 2 mg in 500 mL D5W is infusing at 15 mL/hr.

    Child's weight: 20 kg

    How many micrograms per kilogram per minute is the child receiving? ____________

17. Order: Intropin 5 mcg/kg/min IV for treatment of oliguria after shock

    Supply: Intropin 400 mg/500 mL NS

    Patient's weight: 70 kg

    Calculate milliliters per minute. ____________

18. Order: vancomycin 40 mg/kg/day IV in three divided doses for infection

    Supply: vancomycin 500-mg vial

    Nursing drug reference: Reconstitute each 500-mg vial with 10 mL sterile water and further dilute in 100 mL of 0.9% NS to infuse over 60 minutes.

    Child's weight: 20 lb

    How many milligrams per day is the child receiving? ____________

    How many milligrams per dose is the child receiving? ____________

    How many milliliters will you draw from the vial after reconstitution? ____________

    Calculate milliliters per hour to set the IV pump. ____________

19. Order: gentamicin 2 mg/kg/dose IV every 8 hours for infection

    Supply: gentamicin 40-mg/mL vial

    Nursing drug reference: Further dilute in 50 mL NS and infuse over 30 minutes.

    Child's weight: 40 kg

    How many milligrams per dose is the child receiving? ____________

    How many milliliters will you draw from the vial? ____________

    Calculate milliliters per hour to set the IV pump. ____________

20. Order: Ancef 25 mg/kg/day IV every 8 hours for infection

Supply: Ancef 500-mg vial

Nursing drug reference: Reconstitute each 500-mg vial with 10 mL of sterile water and further dilute in 50 mL NS to infuse over 30 minutes.

Child's weight: 25 kg

How many milligrams per day is the child receiving? ______________

How many milligrams per dose is the child receiving? ______________

How many milliliters will you draw from the vial after reconstitution? ______________

Calculate milliliters per hour to set the IV pump. ______________

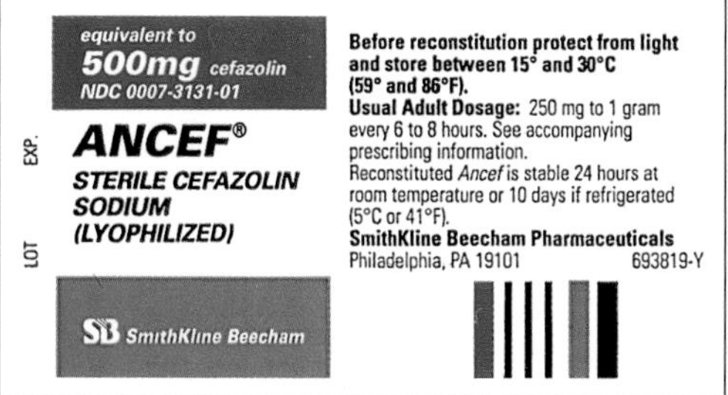

Courtesy of SmithKline Beecham Pharmaceuticals.

Practice Problems — Comprehensive Practice Problems

(See pages 206–208 for answers)

1. Order: digoxin 0.125 mg PO daily for congestive heart failure

   On hand: digoxin 0.25 mg/tablet

   How many tablets will you give? ______________

2. Order: ascorbic acid 0.5 g PO daily for supplemental therapy

   On hand: ascorbic acid 500 mg/tablet

   How many tablets will you give? ______________

3. Order: atropine gr 1/150 IM for on-call preanesthesia

   Supply: atropine 0.4 mg/mL

   How many milliliters will you give? ______________

(Practice problems continue on page 194)

4. Order: Mycostatin oral suspension 500,000 units swish-and-swallow for oral thrush

   On hand: Mycostatin 100,000 units/mL

   How many teaspoons will you give? ______________

5. Order: Demerol 50 mg IM every 4 hours for pain

   Supply: Demerol 100 mg/mL

   How many milliliters will you give? ______________

6. Order: vancomycin 2 mg/kg IV every 12 hours for infection

   Supply: vancomycin 500 mg/10 mL

   Patient's weight: 75 kg

   How many milliliters will you give? ______________

7. Order: ampicillin 2 mg/kg PO every 8 hours for infection

   Supply: ampicillin 500 mg/5 mL

   Patient's weight: 100 lb

   How many milliliters will you give? ______________

8. Order: 1000 mL D5W to infuse in 12 hours

   Drop factor: 15 gtt/mL

   Calculate the number of drops per minute. ______________

9. Order: 500 mL D5W

   Drop factor: 15 gtt/mL

   Infusion rate: 21 gtt/min

   Calculate hours to infuse. ______________

10. Order: heparin 1500 units/hr

    Supply: 250-mL IV bag of D5W with 25,000 units of heparin

    Calculate milliliters per hour to set the IV pump. ______________

11. Order: 1000 mL NS IV

    Drop factor: 15 gtt/mL

    Infusion rate: 50 gtt/min

    Calculate hours to infuse. ______________

12. Order: regular insulin 8 units per hour IV for hyperglycemia

    Supply: 250 mL NS with 100 units of regular insulin

    Calculate milliliters per hour to set the IV pump. ____________

13. Order: 500 mL of 10% lipids to infuse in 8 hours

    Drop factor: 10 gtt/mL

    Calculate the number of drops per minute. ____________

14. Order: KCl 2 mEq/100 mL of D5W for hypokalemia

    On hand: 20 mEq/10-mL vial

    Supply: 500 mL D5W

    How many milliliters of KCl will you add to the IV bag? ____________

15. Order: aminophylline 44 mg/hr IV for bronchodilation

    Supply: 250 mL D5W with 1 g of aminophylline

    Calculate milliliters per hour to set the IV pump. ____________

16. Order: Dilaudid 140 mL/hr

    Supply: 1000 mL D5W/NS with 30 mg of Dilaudid

    Calculate milligrams per hour that the patient is receiving. ____________

17. Order: Staphcillin 750 mg IV every 4 hours for infection

    Supply: Staphcillin 6 g

    Nursing drug reference: Reconstitute with 8.6 mL of sterile water to yield 500 mg/mL and further dilute in 100 mL of NS to infuse over 30 minutes.

    How many milliliters will you draw from the vial after reconstitution? ____________

    Calculate milliliters per hour to set the IV pump. ____________

    Calculate the drops per minute with a drop factor of 10 gtt/mL. ____________

(Practice problems continue on page 196)

18. Order: Pipracil 1.5 g every 6 hours for uncomplicated urinary tract infection

    Supply: Pipracil 3-g vial

    Nursing drug reference: Reconstitute each 3-g vial with 5 mL of sterile water and further dilute in 50 mL of 0.9% NS to infuse over 20 minutes.

    How many milliliters will you draw from the vial after reconstitution? ______________

    Calculate milliliters per hour to set the IV pump. ______________

    Calculate the drops per minute with a drop factor of 20 gtt/mL. ______________

19. Order: dopamine 4 mcg/kg/min IV for decreased cardiac output

    Supply: 250 mL D5W with 400 mg of dopamine

    Patient's weight: 120 lb

    Calculate milliliters per hour to set the IV pump. ______________

20. Order: Nipride 0.8 mcg/kg/min IV for hypertension

    Supply: 500 mL D5W with 50 mg Nipride

    Patient's weight: 143 lb

    Calculate milliliters per hour to set the IV pump. ______________

ANSWER KEY FOR SECTION 2: PRACTICE PROBLEMS

One-Factor Practice Problems

1. Sequential method:

2~~00~~ ~~mg~~	(mL)	2	= 2 mL
	1~~00~~ ~~mg~~	1	

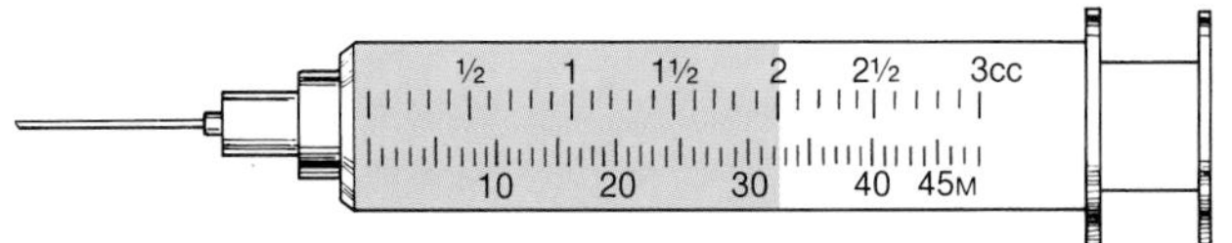

2. Sequential method:

3~~0~~ ~~mg~~	(tablet)	3	= 1 tablet
	3~~0~~ ~~mg~~	3	

3. Sequential method:

7.5 ~~mg~~	(tablet)	7.5	= 3 tablets
	2.5 ~~mg~~	2.5	

4. Sequential method:

~~160 mg~~	~~5 mL~~	1 (tsp)	1	= 1 tsp
	~~160 mg~~	~~5 mL~~		

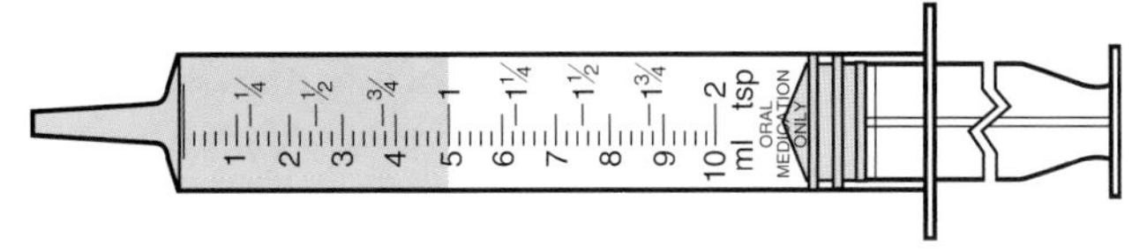

5. Sequential method:

0.5 ~~mg~~	(tablet)	0.5	= 0.5 tablet
	1 ~~mg~~	1	

6. Sequential method:

~~60 mg~~	(tablet)	= 1 tablet
	~~60 mg~~	

7. Sequential method:

0.25 ~~mg~~	(tablet)	0.25	= 2 tablets
	0.125 ~~mg~~	0.125	

8. Sequential method:

8~~0~~ ~~mg~~	(tablet)	8	= 4 tablets
	2~~0~~ ~~mg~~	2	

9. Random method:

1~~0~~ ~~mg~~	(mL)	1 ~~gr~~	1 × 1	1	1	= 1.33 or 1.3 mL
	$\frac{1}{8}$ ~~gr~~	6~~0~~ ~~mg~~	$\frac{1}{8} \times \frac{6}{1}$	$\frac{6}{8}$	0.75	

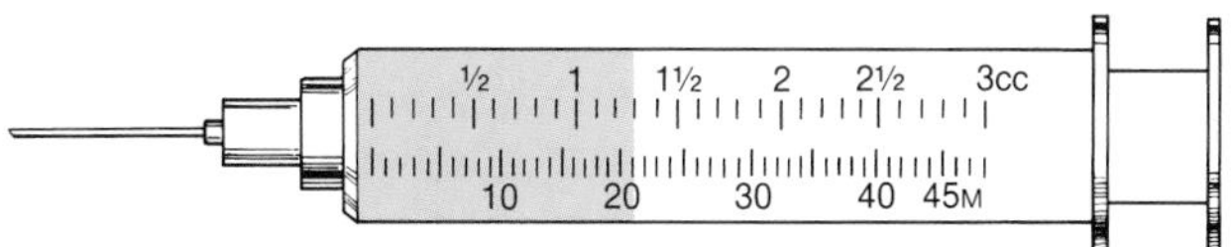

10. Random method:

1~~00~~ ~~mcg~~	(mL)	1 ~~mg~~	1 × 1	1	= 0.25 or 0.3 mL
	0.4 ~~mg~~	1~~000~~ ~~mcg~~	0.4 × 10	4	

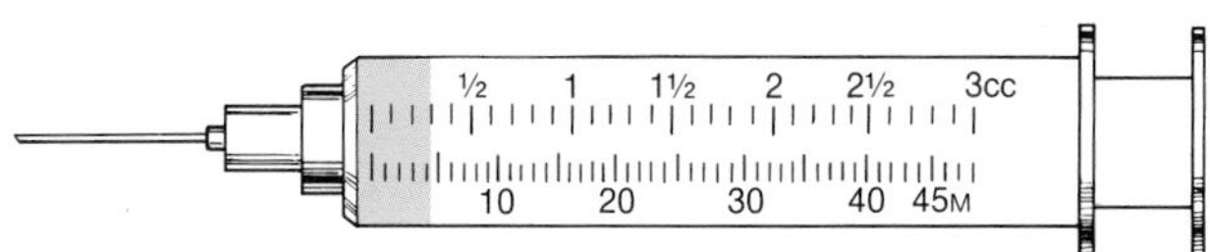

11. Sequential method:

80 ~~mg~~	2 (mL)	80 × 2	160	= 1.28 or 1.3 mL
	125 ~~mg~~	125	125	

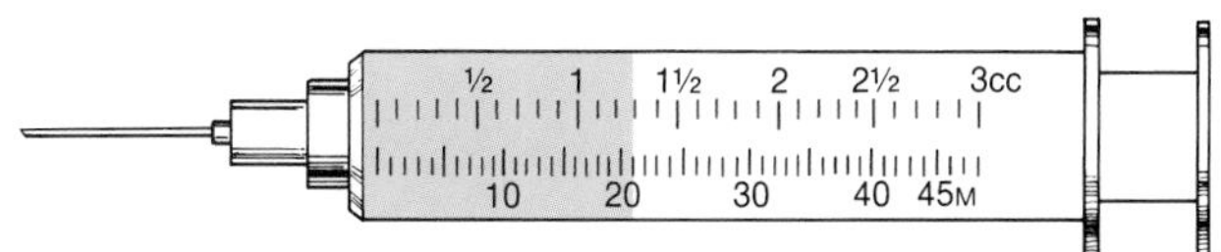

12. Sequential method:

~~20 g~~	15 (mL)	2 × 15	30	= 30 mL
	~~10 g~~	1	1	

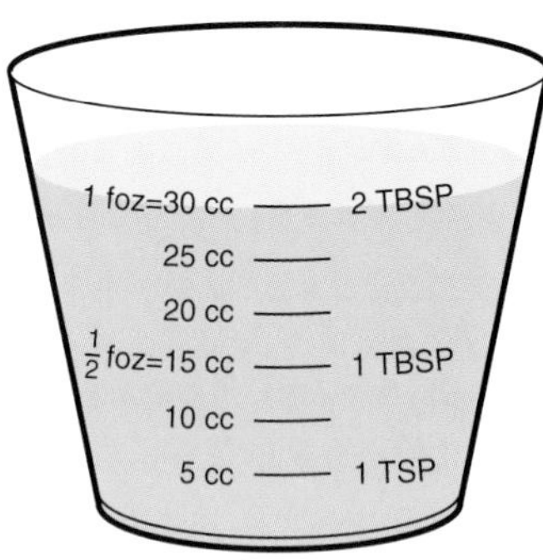

13. Sequential method:

~~5 mg~~	(mL)	= 1 mL
	~~5 mg~~	

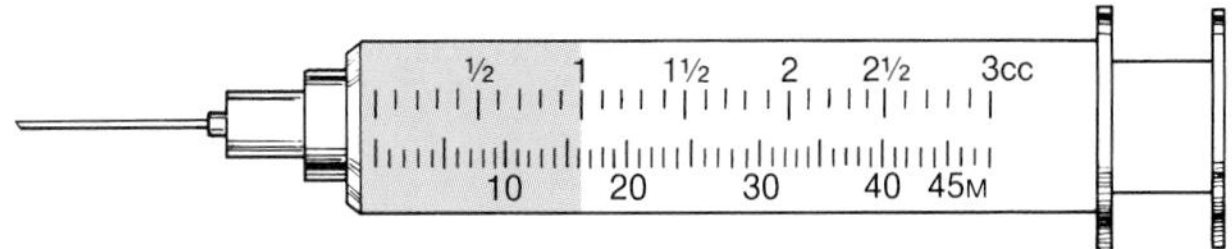

14. Sequential method:

250 ~~mg~~	5 (mL)	250 × 5	1250	= 10 mL
	125 ~~mg~~	125	125	

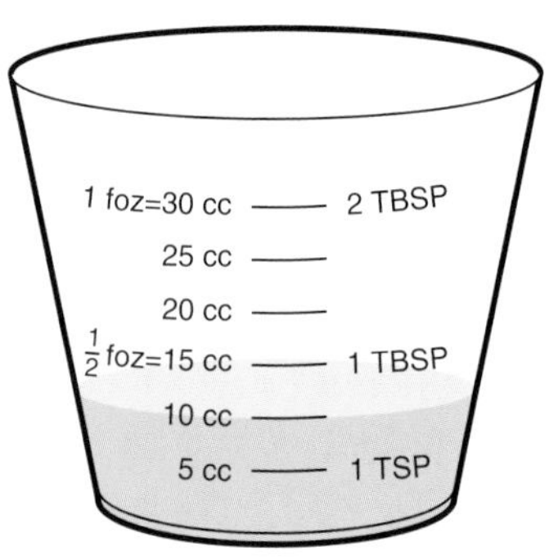

15. Sequential method:

~~200 mg~~	(capsules)	2	= 2 capsules
	~~100 mg~~	1	

16. Sequential method:

10 ~~mg~~	(tablet)	10	= 2 tablets
	5 ~~mg~~	5	

17. Sequential method:

3 ~~mg~~	(mL)	3	= 1.5 mL
	2 ~~mg~~	2	

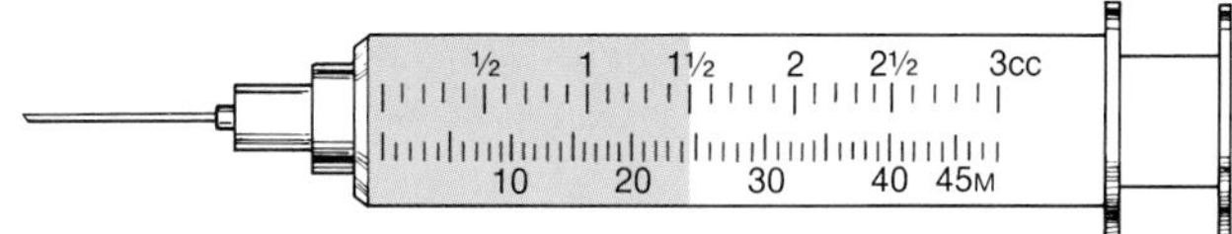

18. Sequential method:

400 ~~mg~~	10.15 (mL)	400 × 10.15	4060	= 12.49 or 12.5 mL
	325 ~~mg~~	325	325	

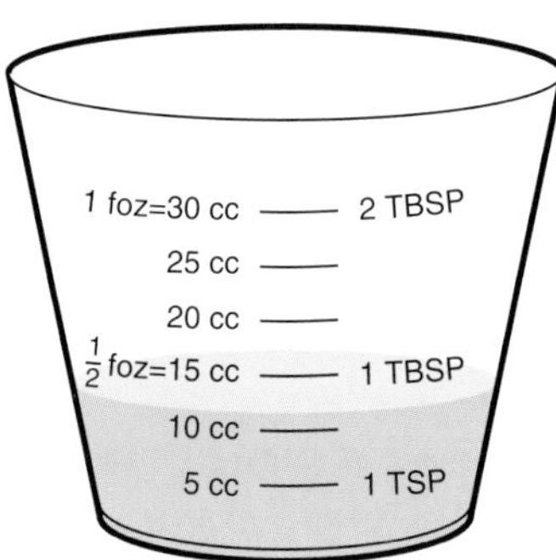

19. Random method:

~~1000 mg~~	2 (mL)	1 ~~g~~	2 × 1	2	= 2 mL
	1 ~~g~~	~~1000 mg~~	1	1	

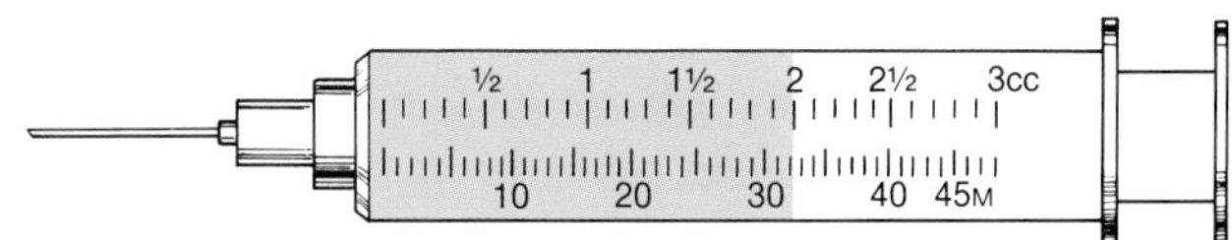

20. Sequential method:

10 ~~mg~~	~~5 mL~~	1 (tsp)	10 × 1	10	= 2 tsp
	~~5 mg~~	5 ~~mL~~	5	5	

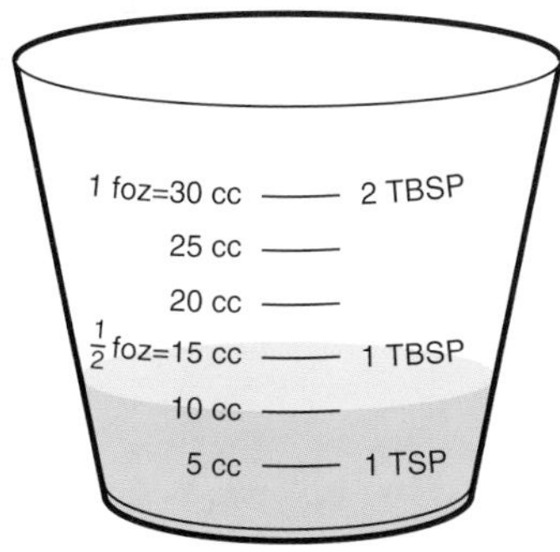

21. Random method:

0.25 ~~mg~~	(mL)	100~~0 mcg~~	0.25 × 100	25	= 1 mL
	25~~0 mcg~~	1 ~~mg~~	25 × 1	25	

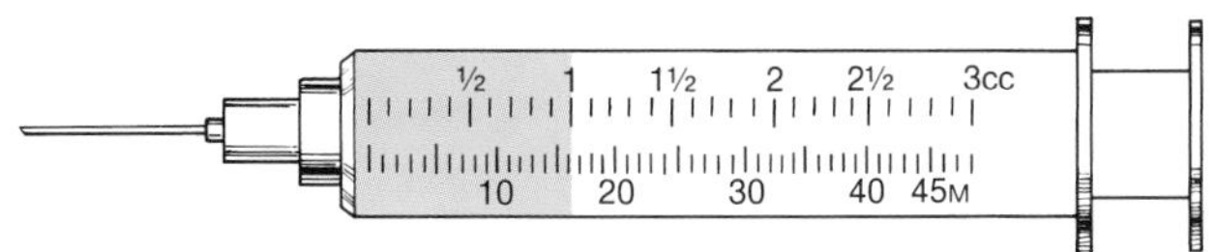

22. Sequential method:

50~~0 mg~~	(mL)	5	= 1.66 or 1.7 mL
	30~~0 mg~~	3	

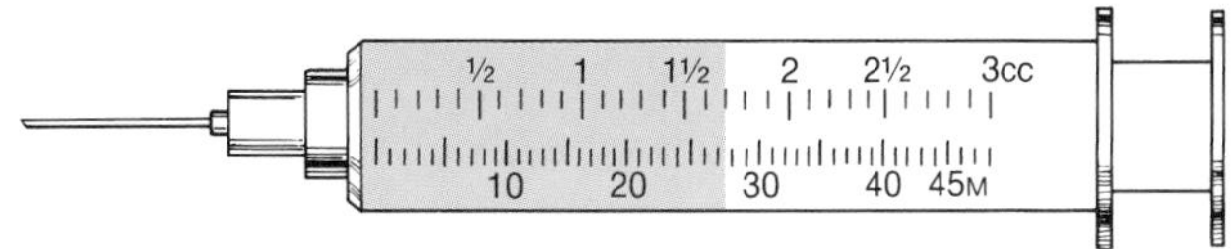

23. Sequential method:

~~2500 IU~~	0.2 (mL)	0.2	= 0.2 mL
	~~2500 IU~~		

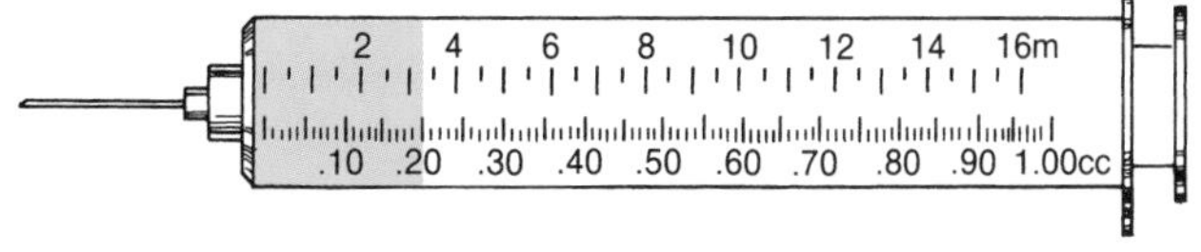

24. Sequential method:

20~~0 mg~~	5 (mL)	20 × 5	100	= 20 mL
	5~~0 mg~~	5	5	

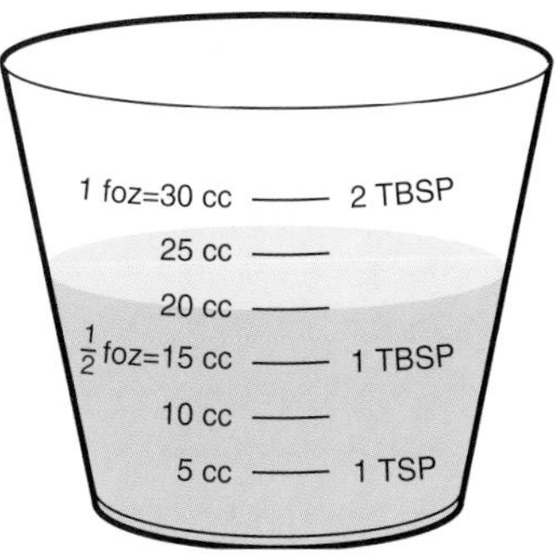

25. Sequential method:

30~~0 mg~~	(capsule)	30	= 2 capsules
	15~~0 mg~~	15	

26. Sequential method:

500 ~~mg~~	(tablets)	500	= 1 tablet
	500 ~~mg~~	500	

27. Sequential method:

0.25 ~~mg~~	(tablets)	0.25	= 2 tablets
	0.125 ~~mg~~	0.125	

28. Sequential method:

25 ~~mg~~	(tablets)	25	= 0.5 tablet
	50 ~~mg~~	50	

29. Sequential method:

5 ~~mg~~	(tablets)	5	= 2 tablets
	2.5 ~~mg~~	2.5	

30. Sequential method:

0.5 ~~mg~~	(tablets)	0.5	= 2 tablets
	0.25 ~~mg~~	0.25	

31. Sequential method:

15~~0~~ ~~mg~~	(mL)	15	= 0.375 or 0.4 mL
	40~~0~~ ~~mg~~	40	

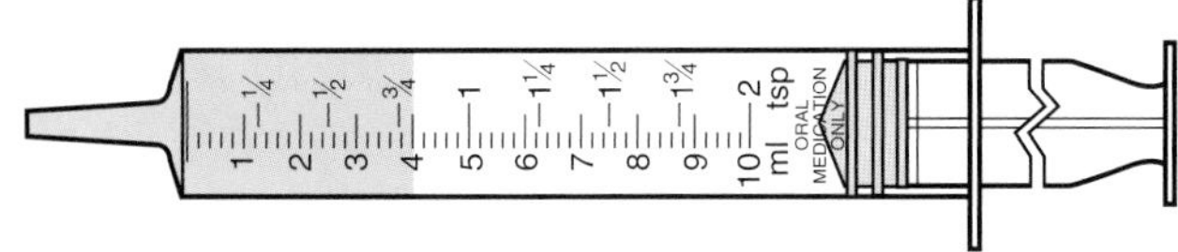

32. Sequential method:

6~~00~~ ~~mg~~	(tablets)	6	= 2 tablets
	3~~00~~ ~~mg~~	3	

Two-Factor Practice Problems

1. Random method:

25 ~~mcg~~	2.5 (mL)	1 ~~kg~~	1 ~~mg~~	25 ~~lb~~	= mL
~~kg~~	0.125 ~~mg~~	2.2 ~~lb~~	1000 ~~mcg~~		

25 × 2.5 × 1 × 1 × 25	1562.5	= 5.68 or 5.7 mL
0.125 × 2.2 × 1000	275	

2. Sequential method:

0.02 ~~mg~~	(mL)	1 ~~kg~~	35 ~~lb~~	0.02 × 1 × 35	0.7	= 3.18 or 3.2 mL
~~kg~~	0.1 ~~mg~~	2.2 ~~lb~~		0.1 × 2.2	0.22	

3. Random method:

~~2 mg~~	50~~0~~ (mL)	~~1 g~~	6~~0~~ ~~min~~	5 × 6	30	= 30 mL/hr
~~min~~	~~2 g~~	1~~000~~ ~~mg~~	~~1~~ (hr)	1	1	

4. Sequential method:

1.5 ~~g~~	10 (mL)	1.5 × 10	15	= 15 mL
	1 ~~g~~	1	1	

5. Sequential method:

1 ~~mg~~	(mL)	1 ~~kg~~	94 ~~lb~~	1 × 1 × 94	94	= 1.068 or 1.1 mL
~~kg~~	40 ~~mg~~	2.2 ~~lb~~		40 × 2.2	88	

6. Sequential method:

15 ~~mg~~	50~~0~~ (mL)	15 × 5	75	= 25 mL/hr
(hr)	3~~00~~ ~~mg~~	3	3	

7. Sequential method:

~~25 mL~~	5~~0~~ (mg)	5	= 5 mg/hr
(hr)	~~25~~0 ~~mL~~		

8. Sequential method:

10 ~~mEq~~	~~20~~ (mL)	10	= 10 mL
	~~20 mEq~~		

9. Sequential method:

3 ~~mL~~	~~50 mg~~	10~~00~~ (mcg)	~~1 hr~~	3 × 10	30	= 5 mcg/min
~~hr~~	~~500 mL~~	~~1 mg~~	6~~0~~ (min)	6	6	

10. Sequential method:

1~~00~~ ~~mL~~	~~10~~ (mEq)	1	= 1 mEq/hr
(hr)	~~1000 mL~~		

11. Sequential method:

250 ~~mL~~	2~~0~~ (gtt)	1 ~~hr~~	250 × 2 × 1	500	= 83.3 or 83 gtt/min
~~hr~~	~~mL~~	6~~0~~ (min)	6	6	

12. Sequential method:

750 ~~mL~~	1~~0~~ (gtt)	1 ~~hr~~	750 × 1 × 1	750	= 25 gtt/min
5 ~~hr~~	~~mL~~	6~~0~~ (min)	5 × 6	30	

13. Sequential method:

500 ~~mL~~	~~60~~ (gtt)	1 ~~hr~~	500 × 1	500	= 62.5 or 63 gtt/min
8 ~~hr~~	~~mL~~	~~60~~ (min)	8	8	

14. Sequential method:

750 ~~mL~~	15 ~~gtt~~	~~min~~	1 (hr)	750 × 15 × 1	11250	= 10.41or 10 hr
	~~mL~~	18 ~~gtt~~	60 ~~min~~	18 × 60	1080	

15. Sequential method:

25~~0~~ ~~mL~~	15 ~~gtt~~	~~min~~	1 (hr)	25 × 15 × 1	375	= 1.25 or
	~~mL~~	50 ~~gtt~~	6~~0~~ ~~min~~	50 × 6	300	1 hr

16. Sequential method:

100~~0~~ ~~mL~~	15 ~~gtt~~	~~min~~	1 (hr)	100 × 15 × 1	1500	= 10 hr
	~~mL~~	25 ~~gtt~~	6~~0~~ ~~min~~	25 × 6	150	

17. Sequential method:

1.25 ~~g~~	10 (mL)	1.25 × 10	12.5	= 12.5 mL
	1 ~~g~~	1	1	

Calculate milliliter per hour to set the IV pump
Sequential method:

$$\frac{112.5\ (mL)}{(hr)} = 112.5 \text{ or } \frac{113\ mL}{hr}$$

Calculate drops per minute with a drop factor of 10 gtt/mL.
Sequential method:

112.5 ~~mL~~	1~~0~~ (gtt)	1 ~~hr~~	112.5 × 1 × 1	112.5	=	18.75 or 19 gtt
~~hr~~	~~mL~~	6~~0~~ (min)	6	6		min

18. How many milliliters will you draw from the vial after reconstitution?
Sequential method:

275 ~~mg~~	1~~0~~ (mL)	275 × 1	275	= 5.5 mL
	50~~0~~ ~~mg~~	50	50	

Calculate milliliters per hour to set the IV pump.
Sequential method:

$$\frac{255.5\ (mL)}{(hr)} = 255.5 \text{ or } \frac{256\ mL}{hr}$$

Calculate drops per minute with a drop factor of 10 gtt/mL.
Sequential method:

255.5 ~~mL~~	1~~0~~ (gtt)	1 ~~hr~~	255.5 × 1 × 1	255.5	=	42.5 or 43 gtt
~~hr~~	~~mL~~	6~~0~~ (min)	6	6		min

19. Random method:

45~~0~~ ~~mg~~	1~~0~~ (mL)	~~1 g~~	45 × 1	45	= 4.5 mL
	~~1 g~~	100~~0~~ ~~mg~~	10	10	

Calculate milliliters per hour to set the IV pump.
Sequential method:

104.5 (mL)	6~~0~~ ~~min~~	104.5 × 6	627	=	209 mL
3~~0~~ ~~min~~	1 (hr)	3 × 1	3		hr

Calculate drops per minute with a drop factor of 10 gtt/mL.
Sequential method:

104.5 ~~mL~~	1~~0~~ (gtt)	104.5 × 1	104.5	=	34.8 or 35 gtt
3~~0~~ (min)	~~mL~~	3	3		min

20. How many milliliters will you draw from the vial?
Sequential method:

23 ~~mg~~	(mL)	23	= 0.57 or 0.6 mL
	40 ~~mg~~	40	

Calculate milliliters per hour to set the IV pump.
Sequential method:

$$\frac{100.6\ (mL)}{(hr)} = 100.6 \text{ or } \frac{101\ mL}{hr}$$

Calculate drops per minute with a drop factor of 15 gtt/mL.

100.6 ~~mL~~	15 (gtt)	1 ~~hr~~	100.6 × 15 × 1	1509	=	25.15 or 25 gtt
~~hr~~	~~mL~~	60 (min)	60	60		min

21. Sequential method:

0.56 ~~mg~~	18 ~~kg~~	5 mL	0.56 × 18 × 5	50.4	= 5.04 or 5 mL
~~kg~~		10 ~~mg~~	10	10	

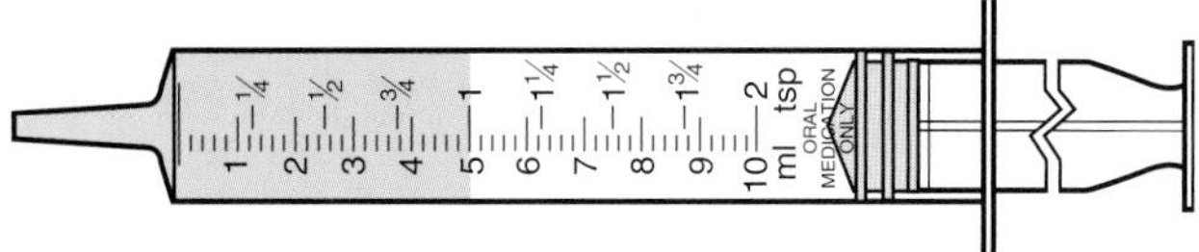

22. Random method:

30 ~~g~~	~~day~~	packet	30	30	= 1.5 packet / dose
~~day~~	4 doses	5 ~~g~~	4 × 5	20	

23. Random method:

10 ~~mcg~~	2 mL	50 ~~kg~~	1 ~~mg~~	1 × 2 × 5 × 1	10	= 0.5 mL
~~kg~~	2 ~~mg~~		1000 ~~mcg~~	2 × 10	20	

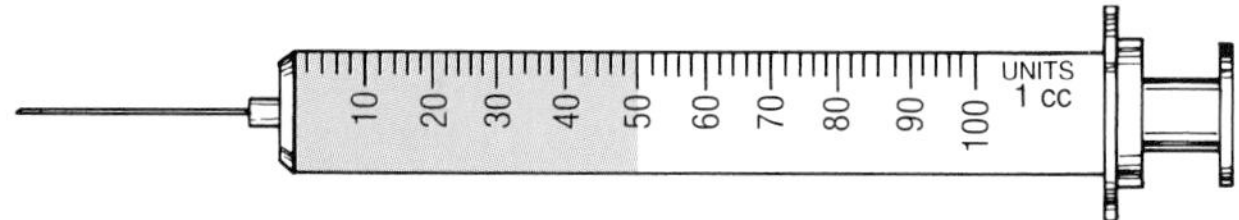

24. Sequential method:

1600 ~~mg~~	tablets	~~day~~	16	16	= 1 tablet / dose
~~day~~	800 ~~mg~~	2 doses	8 × 2	16	

25. Random method:

~~1 g~~	mL	1000 ~~mg~~	~~day~~	10	10	= 3.33 or 3 mL / dose
~~day~~	100 ~~mg~~	~~1 g~~	3 doses	1 × 3		

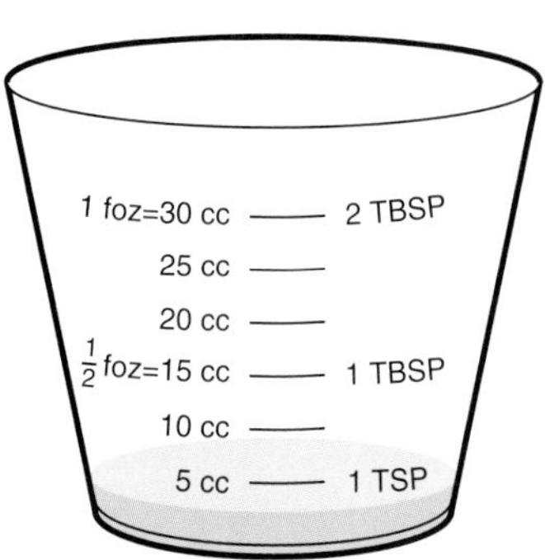

26. Sequential method:

4 ~~mg~~	mL	20 ~~kg~~	4 × 2	8	= 8 mL
~~kg~~	10 ~~mg~~		1	1	

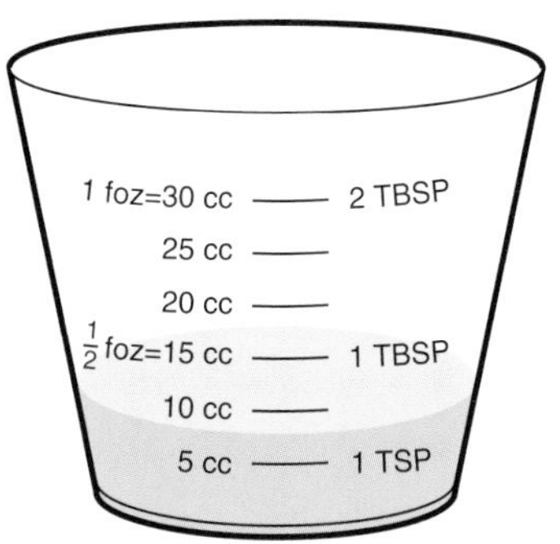

27. Sequential method:

0.15 ~~mg~~	mL	1 ~~kg~~	160 ~~lb~~	0.15 × 1 × 160	24	= 5.45 or 5.5 mL
~~kg~~	2 ~~mg~~	2.2 ~~lb~~		2 × 2.2	4.4	

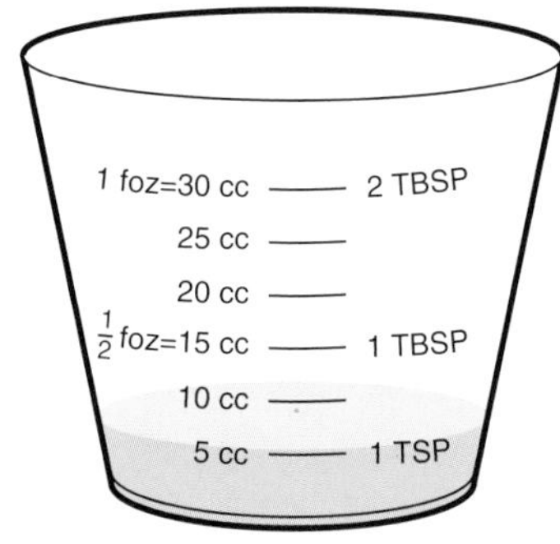

28. Sequential method:

2 ~~mg~~	tablets	40 ~~kg~~	2 × 4	8	= 0.533 or 0.5 tablet
~~kg~~	150 ~~mg~~		15	15	

29. Sequential method:

20 ~~mg~~	tablet	1 ~~kg~~	20 ~~lb~~	2 × 1 × 2	4	= 0.45 or 0.5 tablet
~~kg~~	400 ~~mg~~	2.2 ~~lb~~		4 × 2.2	8.8	

30. Sequential method:

450 ~~mg~~	tablet	~~day~~	45	45	= 1 tablet / dose
~~day~~	150 ~~mg~~	3 doses	15 × 3	45	

31. Random method:

2.4 ~~g~~	(tablet)	~~day~~	10~~00 mg~~	2.4 × 10	24	=	2 tablets
~~day~~	30~~0 mg~~	4 (doses)	1 ~~g~~	3 × 4 × 1	12		dose

32. Sequential method:

50~~0 mg~~	8 (mL)	~~day~~	50 × 8	400	=	2.666 or 2.7 mL
~~day~~	75~~0 mg~~	2 (doses)	75 × 2	150		dose

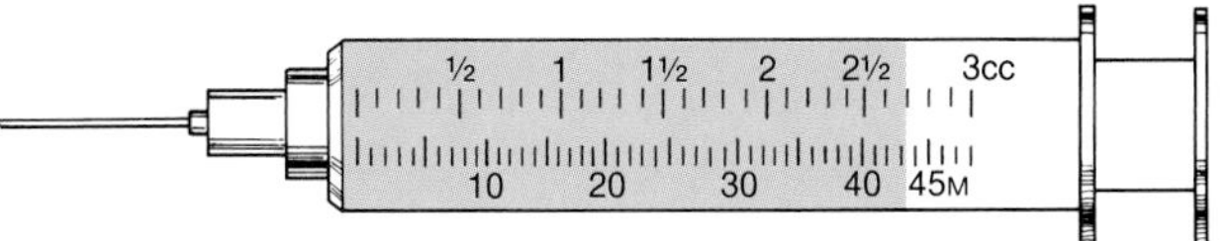

33. Random method:

~~1000 mg~~	20 (mL)	1 ~~g~~	~~day~~	20 × 1	20	=	5 mL
~~day~~	2 ~~g~~	~~1000 mg~~	2 (doses)	2 × 2	4		dose

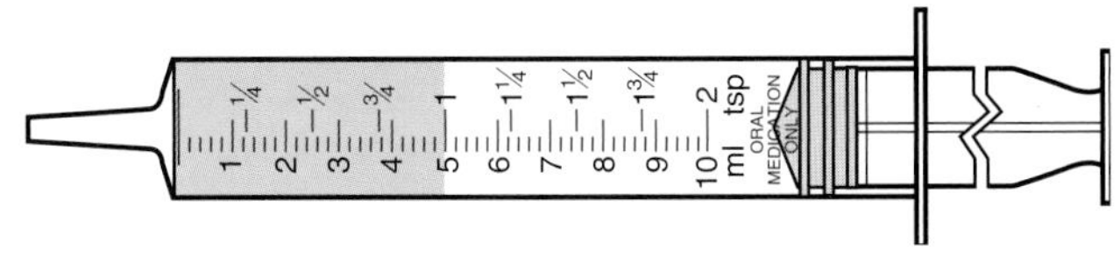

Three-Factor Practice Problems

1. Sequential method:

4~~0 mg~~	5 (mL)	6~~0 kg~~	4 × 5 × 6	120	=	40 mL
~~kg~~/(day)	30~~0 mg~~		3	3		day

How many milliliters per dose will you give?
Sequential method:

4~~0 mg~~	5 (mL)	6~~0 kg~~	~~day~~	4 × 5 × 6	120	=	10 mL
~~kg/day~~	30~~0 mg~~		4 (doses)	3 × 4	12		dose

2. Sequential method:

4 ~~mg~~	(mL)	1 ~~kg~~	6~~0 lb~~	4 × 1 × 6	24	=	10.9 or 11 mL
~~kg~~/(day)	1~~0 mg~~	2.2 ~~lb~~		1 × 2.2	2.2		day

3. Sequential method:

3~~0 mg~~	2 (mL)	5~~0 kg~~	2 × 5	10	=	10 mL
~~kg~~/(day)	30~~0 mg~~					day

How many milliliters per dose will you give?
Sequential method:

3~~0 mg~~	2 (mL)	5~~0 kg~~	~~day~~	2 × 5	10	=	3.33 or 3.3 mL
~~kg/day~~	30~~0 mg~~		3 (doses)	3	3		dose

4. Sequential method:

0.575 ~~mL~~	40 (mg)	2.2 ~~lb~~		3 ~~doses~~	=	mg
~~dose~~	~~mL~~	1 (kg)	45 ~~lb~~	(day)		kg/day

0.575 × 40 × 2.2 × 3	151.8	=	3.37 or 3.4 mg
1 × 45	45		kg/day

5. Sequential method:

0.125 ~~mL~~	5~~0~~ (mg)	2.2 ~~lb~~		3 ~~doses~~	=	mg
~~dose~~	~~mL~~	1 (kg)	2~~0 lb~~	(day)		kg/day

0.125 × 5 × 2.2 × 3	4.125	=	2.06 or 2.1 mg
1 × 2	2		kg/day

6. Sequential method:

~~400 mg~~	10 (mL)	10	= 10 mL
	~~400 mg~~		

Calculate milliliter per hour to set the IV pump.
Random method:

5 ~~mcg~~	26~~0~~ (mL)	1 ~~mg~~	~~1 kg~~	11~~0 lb~~	6~~0 min~~	=	mL
~~kg/min~~	40~~0 mg~~	100~~0 mcg~~	2.2 ~~lb~~		~~1~~ (hr)		hr

5 × 26 × 1 × 11 × 6	8580	=	9.75 or 9.8 mL
4 × 100 × 2.2	880		hr

7. Random method:

$$\frac{0.8\ \cancel{\text{mcg}}}{\cancel{\text{kg/min}}} \left| \frac{500\ \text{mL}}{50\ \cancel{\text{mg}}} \right| \frac{1\ \cancel{\text{mg}}}{1000\ \cancel{\text{mcg}}} \left| \frac{\cancel{1}\ \cancel{\text{kg}}}{2.2\ \cancel{\text{lb}}} \right| \frac{60\ \cancel{\text{min}}}{\cancel{1}\ \text{hr}} \left| \frac{143\ \cancel{\text{lb}}}{\ } \right| = \frac{\text{mL}}{\text{hr}}$$

$$\frac{0.8 \times 5 \times 1 \times 6 \times 143}{5 \times 10 \times 2.2} \left| \frac{3432}{110} \right| = \frac{31.2\ \text{mL}}{\text{hr}}$$

8. Sequential method:

$$\frac{68\ \cancel{\text{mL}}}{\cancel{\text{hr}}} \left| \frac{50\ \cancel{\text{mg}}}{250\ \cancel{\text{mL}}} \right| \frac{1\ \cancel{\text{hr}}}{60\ \text{min}} \left| \frac{2.2\ \cancel{\text{lb}}}{1\ \text{kg}} \right| \frac{1000\ \text{mcg}}{1\ \cancel{\text{mg}}} \left| \frac{\ }{250\ \cancel{\text{lb}}} \right| = \frac{\text{mcg}}{\text{kg/min}}$$

$$\frac{68 \times 5 \times 1 \times 2.2 \times 10}{25 \times 6 \times 1 \times 1 \times 25} \left| \frac{7480}{3750} \right| = 1.99 \text{ or } 2\ \frac{\text{mcg}}{\text{kg/min}}$$

9. Random method:

$$\frac{30\ \cancel{\text{mg}}}{\cancel{\text{kg}}/\text{day}} \left| \frac{1\ \cancel{\text{kg}}}{2.2\ \cancel{\text{lb}}} \right| \frac{157\ \cancel{\text{lb}}}{\ } \left| \frac{1\ \text{g}}{1000\ \cancel{\text{mg}}} \right| \frac{3 \times 1 \times 157 \times 1}{2.2 \times 100} \left| \frac{471}{220} \right| = 2.14 \text{ or } 2.1\ \frac{\text{g}}{\text{day}}$$

10. Random method:

$$\frac{0.01\ \text{mL}}{\cancel{\text{kg/min}}} \left| \frac{1\ \cancel{\text{kg}}}{2.2\ \cancel{\text{lb}}} \right| \frac{180\ \cancel{\text{lb}}}{\ } \left| \frac{60\ \cancel{\text{min}}}{1\ \text{hr}} \right| \frac{0.01 \times 1 \times 180 \times 60}{2.2 \times 1}$$

$$\frac{108}{2.2} = 49.09 \text{ or } 49.1\ \frac{\text{mL}}{\text{hr}}$$

11. Random method:

$$\frac{28\ \cancel{\text{mL}}}{\cancel{\text{hr}}} \left| \frac{400\ \cancel{\text{mg}}}{250\ \cancel{\text{mL}}} \right| \frac{\ }{15\ \text{kg}} \left| \frac{1\ \cancel{\text{hr}}}{60\ \text{min}} \right| \frac{1000\ \text{mcg}}{1\ \cancel{\text{mg}}} = \frac{\text{mcg}}{\text{kg/min}}$$

$$\frac{28 \times 4 \times 1 \times 1000}{25 \times 15 \times 6 \times 1} \left| \frac{112{,}000}{2250} \right| = 49.77 \text{ or } 49.8\ \frac{\text{mcg}}{\text{kg/min}}$$

12. Random method:

$$\frac{3\ \cancel{\text{mcg}}}{\cancel{\text{kg/min}}} \left| \frac{\cancel{100}\ \text{mL}}{\cancel{100}\ \cancel{\text{mg}}} \right| \frac{1\ \cancel{\text{kg}}}{2.2\ \cancel{\text{lb}}} \left| \frac{60\ \cancel{\text{min}}}{1\ \text{hr}} \right| \frac{160\ \cancel{\text{lb}}}{\ } \left| \frac{1\ \cancel{\text{mg}}}{1000\ \cancel{\text{mcg}}} \right| = \frac{\text{r}}{\text{h}}$$

$$\frac{3 \times 1 \times 6 \times 16 \times 1}{2.2 \times 1 \times 10} \left| \frac{288}{22} \right| = 13.09 \text{ or } 13.1\ \frac{\text{mL}}{\text{hr}}$$

13. Random method:

$$\frac{2\ \cancel{\text{mcg}}}{\cancel{\text{kg/min}}} \left| \frac{250\ \text{mL}}{50\ \cancel{\text{mg}}} \right| \frac{1\ \cancel{\text{kg}}}{2.2\ \cancel{\text{lb}}} \left| \frac{250\ \cancel{\text{lb}}}{\ } \right| \frac{\cancel{1}\ \cancel{\text{mg}}}{1000\ \cancel{\text{mcg}}} \left| \frac{60\ \cancel{\text{min}}}{\cancel{1}\ \text{hr}} \right|$$

$$\frac{2 \times 25 \times 1 \times 25 \times 6}{5 \times 2.2 \times 10} \left| \frac{7500}{110} \right| = 68.1 \text{ or } 68\ \frac{\text{mL}}{\text{hr}}$$

14. Random method:

$$\frac{1\ \cancel{\text{mcg}}}{\cancel{\text{kg/min}}} \left| \frac{250\ \text{mL}}{50\ \cancel{\text{mg}}} \right| \frac{\cancel{1}\ \cancel{\text{kg}}}{2.2\ \cancel{\text{lb}}} \left| \frac{60\ \cancel{\text{min}}}{\cancel{1}\ \text{hr}} \right| \frac{160\ \cancel{\text{lb}}}{\ } \left| \frac{\cancel{1}\ \cancel{\text{mg}}}{\cancel{1000}\ \cancel{\text{mcg}}} \right| = \frac{\text{mL}}{\text{hr}}$$

$$\frac{1 \times 25 \times 6 \times 16}{50 \times 2.2} \left| \frac{2400}{110} \right| = 21.81 \text{ or } 21.8\ \frac{\text{mL}}{\text{hr}}$$

15. Random method:

$$\frac{2.5\ \cancel{\text{mcg}}}{\cancel{\text{kg/min}}} \left| \frac{500\ \text{mL}}{400\ \cancel{\text{mg}}} \right| \frac{65\ \cancel{\text{kg}}}{\ } \left| \frac{60\ \cancel{\text{min}}}{1\ \text{hr}} \right| \frac{1\ \cancel{\text{mg}}}{1000\ \cancel{\text{mcg}}} = \frac{\text{mL}}{\text{hr}}$$

$$\frac{2.5 \times 5 \times 65 \times 6 \times 1}{4 \times 1 \times 100} \left| \frac{4875}{400} \right| = 12.18 \text{ or } 12.2\ \frac{\text{mL}}{\text{hr}}$$

16. Random method:

$$\frac{15\ \cancel{\text{mL}}}{\cancel{\text{hr}}} \left| \frac{2\ \cancel{\text{mg}}}{500\ \cancel{\text{mL}}} \right| \frac{1\ \cancel{\text{hr}}}{60\ \text{min}} \left| \frac{\ }{20\ \text{kg}} \right| \frac{1000\ \text{mcg}}{1\ \cancel{\text{mg}}} = \frac{\text{mcg}}{\text{kg/min}}$$

$$\frac{15 \times 2 \times 1 \times 1}{5 \times 6 \times 20 \times 1} \left| \frac{30}{600} \right| = 0.05\ \frac{\text{mcg}}{\text{kg/min}}$$

17. Random method:

5 ~~mcg~~	50~~0~~ mL	7~~0~~ ~~kg~~	1 ~~mg~~	= mL
~~kg~~/min	4~~00~~ ~~mg~~		100~~0~~ ~~mcg~~	min

5 × 5 × 7 × 1	175	= 0.4375 or 0.44 mL
4 × 100	400	min

18. How many milligrams per day is the child receiving?
Sequential method:

40 mg	1 ~~kg~~	20 ~~lb~~	40 x 1 x 20	800	= 363.63 or 363.6 mg
~~kg~~/day	2.2 ~~lb~~		2.2	2.2	day

How many milligrams per dose is the child receiving?
Sequential method:

363.6 mg	~~day~~	363.6	= 121.2 mg
~~day~~	3 doses	3	dose

How many milliliters will you draw from the vial after reconstitution?
Sequential method:

121.2 ~~mg~~	10 mL	121.2 × 10	1212	= 2.424 or 2.4 mL
	500 ~~mg~~	500	500	

Calculate milliliters per hour to set the IV pump.
Sequential method:

102.4 mL	~~60 min~~	102.4	= 102.4 mL
~~60 min~~	1 hr	1	hr

19. How many milligrams per dose is the child receiving?
Random method:

2 mg	40 ~~kg~~	2 × 40	80	= 80 mg
~~kg~~/dose				dose

How many milliliters will you draw from the vial?
Sequential method:

8~~0~~ ~~mg~~	mL	8	= 2 mL
	4~~0~~ ~~mg~~	4	

Calculate milliliters per hour to set the IV pump.
Sequential method:

52 mL	6~~0~~ ~~min~~	52 × 6	312	= 104 mL
3~~0~~ ~~min~~	1 hr	3 × 1	3	hr

20. How many milligrams per day is the child receiving?
Sequential method:

25 mg	25 ~~kg~~	25 × 25	625	= 625 mg
~~kg~~/day				day

How many milligrams per dose is the child receiving?
Sequential method:

625 mg	~~day~~	625	= 208.33 or 208.3 mg
~~day~~	3 doses	3	dose

How many milliliters will you draw from the vial after reconstitution?
Sequential method:

208.3 ~~mg~~	1~~0~~ mL	208.3 × 1	208.3	= 4.166 or 4.2 mL
	50~~0~~ ~~mg~~	50	50	day

Calculate milliliters per hour to set the IV pump.
Sequential method:

54.2 mL	6~~0~~ min	54.2 × 6	325.2	= 108.4 mL
3~~0~~ min	1 hr	3 × 1	3	hr

Comprehensive Practice Problems

1. Sequential method:

0.125 ~~mg~~	(tablet)	0.125	= 0.5 tablet
	0.25 ~~mg~~	0.25	

Answer: 0.5 tablet

2. Random method:

0.5 ~~g~~	(tablet)	10~~00 mg~~	0.5 × 10	5	= 1 tablet
	5~~00 mg~~	1 ~~g~~	5 × 1	5	

Answer: 1 tablet

3. Random method:

$\frac{1}{150}$ ~~gr~~	(mL)	60 ~~mg~~	$\frac{1}{150} \times \frac{60}{1}$	$\frac{60}{150}$	0.4	= 1 mL
	0.4 ~~mg~~	1 ~~gr~~	0.4 × 1	0.4	0.4	

Answer: 1 mL

4. Sequential method:

5~~00,000 units~~	~~mL~~	1 (tsp)	5 × 1	5	= 1 tsp
	1~~00,000 units~~	5 ~~mL~~	1 × 5	5	

Answer: 1 tsp

5. Sequential method:

5~~0 mg~~	(mL)	5	= 0.5 mL
	10~~0 mg~~	10	

Answer: 0.5 mL

6. Sequential method:

2 ~~mg~~	1~~0~~ (mL)	75 ~~kg~~	2 × 1 × 75	150	= 3 mL
~~kg~~	50~~0 mg~~		50	50	

Answer: 3 mL

7. Sequential method:

2 ~~mg~~	5 (mL)	1 ~~kg~~	1~~00 lb~~	2 × 5 × 1 × 1	10	= 0.9 mL
~~kg~~	5~~00 mg~~	2.2 ~~lb~~		5 × 2.2	11	

Answer: 0.9 mL

8. Sequential method:

100~~0 mL~~	15 (gtt)	1 ~~hr~~	100 × 15 × 1	1500	= 20.8 or 21 gtt/min
12 ~~hr~~	~~mL~~	6~~0~~ (min)	12 × 6	72	

Answer: 21 gtt/min

9. Sequential method:

50~~0 mL~~	15 ~~gtt~~	~~min~~	1 (hr)	50 × 15 × 1	750	= 5.9 hr
	~~mL~~	21 ~~gtt~~	6~~0 min~~	21 × 6	126	

Answer: 5.9 hours (Do not round up due to pump)

10. Sequential method:

15~~00 units~~	25~~0~~ (mL)	15 × 25	375	= 15 mL/hr
(hr)	25,~~000 units~~	25	25	

Answer: 15 mL/hr

11. Sequential method:

10~~00 mL~~	15 ~~gtt~~	~~min~~	1 (hr)	10 × 15 × 1	150	= 5 hr
	~~mL~~	5~~0 gtt~~	6~~0 min~~	5 × 6	30	

Answer: 5 hours

12. Sequential method:

8 ~~units~~	25~~0~~ (mL)	8 × 25	200	= 20 mL/hr
(hr)	10~~0 units~~	10	10	

Answer: 20 mL/hr

13. Sequential method:

$$\frac{50\cancel{0}\ \cancel{mL}}{8\ \cancel{hr}}\;\Big|\;\frac{10\ \text{gtt}}{\cancel{mL}}\;\Big|\;\frac{1\ \cancel{hr}}{6\cancel{0}\ \text{min}}\;\Big|\;\frac{50\times 10\times 1}{8\times 6}\;\Big|\;\frac{500}{48}=\frac{10.4\text{ or }10\text{ gtt}}{\text{min}}$$

Answer: 10 gtt/min

14. Random method:

$$\frac{2\ \cancel{mEq}}{1\cancel{00}\ \cancel{mL}}\;\Big|\;\frac{1\cancel{0}\ \text{mL}}{2\cancel{0}\ \cancel{mEq}}\;\Big|\;\frac{5\cancel{00}\ \cancel{mL}}{}\;\Big|\;\frac{2\times 1\times 5}{1\times 2}\;\Big|\;\frac{10}{2}=5\text{ mL}$$

Answer: 5 mL

15. Random method:

$$\frac{44\ \cancel{mg}}{\text{hr}}\;\Big|\;\frac{25\cancel{0}\ \text{mL}}{1\ \cancel{g}}\;\Big|\;\frac{1\ \cancel{g}}{100\cancel{0}\ \cancel{mg}}\;\Big|\;\frac{44\times 25\times 1}{1\times 100}\;\Big|\;\frac{1100}{100}=\frac{11\text{ mL}}{\text{hr}}$$

Answer: 11 mL/hr

16. Sequential method:

$$\frac{14\cancel{0}\ \cancel{mL}}{\text{hr}}\;\Big|\;\frac{3\cancel{0}\ \text{mg}}{10\cancel{00}\ \cancel{mL}}\;\Big|\;\frac{14\times 3}{10}\;\Big|\;\frac{42}{10}=\frac{4.2\text{ mg}}{\text{hr}}$$

Answer: 4.2 mg/hr

17. How many milliliters will you draw from the vial after reconstitution?
Sequential method:

$$\frac{75\cancel{0}\ \cancel{mg}}{}\;\Big|\;\frac{\text{mL}}{50\cancel{0}\ \cancel{mg}}\;\Big|\;\frac{75}{50}=1.5\text{ mL}$$

Calculate the milliliters per hour to set the IV pump.
Sequential method:

$$\frac{101.5\ \text{mL}}{3\cancel{0}\ \cancel{min}}\;\Big|\;\frac{6\cancel{0}\ \cancel{min}}{1\ \text{hr}}\;\Big|\;\frac{101.5\times 6}{3\times 1}\;\Big|\;\frac{609}{3}=\frac{203\text{ mL}}{\text{hr}}$$

Calculate the drops per minute with a drop factor of 10 gtt/mL.
Sequential method:

$$\frac{203\ \cancel{mL}}{\cancel{hr}}\;\Big|\;\frac{1\cancel{0}\ \text{gtt}}{\cancel{mL}}\;\Big|\;\frac{1\ \cancel{hr}}{6\cancel{0}\ \text{min}}\;\Big|\;\frac{203\times 1\times 1}{6}\;\Big|\;\frac{203}{6}=\frac{33.83\text{ or }34\text{ gtt}}{\text{min}}$$

18. How many milliliters will you draw from the vial after reconstitution?
Sequential method:

$$\frac{1.5\ \cancel{g}}{}\;\Big|\;\frac{5\ \text{mL}}{3\ \cancel{g}}\;\Big|\;\frac{1.5\times 5}{3}\;\Big|\;\frac{7.5}{3}=2.5\text{ mL}$$

Calculate the milliliters per hour to set the IV pump.
Sequential method:

$$\frac{52.5\ \text{mL}}{2\cancel{0}\ \cancel{min}}\;\Big|\;\frac{6\cancel{0}\ \cancel{min}}{1\ \text{hr}}\;\Big|\;\frac{52.5\times 6}{2\times 1}\;\Big|\;\frac{315}{2}=\frac{157.5\text{ or }158\text{ mL}}{\text{hr}}$$

Calculate the drops per minute with a drop factor of 20 gtt/mL.
Sequential method:

$$\frac{158\ \cancel{mL}}{\cancel{hr}}\;\Big|\;\frac{2\cancel{0}\ \text{gtt}}{\cancel{mL}}\;\Big|\;\frac{1\ \cancel{hr}}{6\cancel{0}\ \text{min}}\;\Big|\;\frac{158\times 2\times 1}{6}\;\Big|\;\frac{316}{6}=\frac{52.66\text{ or }53\text{ gtt}}{\text{min}}$$

19. Random method:

$$\frac{4\ \cancel{mcg}}{\cancel{kg/min}}\;\Big|\;\frac{25\cancel{0}\ \text{mL}}{40\cancel{0}\ \cancel{mg}}\;\Big|\;\frac{1\ \cancel{mg}}{100\cancel{0}\ \cancel{mcg}}\;\Big|\;\frac{6\cancel{0}\ \cancel{min}}{1\ \text{hr}}\;\Big|\;\frac{1\ \cancel{kg}}{2.2\ \cancel{lb}}\;\Big|\;\frac{12\cancel{0}\ \cancel{lb}}{}=\frac{\text{mL}}{\text{hr}}$$

$$\frac{4\times 25\times 1\times 6\times 1\times 12}{40\times 10\times 1\times 2.2}\;\Big|\;\frac{7200}{880}=\frac{8.1\text{ or }8\text{ mL}}{\text{hr}}$$

Answer: 8 mL/hr

20. Random method:

$$\frac{0.8\ \cancel{mcg}}{\cancel{kg/min}}\left|\frac{5\cancel{00}\ (mL)}{5\cancel{0}\ \cancel{mg}}\right|\frac{1\ \cancel{mg}}{10\cancel{00}\ \cancel{mcg}}\left|\frac{1\ \cancel{kg}}{2.2\ \cancel{lb}}\right|\frac{143\ \cancel{lb}}{}\left|\frac{6\cancel{0}\ \cancel{min}}{1\ (hr)}\right.=\frac{mL}{hr}$$

$$\frac{0.8\times5\times1\times1\times143\times6}{5\times10\times2.2\times1}\left|\frac{3432}{110}\right.=\frac{31.2\text{ or }31\ mL}{hr}$$

Answer: 31 mL/hr

SECTION

3

CASE STUDIES

This section contains case studies simulating typical orders that might be written for patients with selected disorders. In each case, the orders include multiple situations that require the nurse to perform clinical calculations before being able to implement the order. After reading the short scenario, read through the list of orders.

Place a check mark in the box next to the physician's order that probably requires further calculations before implementing.

CASE STUDY 1 Congestive Heart Failure

A patient is admitted to the hospital with a diagnosis of dyspnea, peripheral edema with a 10-lb weight gain, and a history of congestive heart failure. The orders from the physician include:

- ❑ Bed rest in Fowler's position
- ❑ O_2 at 4 L/min per nasal cannula
- ❑ Chest x-ray, complete blood count, electrolyte panel, BUN, serum creatinine levels, and a digoxin level
- ❑ IV of D5W/$\frac{1}{2}$NS at 50 cc/hr
- ❑ Daily AM weight
- ❑ Antiembolism stockings
- ❑ Furosemide 40 mg IV qd
- ❑ Digoxin 0.125 mg PO qd
- ❑ KCl 20 mEq PO tid
- ❑ Low Na diet
- ❑ Restrict PO fluids to 1500 cc/day
- ❑ Vitals q4h
- ❑ Accurate I/O

Identify the orders that require calculations.

Set up and solve each problem using dimensional analysis.

1. Calculate gtt/min using microtubing (60 gtt/mL).

2. Calculate the weight gain in kilograms.

3. Calculate how many mL of Lasix the patient will receive IV from a multidose vial labeled 10 mg/mL.

4. Calculate how many tablets of digoxin the patient will receive from a unit dose of 0.25 mg/tablet.

5. Calculate how many tablets of K-Dur the patient will receive from a unit dose of 10 mEq/tablet.

● CASE STUDY 2 COPD/Emphysema

A patient is admitted to the hospital with dyspnea and COPD exacerbation. The orders from the physician include:

- ❑ Stat ABGs, chest x-ray, complete blood count, and electrolytes
- ❑ IV D5W/$\frac{1}{2}$NS 1000 cc/8 hr
- ❑ Aminophylline IV loading dose of 5.6 mg/kg over 30 minutes followed by 0.5 mg/kg/hr continuous IV
- ❑ O_2 at 2 L/min per nasal cannula
- ❑ Albuterol respiratory treatments q4h
- ❑ Chest physiotherapy q4h
- ❑ Erythromycin 800 mg IV q6h
- ❑ Bed rest
- ❑ Accurate I/O
- ❑ High-calorie, protein-rich diet in six small meals daily
- ❑ Encourage PO fluids to 3 L/day

Identify the orders that require calculations.

Set up and solve each problem using dimensional analysis.

1. Calculate cc/hr to set the IV pump.

2. Calculate cc/hr to set the IV pump for the loading dose of aminophylline for a patient weighing 140 lb. Aminophylline supply: 100 mg/100 mL D5W.

3. Calculate cc/hr to set the IV pump for the continuous dose of aminophylline for a patient weighing 140 lb. Aminophylline supply: 1 g/250 mL D5W.

4. Calculate cc/hr to set the IV pump to infuse erythromycin 800 mg. Erythromycin supply: 1-g vial to be reconstituted with 20 mL sterile water and further diluted in 250 cc NS to infuse over 1 hr.

5. Calculate the PO fluids in mL/shift.

CASE STUDY 3 Small Cell Lung Cancer

A patient with small cell lung cancer is admitted to the hospital with fever and dehydration. The orders from the physician include:

- ❑ O_2 at 2 L/min per nasal cannula
- ❑ Chest x-ray; complete blood count; electrolytes; blood, urine, and sputum cultures; BUN and serum creatinine levels; type and cross for 2 units of PRBCs
- ❑ IV D5W/$\frac{1}{2}$ NS 1000 cc with 10 mEq KCl at 125 cc/hr
- ❑ 2 units of PRBCs if Hg is below 8
- ❑ 6 pack of platelets if < 20,000
- ❑ Neupogen 5 mcg/kg SQ daily
- ❑ Gentamicin 80 mg IV q8h
- ❑ Decadron 8 mg IV daily
- ❑ Fortaz 1 g IV q8h
- ❑ Accurate I/O
- ❑ Encourage PO fluids
- ❑ Vitals q4h (call for temperature > 102°F)

Identify the orders that require calculations.

Set up and solve each problem using dimensional analysis.

1. Calculate gtt/min using macrotubing (20 gtt/mL).

2. Calculate how many mcg of Neupogen will be given SQ to a patient weighing 160 lb.

3. Calculate cc/hr to set the IV pump to infuse gentamicin. The vial is labeled 40 mg/mL and is to be further diluted in 100 cc D5W to infuse over 1 hr.

4. Calculate how many mL of Decadron the patient will receive from a vial labeled dexamethasone 4 mg/mL.

5. Calculate mL/hr to set the IV pump to infuse Fortaz 1 g over 30 minutes. Supply: Fortaz 1 g/50 mL.

CASE STUDY 4 Acquired Immunodeficiency Syndrome (AIDS)

A patient who is HIV+ and a Jehovah's Witness is admitted to the hospital with anemia, fever of unknown origin, and wasting syndrome with dehydration. The orders from the physician include:

- ❑ O_2 at 4 L/min per nasal cannula
- ❑ IV D5W/$\frac{1}{2}$NS at 150 cc/hr
- ❑ CD4 and CD8 T-cell subset counts; erythrocyte sedimentation rate; complete blood count; urine, sputum, and stool cultures; chest x-ray
- ❑ Acyclovir 350 mg IV q8h
- ❑ Neupogen 300 mcg SQ daily
- ❑ Epogen 100 units/kg SQ three times a week
- ❑ Megace 40 mg PO tid
- ❑ Zidovudine 100 mg PO q4h
- ❑ Vancomycin 800 mg IV q6h
- ❑ Respiratory treatments with pentamidine
- ❑ High-calorie, protein-rich diet in six small meals daily
- ❑ Encourage PO fluids to 3 L/day
- ❑ Accurate I/O
- ❑ Daily AM weight

Identify the orders that require calculations.

Set up and solve each problem using dimensional analysis.

1. Calculate gtt/min using macrotubing (20 gtt/mL).

2. Calculate cc/hr to set the IV pump to infuse acyclovir 350 mg. Supply: 500-mg vial to be reconstituted with 10 mL sterile water and further diluted in 100 mL D5W to infuse over 1 hour.

3. Calculate how many mL of Neupogen will be given SQ. The vial is labeled 300 mcg/mL.

4. Calculate how many mL of Epogen will be given SQ to the patient weighing 100 lb. The vial is labeled 4000 units/mL.

5. Calculate how many cc/hr to set the IV pump to infuse vancomycin 800 mg. Supply: 1-g vials to be reconstituted with 10 mL NS and further diluted in 100 mL D5W to infuse over 60 minutes.

● CASE STUDY 5 Sickle Cell Anemia

A patient is admitted to the hospital in sickle cell crisis. The orders from the physician include:

- ❑ Bed rest with joint support
- ❑ O_2 at 2 L/min per nasal cannula
- ❑ Complete blood count, erythrocyte sedimentation rate, serum iron levels, and chest x-ray
- ❑ IV D5W/$\frac{1}{2}$NS at 150 cc/hr
- ❑ Zofran 8 mg IV q8h
- ❑ Morphine sulfate 5 mg IV prn
- ❑ Hydrea 10 mg/kg/day PO
- ❑ Folic acid 0.5 mg daily PO
- ❑ Encourage 3000 cc/daily PO

Identify the orders that require calculations.

Set up and solve each problem using dimensional analysis.

1. Calculate gtt/min using macrotubing (10 gtt/mL).

2. Calculate cc/hr to set the IV pump to infuse Zofran 8 mg. Supply: Zofran 8 mg in 50 cc D5W to infuse over 15 min.

3. Calculate how many mL of morphine sulfate will be given IV. The syringe is labeled 10 mg/mL.

4. Calculate how many mg/day of Hydrea will be given PO to the patient weighing 125 lb.

5. Calculate how many tablets of folic acid will be given PO. Supply: 1 mg/tablet.

● CASE STUDY 6 Deep Vein Thrombosis

A patient is admitted to the hospital with right leg erythema and edema to R/O DVT. The orders from the physician include:

- ❑ Bed rest with right leg elevated
- ❑ Warm, moist heat to right leg with Aqua-K pad
- ❑ Doppler ultrasonography
- ❑ Partial thromboplastin time (PTT) and prothrombin time (PT)
- ❑ IV D5W/$\frac{1}{2}$NS with 20 mEq KCl at 50 cc/hr

- ❑ Heparin 5000 units IV push followed by continuous IV infusion of 1000 units/hr
- ❑ Lasix 20 mg IV bid
- ❑ Morphine 5 mg IV q4h

Identify the orders that require calculations.

Set up and solve each problem using dimensional analysis.

1. Calculate gtt/min using macrotubing (60 gtt/mL).

2. Calculate how many mL of heparin the patient will receive IV from a multidose vial labeled 10,000 units/mL.

3. Calculate mL/hr to set the IV pump for the continuous dose of heparin. Heparin supply: 25,000 units/250 mL D5W.

4. Calculate how many mL of Lasix the patient will receive IV from a multidose vial labeled 10 mg/mL.

5. Calculate how many mL of morphine the patient will receive from a syringe labeled 10 mg/mL.

● CASE STUDY 7 Bone Marrow Transplant

A patient is admitted to the hospital with a rash following an allogeneic bone marrow transplant. The orders from the physician include:

- ❑ IV D5W/$\frac{1}{2}$ NS with 20 mEq KCl/L at 80 cc/hr
- ❑ Complete blood count; electrolytes; sputum, urine, and stool cultures; blood cultures ×3; liver panel; BUN; and creatinine
- ❑ Vitals q4h
- ❑ Strict I/O
- ❑ Fortaz 2 g IV q8h
- ❑ Vancomycin 1 g IV q6h
- ❑ Claforan 1 g IV q12h
- ❑ Erythromycin 800 mg IV q6h

Identify the orders that require calculations.

Set up and solve each problem using dimensional analysis.

1. Calculate how many mEq/hr of KCl the patient will receive IV.

2. Calculate cc/hr to set the IV pump to infuse Fortaz 2 g. Supply: Fortaz 2-g vial to be reconstituted with 10 mL of sterile water and further diluted in 50 cc D5W to infuse over 30 minutes.

3. Calculate cc/hr to set the IV pump to infuse vancomycin 1 g. Supply: vancomycin 500-mg vial to be reconstituted with 10 mL of sterile water and further diluted in 100 cc of D5W to infuse over 60 minutes.

4. Calculate cc/hr to set the IV pump to infuse Claforan 1 g. Supply: Claforan 600 mg/4 mL to be further diluted with 100 cc D5W to infuse over 1 hour.

5. Calculate mL/hr to set the IV pump to infuse erythromycin 800 mg. Supply: Erythromycin 1-g vial to be diluted with 20 mL sterile water and further diluted in 250 mL of NS to infuse over 60 minutes.

● CASE STUDY 8 **Pneumonia**

A patient is admitted to the hospital with fever, cough, chills, and dyspnea to rule out pneumonia. The orders from the physician include:

- ❑ IV 600 cc D5W q8h
- ❑ I/O
- ❑ Vitals q4h
- ❑ Complete blood count, electrolytes, chest x-ray, ABGs, sputum specimen, blood cultures, and bronchoscopy
- ❑ Bed rest
- ❑ Humidified O_2 at 4 L/min per nasal cannula
- ❑ High-calorie diet
- ❑ Encourage oral fluids of 2000 to 3000 mL/day
- ❑ Pulse oximetry qAM
- ❑ Clindamycin 400 mg IV q6h
- ❑ Albuterol respiratory treatments
- ❑ Guaifenesin 200 mg PO q4h
- ❑ Terbutaline 2.5 mg PO tid
- ❑ MS Contrin 30 mg PO q4h prn

Identify the orders that require calculations.

Set up and solve each problem using dimensional analysis.

1. Calculate cc/hr to set the IV pump to infuse clindamycin 400 mg. Supply: Clindamycin 600 mg/4 mL to be further diluted with 50 cc D5W to infuse over 1 hour.

2. Calculate gtt/min to infuse the clindamycin using macrotubing (20 gtt/mL).

3. Calculate how many cc of guaifenesin the patient will receive from a stock bottle labeled 30 mg/tsp.

4. Calculate how many tablets of terbutaline the patient will receive from a unit dose of 5 mg/tablet.

5. Calculate how many tablets of MS Contrin the patient will receive from a unit dose of 30 mg/tablet.

● CASE STUDY 9 Pain

A patient is admitted to the hospital with intractable bone pain secondary to prostate cancer. The orders from the physician include:

- ❑ IV D5W/$\frac{1}{2}$NS with 20 mEq KCl/L at 60 cc/hr
- ❑ IV 500 cc NS with 25 mg Dilaudid and 50 mg Thorazine at 21 cc/hr
- ❑ Heparin 25,000 units/250 cc D5W at 11 cc/hr
- ❑ Bed rest
- ❑ Do not resuscitate
- ❑ O_2 at 2 L/min per nasal cannula
- ❑ Bumex 2 mg IV qAM after albumin infusion
- ❑ Albumin 12.5 g IV qAM

Identify the orders that require calculations.

Set up and solve each problem using dimensional analysis.

1. Calculate how many mEq/hr of KCl the patient is receiving.

2. Calculate how many mg/hr of Dilaudid the patient is receiving.

3. Calculate how many mg/hr of Thorazine the patient is receiving.

4. Calculate how many units/hr of heparin the patient is receiving.

5. Calculate how many mL of Bumex the patient will receive from a stock dose of 0.25 mg/mL.

CASE STUDY 10 Cirrhosis

A patient is admitted to the hospital with ascites, stomach pain, dyspnea, and a history of cirrhosis of the liver. The orders from the physician include:

- ❑ IV D5W/$\frac{1}{2}$ NS with 20 mEq KCl at 125 cc/hr
- ❑ IV Zantac 150 mg/250 cc NS at 11 cc/hr
- ❑ O_2 at 2 L/min per nasal cannula
- ❑ Type and crossmatch for 2 units of packed red blood cells, complete blood count, liver panel, PT/PTT, SMA-12.
- ❑ Carafate 1 g q4h PO
- ❑ Vitamin K 10 mg SQ qAM
- ❑ Spironolactone 50 mg PO bid
- ❑ Lasix 80 mg IV qAM
- ❑ Measure abdominal girth qAM
- ❑ Sodium restriction to 500 mg/day
- ❑ Fluid restriction to 1500 cc/day

Identify the orders that require calculations.

Set up and solve each problem using dimensional analysis.

1. Calculate the gtt/min using macrotubing (20 gtt/mL).

2. Calculate the mg/hr of Zantac the patient is receiving.

3. Calculate how many mL of vitamin K the patient will receive SQ from a unit dose labeled 10 mg/mL.

4. Calculate how many tablets of spironolactone the patient will receive from a unit dose labeled 25 mg/tablet.

5. Calculate how many mL of Lasix the patient will receive from a unit dose labeled 10 mg/mL.

CASE STUDY 11 Hyperemesis Gravidarum

A 14-year-old patient is admitted to the hospital with weight loss and dehydration secondary to hyperemesis gravidarum. The orders from the physician include:

- ❑ Bed rest with bathroom privileges
- ❑ Obtain weight daily
- ❑ Vital q4h
- ❑ Test urine for ketones

- ❑ Urinalysis, complete blood count, electrolytes, liver enzymes, and bilirubin
- ❑ NPO for 48 hours, then advance diet to clear liquid, full liquid, and as tolerated
- ❑ IV D5 $\frac{1}{2}$NS at 150 cc/hr for 8 hours, then decrease to 100 cc/hr
- ❑ Observe for signs of metabolic acidosis, jaundice, or hemorrhage
- ❑ Monitor intake and output
- ❑ Droperidol (Inapsine) 1 mg IV q4h prn for nausea
- ❑ Metoclopramide (Reglan) 20 mg IV in 50 mL of D5W to infuse over 15 minutes
- ❑ Diphenhydramine (Benadryl) 25 mg IV q3h prn for nausea
- ❑ Dexamethasone (Decadron) 4 mg IV q6h

Identify the orders that require calculations.

Set up and solve each problem using dimensional analysis.

1. Calculate gtt/min using macrotubing (20 gtt/mL) to infuse 150 cc/hr, then 100 cc/hr.

2. Calculate how many mL of droperidol the patient will receive IV. Supply: 2.5 mg/mL

3. Calculate mL/hr to set the IV pump to infuse metoclopramide (Reglan) 20 mg in 50 mL of D5W to infuse over 15 minutes.

4. Calculate how many mL of diphenhydramine (Benadryl) the patient will receive IV. Supply: 10 mg/mL.

5. Calculate how many mL of dexamethasone (Decadron) the patient will receive IV. Supply: 4 mg/mL.

● CASE STUDY 12 Preeclampsia

A nulliparous female is admitted to the hospital with pregnancy-induced hypertension. The orders from the physician include:

- ❑ Complete bed rest in left lateral position
- ❑ Insert Foley catheter and check hourly for protein and specific gravity
- ❑ Daily weight
- ❑ Methyldopa (Aldomet) 250 mg PO tid
- ❑ Hydralazine (Apresoline) 5 mg IV every 20 minutes for blood pressure over 160/100
- ❑ Complete blood count, liver enzymes, chemistry panel, clotting studies, type and crossmatch, and urinalysis

- ❑ Magnesium sulfate 4 g in 250 mL D5LR loading dose to infuse over 30 minutes
- ❑ Magnesium sulfate 40 g in 1000 mL LR to infuse at 1 g/hr
- ❑ Keep calcium gluconate and intubation equipment at the bedside
- ❑ Nifedipine (Procardia) 10 mg sublingual for blood pressure over 160/100 and repeat in 15 minutes if needed.
- ❑ Keep lights dimmed and maintain a quiet environment
- ❑ Monitor blood pressure, pulse, and respiratory rate, fetal heart rate (FHR) contractions every 15 to 30 minutes, and deep tendon reflexes (DTR) hourly
- ❑ Monitor intake and output, proteinuria, presence of headache, visual disturbances, and epigastric pain hourly
- ❑ Restrict hourly fluid intake to 100 to 125 mL/hr

Identify the orders that require calculations.

Set up and solve each problem using dimensional analysis.

1. Calculate how many tablets of methyldopa (Aldomet) will be given PO. Supply: 500 mg/tablet.

2. Calculate how many mL of hydralazine (Apresoline) will be given IV. Supply: 20 mg/mL.

3. Calculate mL/hr to set the IV pump to infuse magnesium sulfate 4 g in 250 mL D5W loading dose to infuse over 30 minutes.

4. Calculate mL/hr to set the IV pump to infuse magnesium sulfate 40 g in 1000 mL LR to infuse at 1 g/hr.

5. Calculate how many capsules of nifedipine (Procardia) will be needed to give the sublingual dose. Supply: 10 mg/capsule.

● CASE STUDY 13 Premature Labor

A 35-year-old female in the 30th week of gestation is admitted to the hospital in premature labor. The orders from the physician include:

- ❑ Bed rest in left lateral position
- ❑ Monitor intake and output
- ❑ Daily weights
- ❑ Continuous fetal monitoring
- ❑ Monitor blood pressure, pulse rate, respirations, fetal heart rate, uterine contraction pattern, and neurologic reflexes
- ❑ Keep calcium gluconate at the bedside

- ❑ Initiate magnesium sulfate 4 g in 250 cc LR loading dose over 20 minutes, then 2 g in 250 cc LR at 2 g/hr until contractions stop
- ❑ Continue tocolytic therapy with terbutaline (Brethine) 0.25 mg SQ every 30 minutes for 2 hours after contractions stop
- ❑ Give nifedipine (Procardia) 10 mg sublingual now, then 20 mg PO q6h after infusion of magnesium sulfate and contractions have stopped
- ❑ Betamethasone 12 mg IM × 2 doses 12 hours apart
- ❑ IV LR 1000 cc over 8 hours

Identify the orders that require calculations.

Set up and solve each problem using dimensional analysis.

1. Calculate cc/hr to set the IV pump to infuse the loading dose magnesium sulfate 4 g in 250 cc LR over 20 minutes and the 2 g/hr maintenance dose.

2. Calculate how many mL of terbutaline (Brethine) will be given SQ. Supply: 1 mg/mL.

3. Calculate how many capsules of nifedipine (Procardia) will be given PO q6h. Supply: 10 mg/capsule.

4. Betamethasone 12 mg IM × 2 doses 12 hours apart. Supply: 6 mg/mL.

5. Calculate cc/hr to set the IV pump to infuse LR 1000 cc over 8 hours.

● CASE STUDY 14 Cystic Fibrosis

A 10-year-old child weighing 65 lb is admitted to the hospital with pulmonary exacerbation. The orders from the physician include:

- ❑ Complete blood count with differential, ABGs, chest x-ray, urinalysis, chemistry panel, and sputum culture
- ❑ IV 0.9% normal saline at 75 cc/hr
- ❑ Daily weights
- ❑ Monitor vitals q4h
- ❑ Oxygen at 2 L/min with pulse oximetry checks to maintain oxygen saturation above 92%
- ❑ Pancrease 2 capsules PO with meals and snacks
- ❑ High-calorie, high-protein diet
- ❑ Multivitamin 1 tablet PO daily
- ❑ Tagamet 30 mg/kg/day PO in four divided doses with meals and HS with a snack.
- ❑ Clindamycin 10 mg/kg IV q6h
- ❑ Postural drainage and percussion after aerosolized treatments

- ❑ Albuterol treatments with 2 inhalations q4h to 6h
- ❑ Terbutaline PO 2.5 mg q6h
- ❑ Tobramycin 1.5 mg/kg q6h
- ❑ Tobramycin peak and trough levels after fourth dose

Identify the orders that require calculations.

Set up and solve each problem using dimensional analysis.

1. Calculate gtt/min using macrotubing (15 gtt/mL).

2. Calculate how many tablets of Tagamet will be given PO with meals and HS snack. Supply: 200 mg/tablet.

3. Calculate how many mg of clindamycin the patient will receive, how many mL to draw from the vial, and mL/hr to set the IV pump. Supply: 150 mg/mL vial to be further diluted in 50 mL of NS and infused over 20 minutes.

4. Calculate how many tablets of terbutaline will be given PO. Supply: 2.5 mg/tablet.

5. Calculate how many mg of tobramycin the patient will receive, how many mL to draw from the vial, and cc/hr to set the IV pump. Supply: 40 mg/mL vial to be further diluted in 50 mL of NS and infused over 30 minutes.

CASE STUDY 15 Respiratory Syncytial Virus (RSV)

A 2-year-old child weighing 30 lb is admitted to the hospital for severe respiratory distress. The orders from the physician include:

- ❑ Complete blood count with differential, electrolytes, blood culture, chest x-ray, and nasal washing
- ❑ Humidified oxygen therapy to keep oxygen saturation > 92%
- ❑ Continuous pulse oximetry
- ❑ IV D5W$\frac{1}{2}$NS at 50 cc/hr
- ❑ Elevate HOB
- ❑ Vitals q2h
- ❑ Contact isolation
- ❑ Cardiorespiratory monitor
- ❑ Strict intake and output with urine specific gravities
- ❑ Acetaminophen elixir 120 mg q4h prn for temperature > 101°F
- ❑ Aminophylline loading dose of 5 mg/kg to infuse over 30 minutes and maintenance dose of 0.8 mg/kg/hr

- ❑ Ribavirin (Virazole) inhalation therapy × 12 hr/day
- ❑ NPO with respiratory rate > 60
- ❑ RespiGam 750 mg/kg IV monthly
- ❑ Pediapred 1.5 mg/kg/day in three divided doses
- ❑ Ampicillin 100 mg/kg/day in divided doses q6h

Identify the orders that require calculations.

Set up and solve each problem using dimensional analysis.

1. Calculate how many mL of acetaminophen elixir the patient will receive. Supply: 120 mg/5 mL.

2. Calculate how many mg of aminophylline the patient will receive and the cc/hr to set the IV pump for the loading dose, then calculate the cc/hr to set the IV pump for the maintenance dose. Supply: 250 mg/100 mL.

3. Calculate how many mg of RespiGam the patient will receive IV on a monthly infusion.

4. Calculate how many mL/dose of Pediapred the patient will receive. Supply: 15 mg/5 mL.

5. Calculate how many mg/dose of ampicillin the patient will receive IV, how many mL to draw from the vial, and cc/hr to set the IV pump. Supply: 1-g vials to be diluted with 10 mL of NS and further diluted in 50 cc NS to infuse over 30 minutes.

● CASE STUDY 16 Leukemia

A 14-year-old child is admitted to the hospital with fever of unknown origin (FUO) after chemotherapy administration. The orders from the physician include:

- ❑ Complete blood count with differential, bone marrow aspiration, chemistry panel, PT/PTT, blood cultures, urinalysis, and type and crossmatch
- ❑ Regular diet as tolerated
- ❑ Vitals q4h
- ❑ Daily weights
- ❑ Monitor intake and output
- ❑ Type and cross for 2 units PRBCs
- ❑ Irradiate all blood products
- ❑ Infuse 6 pack of platelets for counts < 20,000
- ❑ IV D5W/NS with 20 mEq KCl 1000 mL/8 hr
- ❑ Allopurinol 200 mg PO tid

- ❏ Fortaz 1 g IV q6h
- ❏ Aztreonam (Azactam) 2 g IV q12h
- ❏ Flagyl 500 mg IV q8h
- ❏ Acetaminophen two tablets q4h prn

Identify the orders that require calculations.

Set up and solve each problem using dimensional analysis.

1. Calculate mL/hr to set the IV pump.

2. Calculate how many tablets of allopurinol will be given PO. Supply: 100 mg/tablet.

3. Calculate how many mL/hr to set the IV pump to infuse Fortaz. Supply: 1-g vial to be diluted with 10 mL of sterile water and further diluted in 50 mL NS to infuse over 30 minutes.

4. Calculate how many mL of aztreonam to draw from the vial. Supply: 2-g vial to be diluted with 10 mL of sterile water and further diluted in 100 mL NS to infuse over 60 minutes.

5. Calculate how many mL/hr to set the IV pump to infuse Flagyl. Supply: 500 mg/100 mL to infuse over 1 hour.

● CASE STUDY 17 **Sepsis**

A neonate born at 32 weeks' gestation (weight 2005 g) is admitted to the Neonatal Intensive Care Unit (NICU) with a diagnosis of sepsis. The orders from the physician include:

- ❏ Admit to NICU with continuous cardiorespiratory monitoring
- ❏ Complete blood counts, blood and urine cultures, chest x-ray, bilirubin, ABGs, theophylline levels, and lumbar puncture
- ❏ Strict intake and output
- ❏ Daily weight
- ❏ Vitals q3h
- ❏ NG breast milk diluted with sterile water 120 cc/day with feedings q3h
- ❏ IV D10 and 20% lipids 120 cc/kg/day
- ❏ Aminophylline 5 mg/kg IV q6h
- ❏ Cefotaxime (Claforan) 50 mg/kg q12h
- ❏ Vancomycin 10 mg/kg/dose q12h

Identify the orders that require calculations.

Set up and solve each problem using dimensional analysis.

1. Calculate how many cc the child will receive with every feeding.

2. Calculate how many mL/hr the child will receive IV.

3. Calculate how many mg of aminophylline the child will receive q6h. Calculate how many mL/hr you will set the IV pump. Supply: 50 mg/10 mL to infuse over 5 minutes.

4. Calculate how many mg of cefotaxime the child will receive every 12 hours. Calculate how many mL/hr you will set the IV pump. Supply: 40 mg/mL to infuse over 30 minutes.

5. Calculate how many mg of vancomycin the child will receive every 12 hours. Calculate how many mL/hr you will set the IV pump. Supply: 5 mg/mL to infuse over 1 hour.

● CASE STUDY 18 Bronchopulmonary Dysplasia

A neonate born at 24 weeks' gestation diagnosed with respiratory distress syndrome and respiratory failure is now 28 weeks' gestation (weight 996 g) with bronchopulmonary dysplasia. This child remains in the Neonatal Intensive Care Unit (NICU) on oxygen therapy and enteral feedings. The orders from the physician include:

- ❑ Complete blood count, chemistry panel, ABGs, chest x-ray, CPPD with nebulizations, glucose monitoring, caffeine citrate levels, and newborn screen
- ❑ NG feedings with Special Care with Iron 120 kcal/kg/day
- ❑ Chlorothiazide (Diuril) 10 mg/kg/day PO
- ❑ Fer-In-Sol 2 mg/kg/day
- ❑ Vitamin E 25 units/kg/day in divided doses q12h
- ❑ Caffeine citrate 5 mg/kg/dose daily

Identify the orders that require calculations.

Set up and solve each problem using dimensional analysis.

1. Calculate how many total calories the child will receive daily. Calculate how many cc/day the child will receive. Supply: 24 kcal/oz.

2. Calculate how many mg of chlorothiazide the child will receive daily. Calculate how many mL/day the child will receive. Supply: 250 mg/5 mL.

3. Calculate how many mg of Fer-In-Sol the child will receive daily. Calculate how many mL/day the child will receive. Supply: 15 mg/0.6 mL.

4. Calculate how many units/dose of vitamin E the child will receive every 12 hours. Calculate how many mL/dose the child will receive. Supply: 67 units/mL.

5. Calculate how many mg of caffeine citrate the child will receive daily. Calculate how many mL/dose the child will receive. Supply: 10 mg/mL.

● CASE STUDY 19 Cerebral Palsy

A 13-year-old child (weight 38 kg) with cerebral palsy being cared for in a children's facility is admitted to the hospital for seizure evaluation. The orders from the physician include:

- ❑ Complete blood count, chemistry panel, urinalysis, dilantin levels, EEG, and CT scan
- ❑ Vitals q4h
- ❑ Seizure precautions
- ❑ Lactulose 3 g PO tid
- ❑ Valproic acid (Depakote) 30 mg/kg/day PO in three divided doses
- ❑ Diazepam (Valium) 2.5 mg PO daily
- ❑ Chlorothiazide (Thiazide) 250 mg PO daily
- ❑ Phenytoin (Dilantin) 5 mg/kg/day PO in three divided doses

Identify the orders that require calculations.

Set up and solve each problem using dimensional analysis.

1. Calculate how many mL of lactulose the child will receive. Supply: 10 g/15 mL.

2. Calculate how many tablets of Depakote the child will receive per dose. Supply: 125 mg/tablet.

3. Calculate how many tablets of diazepam the child will receive per dose. Supply: 5 mg/tablet.

4. Calculate how many tablets of chlorothiazide the child will receive per dose. Supply: 250 mg/tablet.

5. Calculate how many mL of Dilantin the child will receive per dose. Supply: 125 mg/5 mL.

● CASE STUDY 20 Hyperbilirubinemia

A 4-day-old neonate born at 35 weeks' gestation (weight 2210 g) is readmitted to the hospital for treatment of dehydration and jaundice with a bilirubin level of 21 mg/dL. The orders from the physician include:

- ❑ Phototherapy and exchange transfusion through an umbilical venous catheter
- ❑ Total and indirect bilirubin levels, electrolytes, complete blood count, and type and crossmatch
- ❑ Continuous cardiorespiratory monitoring
- ❑ Vitals q2h
- ❑ Monitor intake and output
- ❑ Albumin 5% infusion 1 g/kg 1 hr before exchange
- ❑ Ampicillin 100 mg/kg/dose IV q12h
- ❑ Gentamicin 4 mg/kg/dose IV q12h
- ❑ NPO before exchange, then 120 cc/kg/day formula
- ❑ IV D10W 120 cc/kg/day

Identify the orders that require calculations.

Set up and solve each problem using dimensional analysis.

1. Calculate how many g of albumin the infant will receive before exchange therapy.

2. Calculate how many mg/dose of ampicillin the infant will receive every 12 hours. Calculate how many mL the infant will receive. Supply: 250 mg/5 mL IV push over 5 minutes.

3. Calculate how many mg/dose of gentamicin the infant will receive every 12 hours. Calculate how many mL the infant will receive. Supply: 2 mg/mL.

4. Calculate how many cc/day of formula the infant will receive.

5. Calculate how many cc/hr to set the IV pump.

ANSWER KEY FOR SECTION 3: CASE STUDIES

Case Study 1: Congestive Heart Failure

Orders requiring calculations: IV of D5W/$\frac{1}{2}$ NS at 50 cc/hr; weight gain; Furosemide 40 mg IV qd; Digoxin 0.125 mg PO qd; KCl 20 mEq PO tid

1.

50 ~~cc~~	~~60~~ gtt	1 ~~hr~~	50 × 1	= 50 gtt/min
~~hr~~	~~mL~~	~~60~~ min		

2.

10 ~~lb~~	1 kg	10 × 1	10	= 4.5 kg
	2.2 ~~lb~~	2.2	2.2	

3.

4~~0~~ ~~mg~~	mL	4	= 4 mL
	1~~0~~ ~~mg~~	1	

4.

0.125 ~~mg~~	tablet	0.125	= 0.5 tablet
	0.25 ~~mg~~	0.25	

5.

2~~0~~ ~~mEq~~	tablet	2	= 2 tablets
	1~~0~~ ~~mEq~~	1	

Case Study 2: COPD/Emphysema

Orders requiring calculations: IV of D5W/$\frac{1}{2}$ NS 1000 cc/8 hr; Aminophylline IV loading dose of 5.6 mg/kg over 30 minutes followed by 0.5 mg/kg/hr continuous IV; Erythromycin 800 mg IV q6h; Accurate I/O.

1.

1000 cc	1000	= 125 cc/hr
8 hr	8	

2.

5.6 ~~mg~~	~~100~~ cc	~~1 kg~~	14~~0~~ ~~lb~~	6~~0~~ ~~min~~	5.6 × 14 × 6
~~kg~~/3~~0~~ ~~min~~	~~100 mg~~	2.2 ~~lb~~		~~1~~ hr	3 × 2.2

$\frac{470.4}{6.6} = \frac{71.3 \text{ cc}}{\text{hr}}$ or $\frac{71 \text{ cc}}{\text{hr}}$

3.

0.5 ~~mg~~	25~~0~~ cc	~~1 g~~	~~1 kg~~	14~~0~~ ~~lb~~	0.5 × 25 × 1 × 14
~~kg~~/hr	~~1 g~~	10~~00~~ ~~mg~~	2.2 ~~lb~~		10 × 2.2

$\frac{175}{22} = \frac{7.9 \text{ cc}}{\text{hr}}$ or $\frac{8 \text{ cc}}{\text{hr}}$

4.

8~~00~~ ~~mg~~	2~~0~~ mL	~~1 g~~	8 × 2	= 16 mL
	~~1 g~~	1~~000~~ ~~mg~~	1	

$\frac{266 \text{ cc}}{1 \text{ hr}} = \frac{266 \text{ cc}}{\text{hr}}$

5.

~~3 L~~	~~day~~	1000 mL	1000	= 1000 mL/shift
~~day~~	~~3~~ shifts	~~1 L~~	1	

Case Study 3: Small Cell Lung Cancer

Orders requiring calculations: IV D5W/$\frac{1}{2}$ NS 1000 cc with 10 mEq KCl at 125 cc/hr; Neupogen 5 mcg/kg SQ daily; Gentamicin 80 mg IV q8h; Decadron 8 mg IV daily; Fortaz 1 g IV q8h

1.

125 ~~cc~~	2~~0~~ gtt	1 ~~hr~~	125 × 2 × 1	250	= 41.6 or 42 gtt/min
~~hr~~	~~mL~~	6~~0~~ min	6	6	

2.

5 mcg	1 ~~kg~~	160 ~~lb~~	5 × 1 × 160	800	= 363.6 mcg or 364 mcg
~~kg~~	2.2 ~~lb~~		2.2	2.2	

3.

8~~0~~ ~~mg~~	mL	8	= 2 mL
	4~~0~~ ~~mg~~	4	

$\frac{102 \text{ cc}}{1 \text{ hr}} = \frac{102 \text{ cc}}{\text{hr}}$

4.

8 ~~mg~~	mL	8	= 2 mL
	4 ~~mg~~	4	

5.

50 mL	6~~0~~ ~~min~~	50 × 6	300	= 100 mL/hr
3~~0~~ ~~min~~	1 hr	3 × 1	3	

Case Study 4: Acquired Immunodeficiency Syndrome (AIDS)

Orders requiring calculations: IV D5W/$\frac{1}{2}$ NS at 150 cc/hr; Acyclovir 350 mg IV q8h; Neupogen 300 mcg SQ daily; Epogen 100 units/kg SQ three times a week; Vancomycin 800 mg IV q6h

1. $$\frac{150\ \cancel{cc}}{\cancel{hr}} \Big| \frac{2\cancel{0}\ \text{gtt}}{\cancel{mL}} \Big| \frac{1\ \cancel{hr}}{6\cancel{0}\ \text{min}} \Big| \frac{150 \times 2}{6} \Big| \frac{300}{6} = \frac{50\ \text{gtt}}{\text{min}}$$

2. $$\frac{35\cancel{0}\ \cancel{mg}}{} \Big| \frac{1\cancel{0}\ \text{mL}}{50\cancel{0}\ \cancel{mg}} \Big| \frac{35 \times 1}{5} \Big| \frac{35}{5} = 7\ \text{mL}$$

   $$\frac{107\ \text{cc}}{1\ \text{hr}} \Big| \frac{107}{1} = \frac{107\ \text{cc}}{\text{hr}}$$

3. $$\frac{\cancel{300\ mcg}}{} \Big| \frac{1\ \text{mL}}{\cancel{300\ mcg}} = 1\ \text{mL}$$

4. $$\frac{10\cancel{0}\ \cancel{units}}{\cancel{kg}} \Big| \frac{\text{mL}}{400\cancel{0}\ \cancel{units}} \Big| \frac{1\ \cancel{kg}}{2.2\ \cancel{lb}} \Big| \frac{10\cancel{0}\ \cancel{lb}}{} \Big| \frac{10 \times 1}{4 \times 2.2} \Big| \frac{10}{8.8} = 1.1\ \text{mL or } 1\ \text{mL}$$

5. $$\frac{80\cancel{0}\ \cancel{mg}}{} \Big| \frac{1\cancel{0}\ \text{mL}}{1\ \cancel{g}} \Big| \frac{\cancel{1\ g}}{100\cancel{0}\ \cancel{mg}} \Big| \frac{80 \times 1}{10} \Big| \frac{80}{10} = 8\ \text{mL}$$

   $$\frac{108\ \text{mL}}{\cancel{60\ min}} \Big| \frac{\cancel{60\ min}}{1\ \text{hr}} \Big| \frac{108}{1} = \frac{108\ \text{cc}}{\text{hr}}$$

Case Study 5: Sickle Cell Anemia

Orders requiring calculations: IV D5W/$\frac{1}{2}$ NS at 150 cc/hr; Zofran 8 mg IV q8h; Morphine sulfate 5 mg IV prn; Hydrea 10 mg/kg/day PO; Folic acid 0.5 mg daily PO

1. $$\frac{150\ \cancel{cc}}{\cancel{hr}} \Big| \frac{1\cancel{0}\ \text{gtt}}{\cancel{mL}} \Big| \frac{1\ \cancel{hr}}{6\cancel{0}\ \text{min}} \Big| \frac{150 \times 1 \times 1}{6} \Big| \frac{150}{6} = \frac{25\ \text{gtt}}{\text{min}}$$

2. $$\frac{50\ \text{cc}}{15\ \cancel{min}} \Big| \frac{60\ \cancel{min}}{1\ \text{hr}} \Big| \frac{50 \times 60}{15 \times 1} \Big| \frac{3000}{15} = \frac{200\ \text{cc}}{\text{hr}}$$

3. $$\frac{5\ \cancel{mg}}{} \Big| \frac{\text{mL}}{10\ \cancel{mg}} \Big| \frac{5}{10} = 0.5\ \text{mL}$$

4. $$\frac{10\ \text{mg}}{\cancel{kg}/\text{day}} \Big| \frac{1\ \cancel{kg}}{2.2\ \cancel{lb}} \Big| \frac{125\ \cancel{lb}}{} \Big| \frac{10 \times 1 \times 125}{2.2} \Big| \frac{1250}{2.2} = \frac{568\ \text{mg}}{\text{day}}$$

5. $$\frac{0.5\ \cancel{mg}}{} \Big| \frac{\text{tablet}}{1\ \cancel{mg}} \Big| \frac{0.5}{1} = 0.5\ \text{tablet}$$

Case Study 6: Deep Vein Thrombosis

Orders requiring calculations: IV D5W/$\frac{1}{2}$ NS with 20 mEq KCl at 50 cc/hr; Heparin 5000 units IV push followed by continuous IV infusion of 1000 units/hr; Lasix 20 mg IV bid; Morphine 5 mg IV q4h

1. $$\frac{50\ \cancel{cc}}{\cancel{hr}} \Big| \frac{6\cancel{0}\ \text{gtt}}{\cancel{mL}} \Big| \frac{1\ \cancel{hr}}{\cancel{60}\ \text{min}} \Big| \frac{50 \times 1}{} \Big| \frac{50}{} = \frac{50\ \text{gtt}}{\text{min}}$$

2. $$\frac{5\cancel{000}\ \cancel{units}}{} \Big| \frac{\text{mL}}{10{,}\cancel{000}\ \cancel{units}} \Big| \frac{5}{10} = 0.5\ \text{mL}$$

3. $$\frac{1\cancel{000}\ \cancel{units}}{\text{hr}} \Big| \frac{\cancel{250}\ \text{mL}}{\cancel{25{,}000\ units}} \Big| \frac{10}{} = \frac{10\ \text{mL}}{\text{hr}}$$

4. $$\frac{2\cancel{0}\ \cancel{mg}}{} \Big| \frac{\text{mL}}{1\cancel{0}\ \cancel{mg}} \Big| \frac{2}{1} = 2\ \text{mL}$$

5. $$\frac{5\ \cancel{mg}}{} \Big| \frac{\text{mL}}{10\ \cancel{mg}} \Big| \frac{5}{10} = 0.5\ \text{mL}$$

Case Study 7: Bone Marrow Transplant

Orders requiring calculations: IV D5W/$\frac{1}{2}$ NS with 20 mEq KCl/L at 80 cc/hr; Fortaz 2 g IV q8h; Vancomycin 1 g IV q6h; Claforan 1 g IV q12h; Erythromycin 800 mg IV q6h

1. $$\frac{8\cancel{0}\ \cancel{cc}}{\text{hr}} \Big| \frac{2\cancel{0}\ \text{mEq}}{\cancel{1\ L}} \Big| \frac{\cancel{1\ L}}{100\cancel{0}\ \cancel{mL}} \Big| \frac{8 \times 2}{10} \Big| \frac{16}{10} = \frac{1.6\ \text{mEq}}{\text{hr}}$$

$$2.\ \frac{\cancel{2\,\text{g}}}{\ } \Big| \frac{10\,\text{mL}}{\cancel{2\,\text{g}}} \Big| \frac{10}{\ } = 10\text{ mL}$$

$$\frac{60\,\text{cc}}{3\cancel{0}\,\cancel{\text{min}}} \Big| \frac{6\cancel{0}\,\cancel{\text{min}}}{1\,\text{hr}} \Big| \frac{60 \times 6}{3 \times 1} \Big| \frac{360}{3} = \frac{120\text{ cc}}{\text{hr}}$$

$$3.\ \frac{\cancel{1\,\text{g}}}{\ } \Big| \frac{10\,\text{mL}}{5\cancel{00}\,\cancel{\text{mg}}} \Big| \frac{10\cancel{00}\,\cancel{\text{mg}}}{\cancel{1\,\text{g}}} \Big| \frac{10 \times 10}{5} \Big| \frac{100}{5} = 20\text{ mL}$$

$$\frac{120\,\text{cc}}{\cancel{60\,\text{min}}} \Big| \frac{\cancel{60\,\text{min}}}{1\,\text{hr}} \Big| \frac{120}{1} = \frac{120\text{ cc}}{\text{hr}}$$

$$4.\ \frac{\cancel{1\,\text{g}}}{\ } \Big| \frac{4\,\text{mL}}{6\cancel{00}\,\cancel{\text{mg}}} \Big| \frac{10\cancel{00}\,\cancel{\text{mg}}}{\cancel{1\,\text{g}}} \Big| \frac{4 \times 10}{6} \Big| \frac{40}{6} = 6.7\text{ mL or }7\text{ mL}$$

$$\frac{107\,\text{cc}}{1\,\text{hr}} \Big| \frac{107}{1} = \frac{107\,\text{cc}}{\text{hr}}$$

$$5.\ \frac{8\cancel{00}\,\cancel{\text{mg}}}{\ } \Big| \frac{2\cancel{0}\,\text{mL}}{\cancel{1\,\text{g}}} \Big| \frac{\cancel{1\,\text{g}}}{1\cancel{000}\,\cancel{\text{mg}}} \Big| \frac{8 \times 2}{1} \Big| \frac{16}{1} = 16\text{ mL}$$

$$\frac{266\,\text{mL}}{\cancel{60\,\text{min}}} \Big| \frac{\cancel{60\,\text{min}}}{1\,\text{hr}} \Big| \frac{266}{1} = \frac{266\text{ mL}}{\text{hr}}$$

Case Study 8: Pneumonia

Orders requiring calculations: Clindamycin 400 mg IV q6h; Guaifenesin 200 mg PO q4h; Terbutaline 2.5 mg PO tid; MS Contrin 30 mg PO q4h prn

$$1.\ \frac{4\cancel{00}\,\cancel{\text{mg}}}{\ } \Big| \frac{4\,\text{mL}}{6\cancel{00}\,\cancel{\text{mg}}} \Big| \frac{4 \times 4}{6} \Big| \frac{16}{6} = 2.7\text{ mL or }3\text{ mL}$$

$$\frac{53\,\text{cc}}{\text{hr}} \Big| \frac{53}{\ } = \frac{53\text{ cc}}{\text{hr}}$$

$$2.\ \frac{53\,\cancel{\text{cc}}}{\cancel{\text{hr}}} \Big| \frac{2\cancel{0}\,\text{gtt}}{\cancel{\text{mL}}} \Big| \frac{1\,\cancel{\text{hr}}}{6\cancel{0}\,\text{min}} \Big| \frac{53 \times 2 \times 1}{6} \Big| \frac{106}{6} = \frac{18\text{ gtt}}{\text{min}}$$

$$3.\ \frac{20\cancel{0}\,\cancel{\text{mg}}}{\ } \Big| \frac{\cancel{\text{tsp}}}{3\cancel{0}\,\cancel{\text{mg}}} \Big| \frac{5\,\text{cc}}{1\,\cancel{\text{tsp}}} \Big| \frac{20 \times 5}{3 \times 1} \Big| \frac{100}{3} = 33\text{ cc}$$

$$4.\ \frac{2.5\,\cancel{\text{mg}}}{\ } \Big| \frac{\text{tablet}}{5\,\cancel{\text{mg}}} \Big| \frac{2.5}{5} = 0.5\text{ tablet}$$

$$5.\ \frac{30\,\cancel{\text{mg}}}{\ } \Big| \frac{\text{tablet}}{30\,\cancel{\text{mg}}} \Big| \frac{30}{30} = 1\text{ tablet}$$

Case Study 9: Pain

Orders requiring calculations: IV D5W/$\frac{1}{2}$ NS with 20 mEq KCl/L at 60 cc/hr; IV 500 cc NS with 25 mg Dilaudid and 50 mg Thorazine at 21 cc/hr; Bumex 2 mg IV QAM after albumin infusion

$$1.\ \frac{6\cancel{0}\,\cancel{\text{cc}}}{\text{hr}} \Big| \frac{2\cancel{0}\,\text{mEq}}{\cancel{1\,\text{L}}} \Big| \frac{\cancel{1\,\text{L}}}{10\cancel{00}\,\cancel{\text{mL}}} \Big| \frac{6 \times 2}{10} \Big| \frac{12}{10} = \frac{1.2\text{ mEq}}{\text{hr}}$$

$$2.\ \frac{21\,\cancel{\text{cc}}}{\text{hr}} \Big| \frac{25\,\text{mg}}{500\,\cancel{\text{cc}}} \Big| \frac{21 \times 25}{500} \Big| \frac{525}{500} = \frac{1.05\text{ mg}}{\text{hr}}$$

$$3.\ \frac{21\,\cancel{\text{cc}}}{\text{hr}} \Big| \frac{5\cancel{0}\,\text{mg}}{50\cancel{0}\,\cancel{\text{cc}}} \Big| \frac{21 \times 5}{50} \Big| \frac{105}{50} = \frac{2.1\text{ mg}}{\text{hr}}$$

$$4.\ \frac{11\,\cancel{\text{cc}}}{\text{hr}} \Big| \frac{25{,}00\cancel{0}\,\text{units}}{25\cancel{0}\,\cancel{\text{cc}}} \Big| \frac{11 \times 2500}{25} \Big| \frac{27{,}500}{25} = \frac{1100\text{ units}}{\text{hr}}$$

$$5.\ \frac{2\,\cancel{\text{mg}}}{\ } \Big| \frac{\text{mL}}{0.25\,\cancel{\text{mg}}} \Big| \frac{2}{0.25} = 8\text{ mL}$$

Case Study 10: Cirrhosis

Orders requiring calculations: IV D5W/$\frac{1}{2}$ NS with 20 mEq KCl at 125 cc/hr; IV Zantac 150 mg/250 cc NS at 11 cc/hr; Vitamin K 10 mg SQ QAM; Spironolactone 50 mg PO bid; Lasix 80 mg IV QAM

$$1.\ \frac{125\,\cancel{\text{cc}}}{\cancel{\text{hr}}} \Big| \frac{2\cancel{0}\,\text{gtt}}{\cancel{\text{mL}}} \Big| \frac{1\,\cancel{\text{hr}}}{6\cancel{0}\,\text{min}} \Big| \frac{125 \times 2 \times 1}{6} \Big| \frac{250}{6} = \frac{41.66\text{ or }42\text{ gtt}}{\text{min}}$$

2. $\frac{11\ \cancel{cc}}{hr} \Big| \frac{150\ mg}{250\ \cancel{cc}} \Big| \frac{11 \times 15}{25} \Big| \frac{165}{25} = \frac{6.6\ mg}{hr}$

3. $\frac{10\ \cancel{mg}}{} \Big| \frac{mL}{10\ \cancel{mg}} \Big| \frac{10}{10} = 1\ mL$

4. $\frac{50\ \cancel{mg}}{} \Big| \frac{tablet}{25\ \cancel{mg}} \Big| \frac{50}{25} = 2\ tablets$

5. $\frac{80\ \cancel{mg}}{} \Big| \frac{mL}{10\ \cancel{mg}} \Big| \frac{8}{1} = 8\ mL$

Case Study 11: Hyperemesis Gravidarum

Orders requiring calculations: IV D5$\frac{1}{2}$ NS at 150 cc/hr and 100 cc/hr; Droperidol (Inapsine) 1 mg IV; Metoclopramide (Reglan) 20 mg IV in 50 mL of D5W to infuse over 15 minutes; Diphenhydramine (Benadryl) 25 mg; Dexamethasone (Decadron) 4 mg IV

1. $\frac{150\ \cancel{cc}}{\cancel{hr}} \Big| \frac{20\ gtt}{\cancel{mL}} \Big| \frac{1\ \cancel{hr}}{60\ min} \Big| \frac{150 \times 2 \times 1}{6} \Big| \frac{300}{6} = \frac{50\ gtt}{min}$

   $\frac{100\ \cancel{cc}}{\cancel{hr}} \Big| \frac{20\ gtt}{\cancel{mL}} \Big| \frac{1\ \cancel{hr}}{60\ min} \Big| \frac{100 \times 2 \times 1}{6} \Big| \frac{200}{6} = \frac{33.3\ or\ 33\ gtt}{min}$

2. $\frac{1\ \cancel{mg}}{} \Big| \frac{mL}{2.5\ \cancel{mg}} \Big| \frac{1}{2.5} = 0.4\ mL$

3. $\frac{50\ mL}{15\ \cancel{min}} \Big| \frac{60\ \cancel{min}}{1\ hr} \Big| \frac{50 \times 60}{15 \times 1} \Big| \frac{3000}{15} = \frac{200\ mL}{hr}$

4. $\frac{25\ \cancel{mg}}{} \Big| \frac{mL}{10\ \cancel{mg}} \Big| \frac{25}{10} = 2.5\ mL$

5. $\frac{4\ \cancel{mg}}{} \Big| \frac{mL}{4\ \cancel{mg}} \Big| \frac{4}{4} = 1\ mL$

Case Study 12: Preeclampsia

Orders requiring calculations: Methyldopa (Aldomet) 250 mg; Hydralazine (Apresoline) 5 mg IV; Magnesium sulfate 4 g in 250 mL D5W loading dose to infuse over 30 minutes; Magnesium sulfate 40 g in 1000 mL LR to infuse at 1 g/hr; Nifedipine (Procardia) 10 mg sublingual

1. $\frac{250\ \cancel{mg}}{} \Big| \frac{tablet}{500\ \cancel{mg}} \Big| \frac{25}{50} = 0.5\ tablets$

2. $\frac{5\ \cancel{mg}}{} \Big| \frac{mL}{20\ \cancel{mg}} \Big| \frac{5}{20} = 0.25\ mL$

3. $\frac{250\ mL}{30\ \cancel{min}} \Big| \frac{60\ \cancel{min}}{1\ hr} \Big| \frac{250 \times 6}{3 \times 1} \Big| \frac{1500}{3} = \frac{500\ mL}{hr}$

4. $\frac{1\ \cancel{g}}{hr} \Big| \frac{1000\ mL}{40\ \cancel{g}} \Big| \frac{1 \times 100}{4} \Big| \frac{100}{4} = \frac{25\ mL}{hr}$

5. $\frac{10\ \cancel{mg}}{} \Big| \frac{capsule}{10\ \cancel{mg}} \Big| \frac{10}{10} = 1\ capsule$

Case Study 13: Premature Labor

Orders requiring calculations: Magnesium sulfate at 2 g/hr; Terbutaline (Brethine) 0.25 mg SQ; Nifedipine (Procardia) 20 mg; Betamethasone 12 mg IM; LR 1000 cc over 8 hours

1. $\frac{250\ cc}{20\ \cancel{min}} \Big| \frac{60\ \cancel{min}}{1\ hr} \Big| \frac{250 \times 6}{2 \times 1} \Big| \frac{1500}{2} = \frac{750\ cc}{hr}$

   $\frac{2\ \cancel{g}}{hr} \Big| \frac{250\ cc}{4\ \cancel{g}} \Big| \frac{2 \times 250}{4} \Big| \frac{500}{4} = \frac{125\ cc}{hr}$

2. $\frac{0.25\ \cancel{mg}}{} \Big| \frac{mL}{1\ \cancel{mg}} \Big| \frac{0.25}{1} = 0.25\ mL$

3. $\frac{20\ \cancel{mg}}{} \Big| \frac{capsule}{10\ \cancel{mg}} \Big| \frac{2}{1} = 2\ capsules$

4. $$\frac{12\ \cancel{\text{mg}}}{\ } \,\Big|\, \frac{\text{mL}}{6\ \cancel{\text{mg}}} \,\Big|\, \frac{12}{6} = 2\text{ mL}$$

5. $$\frac{1000\ \text{cc}}{8\ \text{hr}} \,\Big|\, \frac{1000}{8} = \frac{125\text{ cc}}{\text{hr}}$$

Case Study 14: Cystic Fibrosis

Orders requiring calculations: IV 0.9% normal saline at 75 cc/hr; Tagamet 30 mg PO; Clindamycin 10 mg/kg IV; Terbutaline 2.5 mg PO; Tobramycin 1.5 mg/kg IV

1. $$\frac{75\ \cancel{\text{cc}}}{\cancel{\text{hr}}} \,\Big|\, \frac{15\ \text{gtt}}{\cancel{\text{mL}}} \,\Big|\, \frac{1\ \cancel{\text{hr}}}{60\ \text{min}} \,\Big|\, \frac{75\times 15\times 1}{60} \,\Big|\, \frac{1125}{60} = \frac{18.75\text{ or }19\text{ gtt}}{\text{min}}$$

2. $$\frac{30\ \cancel{\text{mg}}}{\cancel{\text{kg/day}}} \,\Big|\, \frac{\text{tablet}}{200\ \cancel{\text{mg}}} \,\Big|\, \frac{1\ \cancel{\text{kg}}}{2.2\ \cancel{\text{lb}}} \,\Big|\, \frac{65\ \cancel{\text{lb}}}{\ } \,\Big|\, \frac{\cancel{\text{day}}}{4\ \text{doses}} \,\Big|\, \frac{3\times 1\times 65}{20\times 2.2\times 4} \,\Big|\, \frac{195}{176} = 1.1\text{ or }1\text{ tablet}$$

3. $$\frac{10\ \text{mg}}{\cancel{\text{kg}}} \,\Big|\, \frac{1\ \cancel{\text{kg}}}{2.2\ \cancel{\text{lb}}} \,\Big|\, \frac{65\ \cancel{\text{lb}}}{\ } \,\Big|\, \frac{10\times 1\times 65}{2.2} \,\Big|\, \frac{650}{2.2} = 295.45\text{ or }295\text{ mg}$$

$$\frac{295\ \cancel{\text{mg}}}{\ } \,\Big|\, \frac{\text{mL}}{150\ \cancel{\text{mg}}} \,\Big|\, \frac{295}{150} = 1.96\text{ or }2\text{ mL}$$

$$\frac{52\ \text{mL}}{20\ \cancel{\text{min}}} \,\Big|\, \frac{60\ \cancel{\text{min}}}{1\ \text{hr}} \,\Big|\, \frac{52\times 6}{2\times 1} \,\Big|\, \frac{312}{2} = \frac{156\text{ mL}}{\text{hr}}$$

4. $$\frac{2.5\ \cancel{\text{mg}}}{\ } \,\Big|\, \frac{\text{tablet}}{2.5\ \cancel{\text{mg}}} \,\Big|\, \frac{2.5}{2.5} = 1\text{ tablet}$$

5. $$\frac{1.5\ \text{mg}}{\cancel{\text{kg}}} \,\Big|\, \frac{1\ \cancel{\text{kg}}}{2.2\ \cancel{\text{lb}}} \,\Big|\, \frac{65\ \cancel{\text{lb}}}{\ } \,\Big|\, \frac{1.5\times 1\times 65}{2.2} \,\Big|\, \frac{97.5}{2.2} = 44.31\text{ or }44\text{ mg}$$

$$\frac{44\ \cancel{\text{mg}}}{\ } \,\Big|\, \frac{\text{mL}}{40\ \cancel{\text{mg}}} \,\Big|\, \frac{44}{40} = 1.1\text{ or }1\text{ mL}$$

$$\frac{51\ \text{mL}}{30\ \cancel{\text{min}}} \,\Big|\, \frac{60\ \cancel{\text{min}}}{1\ \text{hr}} \,\Big|\, \frac{51\times 6}{3\times 1} \,\Big|\, \frac{306}{3} = \frac{102\text{ mL}}{\text{hr}}$$

Case Study 15: Respiratory Syncytial Virus (RSV)

Orders requiring calculations: Acetaminophen elixir 120 mg PO; Aminophylline 5 mg/kg to infuse over 30 minutes and 0.8 mg/kg/hr IV; RespiGam 750 mg/kg IV; Pediapred 1.5 mg/kg/day in three divided doses PO; Ampicillin 100 mg/kg/day in divided doses q6h IV

1. $$\frac{\cancel{120\ \text{mg}}}{\ } \,\Big|\, \frac{5\ \text{mL}}{\cancel{120\ \text{mg}}} \,\Big|\, \frac{5}{\ } = 5\text{ mL}$$

2. $$\frac{5\ \text{mg}}{\cancel{\text{kg}}} \,\Big|\, \frac{1\ \cancel{\text{kg}}}{2.2\ \cancel{\text{lb}}} \,\Big|\, \frac{30\ \cancel{\text{lb}}}{\ } \,\Big|\, \frac{5\times 1\times 30}{2.2} \,\Big|\, \frac{150}{2.2} = 68.18\text{ or }68.2\text{ mg}$$

$$\frac{68.2\ \cancel{\text{mg}}}{30\ \cancel{\text{min}}} \,\Big|\, \frac{100\ \text{mL}}{250\ \cancel{\text{mg}}} \,\Big|\, \frac{60\ \cancel{\text{min}}}{1\ \text{hr}} \,\Big|\, \frac{68.2\times 10\times 6}{3\times 25\times 1} \,\Big|\, \frac{4092}{75} = \frac{54.56\text{ or }54.6\text{ mL}}{\text{hr}}$$

$$\frac{0.8\ \cancel{\text{mg}}}{\cancel{\text{kg}}/\text{hr}} \,\Big|\, \frac{100\ \text{mL}}{250\ \cancel{\text{mg}}} \,\Big|\, \frac{1\ \cancel{\text{kg}}}{2.2\ \cancel{\text{lb}}} \,\Big|\, \frac{30\ \cancel{\text{lb}}}{\ } \,\Big|\, \frac{0.8\times 100\times 1\times 3}{25\times 2.2} \,\Big|\, \frac{240}{55} = \frac{4.36\text{ or }4.4\text{ mL}}{\text{hr}}$$

3. $$\frac{750\ \text{mg}}{\cancel{\text{kg}}} \,\Big|\, \frac{1\ \cancel{\text{kg}}}{2.2\ \cancel{\text{lb}}} \,\Big|\, \frac{30\ \cancel{\text{lb}}}{\ } \,\Big|\, \frac{750\times 1\times 30}{2.2} \,\Big|\, \frac{22{,}500}{2.2} = 10{,}227.27\text{ or }10{,}227.3\text{ mg}$$

4. $$\frac{1.5\ \cancel{\text{mg}}}{\cancel{\text{kg/day}}} \,\Big|\, \frac{5\ \text{mL}}{15\ \cancel{\text{mg}}} \,\Big|\, \frac{1\ \cancel{\text{kg}}}{2.2\ \cancel{\text{lb}}} \,\Big|\, \frac{30\ \cancel{\text{lb}}}{\ } \,\Big|\, \frac{\cancel{\text{day}}}{3\ \text{doses}} \,\Big|\, \frac{1.5\times 5\times 1\times 30}{15\times 2.2\times 3} \,\Big|\, \frac{225}{99} = \frac{2.27\text{ or }2.3\text{ mL}}{\text{dose}}$$

5. $$\frac{100\ \text{mg}}{\cancel{\text{kg/day}}} \,\Big|\, \frac{1\ \cancel{\text{kg}}}{2.2\ \cancel{\text{lb}}} \,\Big|\, \frac{30\ \cancel{\text{lb}}}{\ } \,\Big|\, \frac{\cancel{\text{day}}}{4\ \text{doses}} \,\Big|\, \frac{100\times 1\times 30}{2.2\times 4} \,\Big|\, \frac{3000}{8.8} = \frac{340.9\text{ or }341\text{ mg}}{\text{dose}}$$

$$\frac{341\ \cancel{\text{mg}}}{\ } \,\Big|\, \frac{10\ \text{mL}}{1\ \cancel{\text{g}}} \,\Big|\, \frac{1\ \cancel{\text{g}}}{1000\ \cancel{\text{mg}}} \,\Big|\, \frac{341\times 1\times 1}{1\times 100} \,\Big|\, \frac{341}{100} = 3.41\text{ or }3.4\text{ mL}$$

$$\frac{53\ \text{cc}}{30\ \cancel{\text{min}}} \,\Big|\, \frac{60\ \cancel{\text{min}}}{1\ \text{hr}} \,\Big|\, \frac{53\times 6}{3\times 1} \,\Big|\, \frac{318}{3} = \frac{106\text{ cc}}{\text{hr}}$$

Case Study 16: Leukemia

Orders requiring calculations: IV D5W/NS with 20 mEq KCl 1000 mL over 8 hours; Allopurinol 200 mg PO; Fortaz 1 g IV; Aztreonam 2 g IV; Flagyl 500 mg IV

1. $$\frac{1000\text{ mL}}{8\text{ hr}} \;\Big|\; \frac{1000}{8} = \frac{125\text{ mL}}{\text{hr}}$$

2. $$\frac{2\cancel{00}\ \cancel{\text{mg}}}{} \;\Big|\; \frac{\text{tablet}}{1\cancel{00}\ \cancel{\text{mg}}} \;\Big|\; \frac{2}{1} = 2\text{ tablets}$$

3. $$\frac{\cancel{1\text{ g}}}{} \;\Big|\; \frac{10\text{ mL}}{\cancel{1\text{ g}}} = 10\text{ mL}$$

$$\frac{60\text{ mL}}{3\cancel{0}\ \cancel{\text{min}}} \;\Big|\; \frac{6\cancel{0}\ \cancel{\text{min}}}{1\text{ hr}} \;\Big|\; \frac{60\times 6}{3\times 1} \;\Big|\; \frac{360}{3} = \frac{120\text{ mL}}{\text{hr}}$$

4. $$\frac{\cancel{2\text{ g}}}{} \;\Big|\; \frac{10\text{ mL}}{\cancel{2\text{ g}}} = 10\text{ mL}$$

$$\frac{110\text{ mL}}{\cancel{60\text{ min}}} \;\Big|\; \frac{\cancel{60\text{ min}}}{1\text{ hr}} \;\Big|\; \frac{110}{1} = \frac{110\text{ mL}}{\text{hr}}$$

5. $$\frac{\cancel{500\text{ mg}}}{1\text{ hr}} \;\Big|\; \frac{100\text{ mL}}{\cancel{500\text{ mg}}} \;\Big|\; \frac{100}{1} = \frac{100\text{ mL}}{\text{hr}}$$

Case Study 17: Sepsis

Orders requiring calculations: NG breast milk with sterile water 120 cc per feeding; IV D1O and 20% lipids 120 cc/kg/day; Aminophylline 5 mg/kg IV q6h; Cefotaxime 50 mg/kg q12h; Vancomycin 10 mg/kg/dose q12h

1. $$\frac{120\text{ cc}}{\cancel{\text{day}}} \;\Big|\; \frac{\cancel{\text{day}}}{24\ \cancel{\text{hr}}} \;\Big|\; \frac{3\ \cancel{\text{hr}}}{\text{feeding}} \;\Big|\; \frac{120\times 3}{24} \;\Big|\; \frac{360}{24} = \frac{15\text{ cc}}{\text{feeding}}$$

2. $$\frac{12\cancel{0}\text{ mL}}{\cancel{\text{kg}}/\cancel{\text{day}}} \;\Big|\; \frac{\cancel{\text{day}}}{24\text{ hr}} \;\Big|\; \frac{1\ \cancel{\text{kg}}}{100\cancel{0}\ \cancel{\text{g}}} \;\Big|\; \frac{2005\ \cancel{\text{g}}}{} \;\Big|\; \frac{12\times 1\times 2005}{24\times 100} \;\Big|\; \frac{24{,}060}{2400} = \frac{10.025\text{ or }10\text{ mL}}{\text{hr}}$$

3. $$\frac{5\text{ mg}}{\cancel{\text{kg}}} \;\Big|\; \frac{1\ \cancel{\text{kg}}}{1000\ \cancel{\text{g}}} \;\Big|\; \frac{2005\ \cancel{\text{g}}}{} \;\Big|\; \frac{5\times 1\times 2005}{1000} \;\Big|\; \frac{10025}{1000} = 10.025\text{ or }10\text{ mg}$$

$$\frac{10\ \cancel{\text{mg}}}{5\ \cancel{\text{min}}} \;\Big|\; \frac{10\text{ mL}}{5\cancel{0}\ \cancel{\text{mg}}} \;\Big|\; \frac{6\cancel{0}\ \cancel{\text{min}}}{1\text{ hr}} \;\Big|\; \frac{10\times 10\times 6}{5\times 5\times 1} \;\Big|\; \frac{600}{25} = \frac{24\text{ mL}}{\text{hr}}$$

4. $$\frac{5\cancel{0}\text{ mg}}{\cancel{\text{kg}}} \;\Big|\; \frac{1\ \cancel{\text{kg}}}{100\cancel{0}\ \cancel{\text{g}}} \;\Big|\; \frac{2005\ \cancel{\text{g}}}{} \;\Big|\; \frac{5\times 1\times 2005}{100} \;\Big|\; \frac{10025}{100} = 100.25\text{ or }100\text{ mg}$$

$$\frac{10\cancel{0}\ \cancel{\text{mg}}}{3\cancel{0}\ \cancel{\text{min}}} \;\Big|\; \frac{\text{mL}}{4\cancel{0}\ \cancel{\text{mg}}} \;\Big|\; \frac{6\cancel{0}\ \cancel{\text{min}}}{1\text{ hr}} \;\Big|\; \frac{10\times 6}{3\times 4\times 1} \;\Big|\; \frac{60}{12} = \frac{5\text{ mL}}{\text{hr}}$$

5. $$\frac{1\cancel{0}\text{ mg}}{\cancel{\text{kg}}/\text{dose}} \;\Big|\; \frac{1\ \cancel{\text{kg}}}{100\cancel{0}\ \cancel{\text{g}}} \;\Big|\; \frac{2005\ \cancel{\text{g}}}{} \;\Big|\; \frac{1\times 1\times 2005}{100} \;\Big|\; \frac{2005}{100} = \frac{20.05\text{ or }20\text{ mg}}{\text{dose}}$$

$$\frac{20\ \cancel{\text{mg}}}{1\text{ hr}} \;\Big|\; \frac{1\text{ mL}}{5\ \cancel{\text{mg}}} \;\Big|\; \frac{20\times 1}{1\times 5} \;\Big|\; \frac{20}{5} = \frac{4\text{ mL}}{\text{hr}}$$

Case Study 18: Bronchopulmonary Dysplasia

Orders requiring calculations: NG feedings with Special Care with Iron 120 KCal/kg/day; Chlorothiazide 10 mg/kg/day; Fer-In-Sol 2 mg/kg/day; Vitamin E 25 units/kg/day in divided doses q12h; Caffeine citrate 5 mg/kg/dose daily

1. $$\frac{12\cancel{0}\text{ kcal}}{\cancel{\text{kg}}/\text{day}} \;\Big|\; \frac{1\ \cancel{\text{kg}}}{100\cancel{0}\ \cancel{\text{g}}} \;\Big|\; \frac{996\ \cancel{\text{g}}}{} \;\Big|\; \frac{12\times 1\times 996}{100} \;\Big|\; \frac{11{,}952}{100} = \frac{119.52\text{ or }120\text{ kcal}}{\text{day}}$$

$$\frac{120\ \cancel{\text{kcal}}}{\text{day}} \;\Big|\; \frac{\cancel{\text{oz}}}{24\ \cancel{\text{kcal}}} \;\Big|\; \frac{30\text{ cc}}{1\ \cancel{\text{oz}}} \;\Big|\; \frac{120\times 30}{24\times 1} \;\Big|\; \frac{3600}{24} = \frac{150\text{ cc}}{\text{day}}$$

2. $$\frac{1\cancel{0}\text{ mg}}{\cancel{\text{kg}}/\text{day}} \;\Big|\; \frac{1\ \cancel{\text{kg}}}{100\cancel{0}\ \cancel{\text{g}}} \;\Big|\; \frac{996\ \cancel{\text{g}}}{} \;\Big|\; \frac{1\times 1\times 996}{100} \;\Big|\; \frac{996}{100} = \frac{9.96\text{ or }10\text{ mg}}{\text{day}}$$

$$\frac{1\cancel{0}\ \cancel{\text{mg}}}{\text{day}} \;\Big|\; \frac{5\text{ mL}}{25\cancel{0}\ \cancel{\text{mg}}} \;\Big|\; \frac{1\times 5}{25} \;\Big|\; \frac{5}{25} = \frac{0.2\text{ mL}}{\text{day}}$$

3. $$\frac{2\text{ mg}}{\cancel{\text{kg}}/\text{day}} \;\Big|\; \frac{1\ \cancel{\text{kg}}}{1000\ \cancel{\text{g}}} \;\Big|\; \frac{996\ \cancel{\text{g}}}{} \;\Big|\; \frac{2\times 1\times 996}{1000} \;\Big|\; \frac{1992}{1000} = \frac{1.99\text{ or }2\text{ mg}}{\text{day}}$$

$$\frac{2\ \cancel{\text{mg}}}{\text{day}} \;\Big|\; \frac{0.6\text{ mL}}{15\ \cancel{\text{mg}}} \;\Big|\; \frac{2\times 0.6}{15} \;\Big|\; \frac{1.2}{15} = \frac{0.08\text{ mL}}{\text{day}}$$

4.

25 units	1 ~~kg~~	996 ~~g~~	~~day~~	25 × 1 × 996	24,900	= 12.45 or 12.5 units
~~kg/day~~	1000 ~~g~~		2 doses	1000 × 2	2000	dose

12.5 ~~units~~	mL	12.5	= 0.18 or 0.2 mL
dose	67 ~~units~~	67	dose

5.

5 mg	1 ~~kg~~	996 ~~g~~	~~day~~	5 × 1 × 996	4980	= 1.24 or 1.2 mg
~~kg/day~~	1000 ~~g~~		4 doses	1000 × 4	4000	dose

1.2 ~~mg~~	mL	1.2	= 0.12 or 0.1 mL
dose	10 ~~mg~~	10	dose

Case Study 19: Cerebral Palsy

Orders requiring calculations: Lactulose 3 g PO tid; Depakote 30 mg/kg/day PO in three divided doses; Diazepam 2.5 mg PO daily; Chlorothiazide 250 mg PO daily; Dilantin 5 mg/kg/day PO in three divided doses

1.

3 ~~g~~	15 mL	3 × 15	45	= 4.5 or 5 mL
	10 ~~g~~	10	10	

2.

30 mg	38 ~~kg~~	~~day~~	30 × 38	1140	= 380 mg
~~kg/day~~		3 doses	3	3	dose

380 ~~mg~~	tablet	380	= 3.04 or 3 tablets
	125 ~~mg~~	125	

3.

2.5 ~~mg~~	tablet	2.5	= 0.5 tablet
	5 ~~mg~~	5	

4.

250 ~~mg~~	tablet	250	= 1 tablet
	250 ~~mg~~	250	

5.

5 ~~mg~~	38 ~~kg~~	~~day~~	5 mL	5 × 38 × 5	950	= 2.53 or 2.5 mL
~~kg/day~~		3 dose	125 ~~mg~~	3 × 125	375	dose

Case Study 20: Hyperbilirubinemia

Orders requiring calculations: Albumin 5% infusion 1 g/kg 1 hr before exchange; Ampicillin 100 mg/kg/dose IV q12h; Gentamicin 2.5 mg/kg/dose IV q12h; 120 cc/kg/day formula; IV D10W 120 cc/kg/day

1.

1 g	1 ~~kg~~	221~~0~~ ~~g~~	1 × 1 × 221	221	= 2.21 or 2.2 g
~~kg~~	100~~0~~ ~~g~~		100	100	

2.

~~100~~ mg	1 ~~kg~~	221~~0~~ ~~g~~	1 × 221	221	= 221 mg
~~kg~~/dose	~~1000~~ ~~g~~		1	1	dose

221 ~~mg~~	5 mL	221 × 5	1105	= 4.42 or 4.4 mL
	250 ~~mg~~	250	250	

3.

4 mg	1 ~~kg~~	221~~0~~ ~~g~~	4 × 1 × 221	884	= 8.84 or 8.8 mg
~~kg~~/dose	100~~0~~ ~~g~~		100	100	dose

8.8 ~~mg~~	mL	8.8	= 4.4 mL
	2 ~~mg~~	2	

4.

12~~0~~ cc	1 ~~kg~~	221~~0~~ ~~g~~	12 × 1 × 221	2652	= 265.2 or 265 cc
~~kg~~/day	10~~00~~ ~~g~~		10	10	day

5.

12~~0~~ cc	1 ~~kg~~	221~~0~~ ~~g~~	~~day~~	12 × 1 × 221	2652	= 11.05 or 11 cc
~~kg/day~~	10~~00~~ ~~g~~		24 hr	10 × 24	240	hr

SECTION

4

COMPREHENSIVE POST-TEST

COMPREHENSIVE POST-TEST

Name ______________________ **Date** ____________

1. Order: Phenobarbital 60 mg PO daily for seizures

   Supply on hand: Phenobarbital 30 mg/tablet

   How many tablets will you give? ____________

2. Order: Chloral hydrate 250 mg PO 30 minutes before hs as sedative

   Supply on hand: Chloral hydrate 250 mg/5 mL

   How many milliliters will you give? ____________

3. Order: Digitoxin 0.3 mg PO daily for maintenance dose after digitalization

   Supply on hand: Digitoxin 100 mcg/tablets

   How many tablets will you give? ____________

4. Order: Potassium chloride 20 mEq PO tid for hypokalemia

   Supply: Potassium chloride 40 mEq/15 mL

   How many teaspoons will you give? ____________

5. Order: 500 mL D5W to infuse over 12 hours

   Drop factor: 60 gtt/mL

   Calculate the number of drops per minute. ____________

6. Order: Heparin 1500 units/hr for thrombophlebitis

   Supply: Heparin 25,000 units/500 cc

   Calculate cc/hr to set the IV pump. ____________

7. Order: Infuse heparin at 20 cc/hr for thrombophlebitis

   Supply: Heparin 25,000 units in 250 cc

   How many units/hr is the patient receiving? ____________

8. Order: Infuse bolus of 0.9% NS at 100 gtt/min

   Supply: 250 mL 0.9% NS with 60 gtt/mL tubing

   How many hours will it take to infuse the IV bolus? ____________

9. Order: Fluconazole 200 mg IVPB over 60 minutes for systemic candidal infections

   Supply: Fluconazole 200 mg/100 mL with 20 gtt/mL tubing

   Calculate the number of drops per minute. ______________

10. Order: Furosemide 2 mg/kg PO daily for congestive heart failure

    Supply: Furosemide 10 mg/mL oral solution

    How many milliliters will you give a child weighing 10 lb? ______________

11. Order: Neupogen 6 mcg/kg SQ twice daily for chronic neutropenia

    Supply: Neupogen 300 mcg/mL

    How many milliliters will you give a patient weighing 175 lb? ______________

12. Order: Ampicillin 500 mg IV every 6 hours for urinary tract infection

    Supply: Ampicillin 1-g vial

    Nursing drug reference: Reconstitute each 1-g vial with 10 mL of sterile water and further dilute in 50 mL of 0.9% NS and infuse over 15 minutes.

    How many milliliters will you draw from the vial after reconstitution? ______________

    Calculate milliliters per hour to set the IV pump. ______________

    Calculate the drops per minute with a drop factor of 10 gtt/mL. ______________

13. Order: Acyclovir 10 mg/kg IV every 8 hours for varicella zoster in immunosuppressed patient weighing 140 lb

    Supply: Acyclovir 1-g vial.

    Nursing drug reference: Reconstitute each 1-g vial with 10 mL of sterile water and further dilute in 100 mL of 0.9% NS and infuse over 1 hour.

    How many milliliters will you draw from the vial after reconstitution? ______________

    Calculate milliliters per hour to set the IV pump. ______________

    Calculate the drops per minute with a drop factor of 10 gtt/mL. ______________

14. Order: Epinephrine 1 mcg/min IV for bradycardia

Supply: Epinephrine 1 mg/250 mL 0.9% NS

Calculate milliliters per hour to set the IV pump. ____________

15. Order: Isuprel 5 mcg/min IV for heart block

Supply: Isuprel 2 mg in 500 mL D5W

Calculate milliliters per hour to set the IV pump. ____________

16. Order: Dobutamine 2.5 mcg/kg/min IV for management of heart failure for a patient weighing 130 lb

Supply: Dobutamine 250 mg in 1000 mL of 0.9% NS

Calculate milliliters per hour to set the IV pump. ____________

17. Order: Dopamine 10 mcg/kg/min IV for management of hypotension secondary to decreased cardiac output for a patient weighing 120 lb

Supply: Dopamine 400 mg in 500 mL D5W

Calculate milliliters per hour to set the IV pump. ____________

18. Order: Aminophylline is infusing at 24 mL/hr for respiratory distress for a patient weighing 80 kg

Supply: Aminophylline is 250 mg in 250 mL in D5W

How many mg/kg/hr is the patient receiving? ____________

19. Order: Amrinone infusing at 47 mL/hr for a patient weighing 100 kg for short-term treatment of congestive heart failure

Supply: Amrinone 100 mg/100 mL 0.45% NS

How many mcg/kg/min is the patient receiving? ____________

20. Order: Aminophylline loading dose of 5.6 mg/kg to infuse over 30 minutes for a patient weighing 50 kg followed by 0.6 mg/kg/hr maintenance dose for COPD

Supply: Aminophylline 500 mg in 500 mL of D5W

How many milliliters per hour will you set the IV pump for the loading dose? ____________

How many milliliters per hour will you set the IV pump for the maintenance dose? ____________

APPENDIX

EDUCATIONAL THEORY OF DIMENSIONAL ANALYSIS

Dimensional analysis is a problem-solving method based on the principles of cognitive theory. Bruner (1960) theorized that learning is dependent on how information is structured, organized, and conceptualized. He proposed a cognitive learning model that emphasized the acquisition, organization (structure), understanding, and transfer of knowledge—focusing on "how" to learn, rather than "what" to learn. Learning involves associations established according to the principles of continuity and repetition.

Dimensional analysis (also called factor-label method, conversion-factor method, units analysis, and quantity calculus) provides a systematic way to set up problems and helps to organize and evaluate data. Hein (1983) emphasized that dimensional analysis gives a clear understanding of the principles of the problem-solving method that correlates with the ability to verbalize what steps are taken leading to critical thinking. He described dimensional analysis as a useful method for solving a variety of chemistry, physics, mathematics, and daily life problems. He identified that dimensional analysis is often the problem-solving method of choice because it provides a straightforward way to set up problems, gives a clear understanding of the principles of the problem, helps the learner to organize and evaluate data, and assists in identifying errors if the setup of the problem is incorrect.

Goodstein (1983) described dimensional analysis as a problem-solving method that is very simple to understand, reduces errors, and requires less conceptual reasoning power to understand than does the ratio–proportion method. She expressed that "even though the ratio–proportion method was at one time the primary problem-solving method, it has been largely replaced by a dimensional analysis approach in most introductory chemistry textbooks . . . this method condenses multi-step problems into one orderly extended solution."

Peters (1986) identified dimensional analysis as a method used for solving not only chemistry problems but also a variety of other mathematical problems that require conversions. He defined dimensional analysis as a method that can be used whenever two quantities are directly proportional to each other and one quantity must be converted to the other using a conversion factor or conversion relationship.

Literature that has examined the quality of higher education and professional education in the United States (National Institute of Education, 1984) recommends that educators increase the emphasis of the intellectual skills of problem solving and critical thinking. Also recommended is an increased emphasis on the mastery of concepts rather than specific facts. Other literature on curriculum revolution in nursing (Bevis, 1988; Lindeman, 1989; Tanner, 1988) recommends that learning not be characterized merely as a change in behavior or the acquisition of facts, but in seeing and *understanding* the significance of the whole. Because it focuses on "how" to learn, rather than "what" to learn, dimensional analysis supports conceptual mastery and higher-level thinking skills that have become the core of the curriculum change that is sweeping through all levels of education and, most importantly, nursing education.

BIBLIOGRAPHY

Bevis, E. (1988). New directions for a new age. In National League for Nursing, *Curriculum revolution: Mandate for change* (pp. 27–52). New York: National League for Nursing (Pub. No. 15–2224).

Bruner, J. (1960). *The process of education*. New York: Random House.

Craig, G. (1995). The effects of dimensional analysis on the medication dosage calculation abilities of nursing students. *Nurse Educator, 20*(3), 14–18.

Craig, G. P. (1997). The effectiveness of dimensional analysis as a problem-solving method for medication calculations from the nursing student perspective. Unpublished doctoral dissertation, Drake University, Des Moines, IA.

Goodstein, M. (1983). Reflections upon mathematics in the introductory chemistry course. *Journal of Chemical Education, 60*(8), 665–667.

Hein, M. (1983). *Foundations of chemistry* (4th ed.). Encino, CA: Dickenson Publishing Company.

Lindeman, C. (1989). Curriculum revolution: Reconceptualizing clinical nursing education. *Nursing and Health Care, 10*(1), 23–28.

National Institute of Education. (1984). *Involvement in learning: Realizing the potential of American higher education*. Washington, DC: National Institute of Education.

Peters, E. (1986). *Introduction to chemical principles* (4th ed.). Saratoga, CA: Saunders College Publishing.

Tanner, C. (1988). Curriculum revolution: The practice mandate. *Nursing and Health Care, 9*(8), 426–430.

Page numbers followed by *f* refer to figures; page numbers followed by *t* refer to tables.

A

B

C

D

E

F

N

O

P

Q

R

S

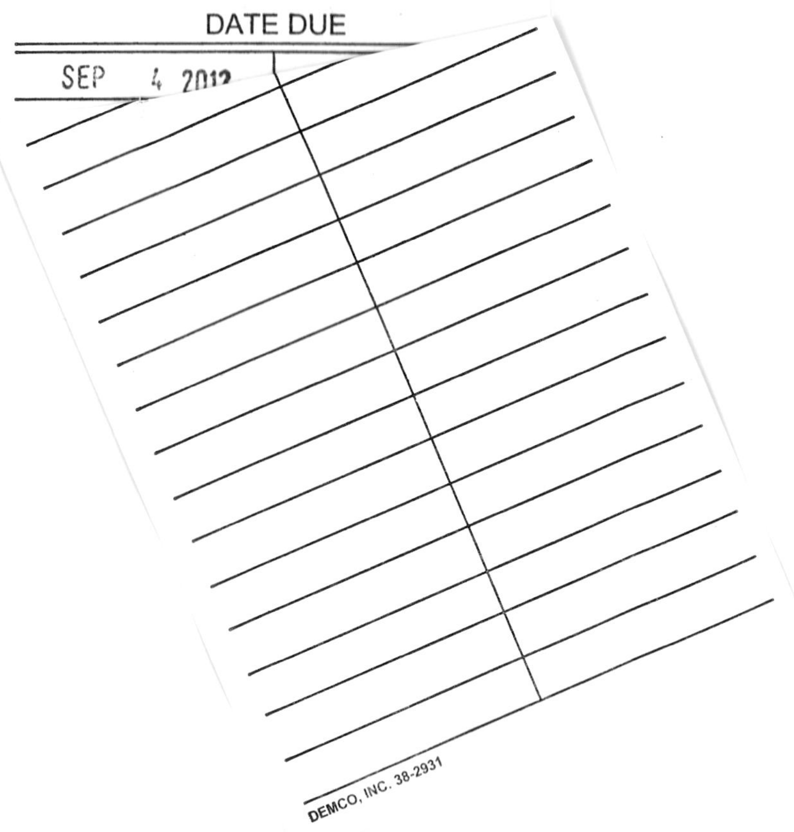
DATE DUE
SEP 4 201
DEMCO, INC. 38-2931